PHLEBOTOMY TECHNICIAN
SPECIALIST
A Practical Guide to Phlebotomy

Kathryn A. Kalanick, CMA, NCPT
Director of Education
Career Academy
Anchorage, Alaska

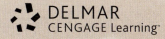

DELMAR
CENGAGE Learning

Australia • Brazil • Japan • Korea • Mexico • Singapore • Spain • United Kingdom • United States

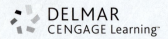
DELMAR
CENGAGE Learning

Phlebotomy Technician Specialist:
A Practical Guide to Phlebotomy
Kathryn A. Kalanick

Vice President, Health Care Business
   Unit: William Brottmiller

Editorial Director: Cathy L. Esperti

Acquisitions Editor: Maureen Rosener

Editorial Assistant: Matthew Thouin

Marketing Director: Jennifer McAvey

Channel Manager: Lisa M. Osgood

Production Editor: Mary Colleen Liburdi

For product information and technology assistance, contact us at
Cengage Learning Customer & Sales Support, 1-800-354-9706

For permission to use material from this text or product,
submit all requests online at **www.cengage.com/permissions**
Further permissions questions can be emailed to
permissionrequest@cengage.com

ISBN-13: 978-0-7668-2346-4
ISBN-10: 0-7668-2346-6

Delmar
Executive Woods
5 Maxwell Drive
Clifton Park, NY 12065
USA

Cengage Learning is a leading provider of customized learning solutions with office locations around the globe, including Singapore, the United Kingdom, Australia, Mexico, Brazil, and Japan. Locate your local office at **international.cengage.com/region**

Cengage Learning products are represented in Canada by Nelson Education, Ltd.

For your lifelong learning solutions, visit **delmar.cengage.com**

Visit our corporate website at **www.cengage.com**

Printed in China by China Translation & Printing Services Limited
8 9 10 11 12 12 11 10

Dedication

This book is dedicated to every student who has touched my life and over the years taught me the true meaning and value of education.

A special note of appreciation to:

Jennifer Deitz, Owner and President of Career Academy, Anchorage, Alaska for her endless supply of support, encouragement, and red pens.

Valerie Anwari, Inside Sales Manager at Delmar Cengage Learning, for being the reason that this project was started in the first place.

Matt Thouin, Editorial Assistant, who worked beyond my expectations to make this book a reality.

Mary Colleen Liburdi, Production Editor, who was there in the very beginning and stayed to the very end. Thank you.

Diane Caudill, for her friendship, her belief in my abilities, and her long hours of research and proofreading.

Each individual who reviewed this text and provided me with their insight and tremendous knowledge and who kept me informed on "the latest regs."

And, most importantly, thank you to my husband, Geno, my daughter, Anishia, and my mother. Without their support, encouragement, and patience this project would not have been possible.

Kathryn A. Kalanick

Acknowledgment

Gratitude and thanks to Geno Kalanick for his photography services for some of the images in this book.

Contents

Preface

Phlebotomy is a critical practice in the world of medicine. Professional phlebotomists perform their skills with efficiency and accuracy, within the parameters of OSHA and CLIA guidelines, and treat every patient with consideration and respect. That is why *Phlebotomy Technician Specialist* is designed to address the wide range of knowledge and skills that are required of a successful phlebotomist. This comprehensive text is for use in the Allied Health educational system at a post-secondary level. It may be utilized in a stand-alone program which trains students to be nationally-certified entry-level phlebotomists; one-semester college courses teaching phlebotomy as a core program requirement; or adopted into any Allied Health program that teaches phlebotomy as part of its core curriculum. This text may also be used as a reference text for cross training of lab personnel or nursing staff, or as a quick reference for use in any laboratory.

As an Allied Health professional and educator for over 25 years, I have extensive experience working with thousands of medical assistants and phlebotomists in classrooms, laboratories, clinics, and hospitals. My goal in writing this textbook was born out of frustration due to an inability to find a textbook that provided students with sufficient technical education. *Phlebotomy Technician Specialist* has been organized based on methods and techniques presented in the classroom for years.

This book was written with two goals in mind. The first goal is to provide the best educational training tool in phlebotomy. The second goal is to offer a valuable resource for use in both the classroom and the workplace. This text is organized sequentially, building from one skill to the next. The topics covered in the text are presented in a concise and systematic format, and the concepts consist of the competency-based essentials students need to become a phlebotomy technician.

Because the field of phlebotomy is ever-expanding and updated technology and regulations are of great concern, this book includes the most up-to-date information based on national standards set by The National Committee for Clinical Laboratory Standards (NCCLS) and The Occupational Safety and Health Administration (OSHA).

One of the main focuses of any Allied Health textbook needs to be medical terminology. Medical terms should be the building blocks for all medical courses of study. This text provides a concise and solid foundation of medical terminology by broadening the scope of terms presented in this text. An entire chapter devoted to medical terminology allows the student to develop skills and understand the basics of medical terminology. This skill building emphasizes word parts and includes prefixes, suffixes, and combining forms.

The Anatomy and Physiology chapter provides an overview of each body system, which every Allied Health professional needs to know in order to form a solid foundation for further study. Knowing how each body system is constructed, how it works, and what tests can be performed to determine a diagnosis, will provide students with the information they need to accomplish their objectives.

Nationally, employers are requiring phlebotomy technicians to be proficient in a variety of point-of-care testing, so a chapter is dedicated to these enhanced skills. Specialized testing such as hematocrits, hemoglobins, blood glucose, coagulation studies, bleeding time, chemistry panels, pregnancy testing, and other point-of-care tests are also included in a chapter of their own.

While the correct techniques for obtaining blood specimens are the main focus of this text, there are many other areas of the profession that are of equal importance. OSHA regulations and CLIA guidelines are two areas of critical concern and boxed "OSHA Alerts" are presented throughout the text to emphasize their importance. Other crucial areas of study are professional communication skills; law and ethics; and cultural diversity, to include the non-traditional patient and the non-English speaking patient. Finally, since the goal of every student is to find suitable employment in the field they have trained for, a chapter addressing employment skills has been included to give the phlebotomist that extra edge.

Phlebotomy Technician Specialist's dynamic full color images enhance the presentation of material and visually engage the reader in the content. Each chapter lists learning objectives, key terms, and a chapter outline. Key terms also appear in the chapter margins along with their phonetic spelling and definition to reinforce this critical information. Chapter summaries review the main points of the chapter content, bringing the objectives of the chapter back to the surface, and study and review questions follow the summary, to test the students' grasp of the material. Chapters with hands-on applications include sheets at the end of the chapter for competency based skills check-offs.

An accompanying instructor manual is also available, and includes lecture outlines and answers to the study and review questions found in each chapter.

Kathryn A. Kalanick, CMA, NCPT

Reviewers

Cynthia Boles, MT(ASCP), MBA
Sawyer School
Pittsburgh, PA

Mary Ellen Brown
Stone Academy
Hamden, CT

Deb Grieneisen
Harrisburg Area Community College
Carlisle, PA

Lynette Hobbs
Tyler Junior College
Tyler, TX

Chris Hollander
Westwood College
Denver, CO

Karen Ingham
Dutchess Community College
Poughkeepsie, NY

Bernice Lewis, RN
Brunswick Community College
Supply, NC

Mary Marks, MSN, RN-C
Mitchell Community College
Mooresville, NC

Nancy Mitchell, MS, MT(ASCP), DLM
Rochester General Hospital
Rochester, NY

Lucia D. Roncalli, CDM
Anchorage, AK

Peggy White
Sauk Valley Community College
Dixon, IL

Procedure Icons

Taking the correct precautions, when performing any medical procedure, is imperative to your safety and the safety of your patient. OSHA has set specific standards that must be followed. Icons have been incorporated into this text, at the beginning of each procedure, to assist you in meeting these standards. These icons are described and illustrated below.

 Handwashing is the first line of defense in the fight against the spread of infection. Handwashing is performed before and after *every* patient contact, between different procedures on the same patient, whenever hands are visibly contaminated, before and after using the lavatory, and before leaving the laboratory, before and after breaks and lunch, and before and after wearing and removing gloves. Handwashing involves the use of running warm water and antibacterial or antimicrobial soap and is considered an aseptic practice.

The phlebotomy technician must wear intact, clean, disposable gloves every time contact is made with a potentially infectious material, such as blood, body fluids, nonintact skin, or mucous membranes. Gloves must be worn for collection of all specimens. If the phlebotomist has cuts, scratches, or other breaks in his or her skin, they must be bandaged prior to wearing gloves. Torn or damaged gloves must be replaced immediately. Disposable gloves are never washed and reused. They are appropriately removed and disposed of in a biohazardous waste container. Gloves must be changed between patient contacts and hands washed immediately or as soon as patient safety permits after gloves are removed.

Lab coats are worn to prevent contamination of the phlebotomist's clothing during laboratory procedures. Lab coats are never worn when the phlebotomist is on break or lunch, or outside of the clinical setting. Most laboratories provide a coat, which remains at the laboratory and is either laundered on the premises or disposable.

Wearing masks, protective eye wear (goggles), and face shields any time there is an anticipated exposure to splashes or sprays of blood or other infectious material, is mandated by the OSHA blood-borne pathogens final rule to reduce the risk of exposures to blood-borne pathogens.

All contaminated items otherwise considered infectious waste must be disposed of in a biohazardous waste container. The container must be appropriately labeled with the biohazardous waste symbol and color-coded (typically red) for easy recognition. The biohazardous waste container must be sturdily constructed, close-able, and leak-proof.

All health care workers should take precautions to prevent injuries caused by needles, glass slides, and other sharp instruments during procedures, while cleaning used instruments, and when disposing of used needles. To prevent needle-stick injuries, needles should not be recapped by hand, purposely bent or broken by hand, removed from disposable syringes, or otherwise manipulated by hand. After they are used, disposable syringes and needles, glass slides, and other sharps should be placed in puncture-resistant containers (called "sharps" containers) for disposal. The puncture-resistant containers should be located as close as practical to the area of use.

Introduction to Phlebotomy

KEY TERMS

abandonment
antisepsis (**an**-ti-**SEP**-sis)
assault (a-**SAWLT**)
battery
biohazardous waste
blood-borne pathogen
burden of proof
chain of custody
duty of care
false imprisonment
felony
fraud
hemochromatosis
   (**he**-mo-**kro**-ma-**TO**-sis)
hemolysis (he-**MOL**-ih-sis)
informed consent
intentional infliction of
   emotional distress
invasion of privacy
libel
malpractice
misdemeanor
negligence
personal protective
   equipment
polycythemia
   (**pol**-ee-si-**THE**-me-a)
respondeat superior
slander
tort

OBJECTIVES

Upon completion of this chapter the student should be able to:

- Define and correctly spell each of the key terms.
- Understand the history and advancements of phlebotomy as a profession.
- Describe the purpose of certification and methods of recertification.
- List the responsibilities of a phlebotomy technician.
- List the personal characteristics that employers look for when hiring a phlebotomy technician.
- Identify national organizations supporting the profession of phlebotomy.
- Describe the phlebotomy technician's role as a member of the health care team.
- Identify the organization and responsibilities of the employees of a clinical laboratory.
- Identify the various health care personnel affiliated with hospitals and independent laboratories.
- List the main points of "The Patient Care Partnership."
- Contrast the two main divisions of law as they affect health care providers.
- Describe the three basic divisions of tort law and provide examples of intentional torts.
- Describe malpractice and negligence.
- Identify the regulatory agencies involved with health care.
- Describe Total Quality Management, Quality Control, Quality Assurance, and Risk Management.
- Describe the organizations OSHA and CLIA.

THE HISTORY OF PHLEBOTOMY

The practice of phlebotomy was employed as a medical practice long before Hippocrates (460–377 BC) provided written documentation of its benefits. Ancient Mayan hieroglyphics discovered on temple walls illustrated the performance of bloodletting. Ancient bloodletting, it was believed, ensured the blessings of the gods to favor health and prosperity. In Mayan cultures bloodletting might have been accomplished by a female running a rope through her tongue, by a male cutting his penis, or by either sex driving sharp objects through their ears.

In approximately 1400 BC a representation of bloodletting was depicted in an Egyptian tomb. The glyph depicted the application of a leech to a patient. It has even been suggested that bloodletting dates back to the Stone Age, when crude tools such as pointed sticks and sharp stones were used to puncture vessels and allow blood to drain out.

Early phlebotomies were more therapeutic and religious in nature. For example, in medieval times, bloodletting was used to "bleed out" evil spirits, which were said to be making the patient ill (see Figure 1-1).

Hippocrates provided the first written documentation of the practice of bloodletting. He theorized that man was "made" of four body "humors": blood, phlegm, yellow bile, and black bile. His theory stated that when any of the four humors was found in excess it caused disease. The offending humor had to be immediately removed from the patient to bring the body back into proper balance.

Hippocrates was very familiar with phlebotomy, which was then called venesection. He also practiced scarification, another method of bloodletting. He believed that large amounts of blood should be quickly removed from the body in order to produce syncope (fainting). Often, the amount of blood let was too great, and the patient would die. This, however, was blamed on the disease and not the bloodletting.

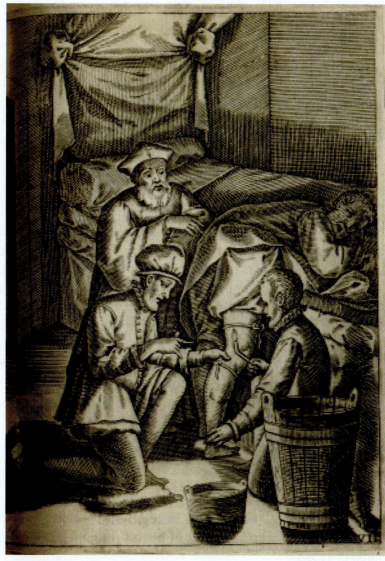

FIGURE 1-1: Early bloodletting

Galen, a student of Hippocrates, continued to study and improve upon Hippocrates' work. He was the first to record that specific amounts of blood should be extracted for certain ailments. In routine cases Galen stated that the amount of blood removed should not exceed 1 to 1½ pounds and should be no less than 6 to 7 ounces. The average amount of blood drained was 16 to 30 ounces. The rule of thumb was to take just enough blood to cause the patient to faint.

During the 17th and 18th centuries, bloodletting was considered to be a major therapeutic medical treatment. It has been said that George Washington died in 1799 from complications of bloodletting. He had four bloodlettings in less than two days for a throat infection. In the 19th century the practice of bloodletting was widespread in America and was used to treat ailments ranging from the common cold to convulsions and mental illness. The standard pioneer doctor's tool kit contained one major implement—the lancet, or knife, used for bloodletting, in addition to cups and leeches.

It was not until the late 19th century, with the widespread use of the microscope, along with a more accurate description of physiological chemistry and cellular physiology, that phlebotomy became a diagnostic tool. By the end of the 19th century, the use of bloodletting as therapeutic medicine began to diminish and was quickly branded as quackery.

Today, phlebotomy has become a valuable diagnostic tool with the improvement in technology and the development of computerized blood testing. However, therapeutic bloodletting is resurfacing. Leeching is once again being performed as a means of reducing swelling and promoting healing after surgery, and is one of the newest therapies for hepatitis C. Bloodletting is also a viable treatment for **polycythemia** and **hemochromatosis**.

Bloodletting Devices and Methods

Bleeding was often performed over large areas of the body by multiple incisions, which were made by a variety of devices that went in and out of favor over the years.

Lancets

Lancets were first used around 400 BC and were often made of stone or wood.

Lancets were often used on more than one patient. As there was no concept of **antisepsis**, infections passed from patient to patient.

Spring-Loaded Lancets

Spring-loaded lancets became popular during the early 18th century. The device was cocked and a trigger fired the spring-driven blade into the vein (see Figure 1-2). Today spring-loaded lancets are one of the most commonly used lancing devices. Although the design has been modernized, the technique is much the same as it was in the 18th century. Lancets are discussed in further detail in Chapters 8 and 9.

Fleam

The fleam was widely used during the 18th and 19th centuries. The basic design was similar to that of the lancet. Sometimes wooden "fleam sticks" would be used to hit the back of the blade and drive it into the vein. Veterinarians often used this method.

POLYCYTHEMIA

A disease characterized by an overproduction of red blood cells.

HEMOCHROMATOSIS

A genetic disease marked by excessive absorption and accumulation of iron in the body.

ANTISEPSIS

The prevention of sepsis by preventing or inhibiting the growth of a causative microorganism.

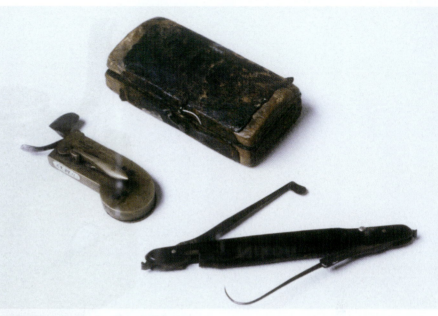

FIGURE 1-2: Spring-loaded lancets

Scarificator

The scarificator was very popular in the 18th century. The device consisted of a small box that contained 12 small spring-driven rotary blades. The device would be cocked and the trigger released, causing many shallow cuts of a section of skin (see Figure 1-3).

Flint Glass Cups

Cups were used to bring the blood to the surface of the skin prior to making the incision. This was called dry cupping. A flint glass cup would be heated and then placed on the patient's skin. After a few minutes the incision was made. The cup could also be heated and placed on a localized area of the skin after the incision had been made. The heated air would create a vacuum causing the blood to flow into the cup—the first version of today's evacuated tube system. This was called wet cupping. Around the 1800s glass cups with brass syringes were marketed, thereby eliminating the need to heat the cup. Air could be removed via the attached syringe, allowing blood to collect in the cup.

Leeches

The medicinal leech, *Hirudo medicinalis,* has been used as a method of bloodletting for thousands of years and has been traced back to eastern Asia long before traders brought knowledge of this method to Europe. The medicinal leech was used extensively in the 19th

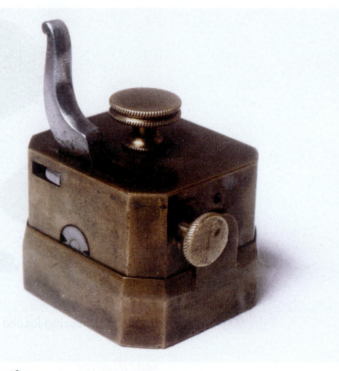

FIGURE 1-3: Scarificator

century for a wide variety of conditions. Leeches are increasingly being used today as surgical tools in tissue grafts and reattachment surgery because of their ability to prevent blood clots from forming. Leeches secrete an anticoagulant into the wound, which delays the formation of a scab and prevents the skin from sealing over too quickly. The lack of a delay in the formation of a scab promotes wound healing from the inside out. Internal healing first is especially important where very delicate repairs such as reconstructive facial surgery have been made. Research is continuing to isolate the specific properties of the leeches' natural anticoagulant.

The medicinal leech is typically 3 to 6 inches in length and, when full, contains from one-half an ounce to an ounce of blood (see Figure 1-4). During the 19th century, physicians and pharmacists stored leeches in decorative jars with tiny air holes in the lids. At one point leeches were in such high demand they nearly became extinct. Biopharm, located in Wales (United Kingdom) is a commercial leech breeding company. Biopharm is one of a very few research companies who also ship leeches to health care practitioners and facilities around the world.

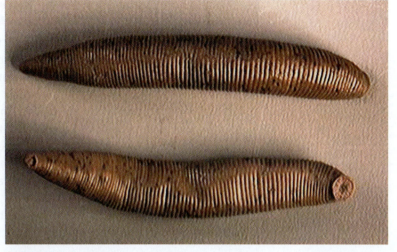

FIGURE 1-4: Leeches

Box 1-1: Leeches

Did you know?

● There are 650 known species of leeches.
● The largest leech discovered measured 18 inches.
● The leech has 32 brains—31 more than humans.
● The *Hirudo* leech has three jaws with 100 teeth per jaw—with 300 teeth in all.
● The bite of a leech is painless because of its own anesthetic.
● The leech will gorge itself up to five times its body weight.
● The leech will gorge itself until full and will then fall off.
● After the leech falls off, the wound it leaves will bleed, on average, for 10 hours.
● The nearest relatives of leeches are earthworms.
● The nervous system of the leech is very similar to the human nervous system.
● In the past, women and children were paid to wade barelegged into ponds to gather leeches for use in medicine.

Box 1-2: History of the Barber Pole

The legacy of the barber pole can be traced to the local barbers of the Middle Ages. In the Middle Ages, the barber not only cut hair, but performed surgery, tooth extraction, and bloodletting. The father of modern surgery, Ambroise Pare, the greatest surgeon of the Renaissance, began as a barber surgeon. The tools of the barber surgeon included a staff for the patient to grasp during the procedure so that the veins of the arm would stand out, a basin to hold leeches and catch the "let"

(continues)

Box 1-2: History of the Barber Pole *(continued)*

blood, and an adequate supply of linen bandages. After the bloodletting procedure was completed, the bandages would be hung on the staff. The staff would then be placed outside the establishment as an advertisement. The bandages, blown by the wind, would twirl around the staff in a red and white spiral pattern. Subsequently, when in need of a barber's services, you only had to locate the barber's pole. Frequently the leech basin would be placed on top of the pole as further identification. The "barber pole" later was painted with red, white, and blue stripes, and the leech basin became a ball.

One interpretation of the colors of the barber pole was red for blood, blue for veins, and white for the bandages. This symbol is still used today by the modern barber, now a stylist rather than a surgeon.

PHLEBOTOMY EDUCATION AND CERTIFICATION

It is no longer adequate to simply be trained as a lay person in the field of medicine. Every discipline requires a standardized formal education and either licensure or certification. As little as 10 years ago these requirements would have been inaccurate. In today's society of specialists, the standard is education. In the field of phlebotomy as well as in other health care fields, the provider or technician who performs phlebotomy techniques must be formerly trained to be employed. Many of the licensed health care professions require phlebotomy certification, as well as licensure when phlebotomy is not a direct requirement of the profession. For example, a certified nursing assistant working in a hospital setting and performing phlebotomy procedures as part of the routine job requirements must also become certified as a phlebotomist. Certification sets a standard of demonstrated competency. Certification is evidence that an individual has mastered the skills required to perform in a specific technical area—in this case, phlebotomy.

The purpose of certification is twofold: First, it establishes that the individual has met the required competencies with the skills to perform as a credentialed phlebotomist. Second, upon successful completion of the certification exam, the phlebotomist is given credentials and/or a title. Certified phlebotomists are authorized to use the appropriate initials after their names. Certification exams are generally given on a national level in conjunction with an educational program and are affiliated with the program's approval or the schools accrediting organization. Agencies that administer certification examinations in phlebotomy and the credentials that are awarded are listed in Table 1-1.

Table 1-1: List of Agencies That Certify Phlebotomy Technicians
● American Association of Allied Health Professionals, Inc. (AAAHP): Certified Phlebotomy Technician, CPT (AAAHP)
● American Medical Technologists (AMT): Registered Phlebotomy Technician, RPT (AMT)
● American Society for Phlebotomy Technicians (ASPT): Certified Phlebotomy Technician, CPT (ASPT)
● American Society of Clinical Pathologists (ASCP): Phlebotomy Technician, PBT (ASCP)
● National Center for Competency Testing (NCCT): Nationally Certified Phlebotomy Technician, NCPT (NCCT)
● National Certification Agency for Medical Laboratory Personnel (NCA): Clinical Laboratory Phlebotomist, CLPlb (NCA)
● National Phlebotomy Association (NPA): Certified Phlebotomy Technician, CPT (NPA)

Continuing education is required by most certifying agencies in order to maintain certification. Continuing education ensures that the phlebotomist remains current with the latest technology and medical advances while maintaining a proficient skill level. Each agency has specific requirements for recertification, including continuing education and/or retesting in a prescribed time frame. Continuing education units (CEUs) may be obtained in a variety of ways, such as workshops and seminars offered by phlebotomy associations, in-service training by laboratories, hospitals, and national conferences. Often the phlebotomist's employer provides compensation for attending continuing education functions. In order to remain current, the phlebotomist should participate in as many workshops and seminars as possible.

There are several sources offering phlebotomy technician training, education, and certification. Many hospitals offer in-house training programs, which are available to their employees. Independently owned and operated phlebotomy programs provide another source. Career colleges, community colleges, and universities offer independent phlebotomy technician programs, as well as offering phlebotomy training as a component of other curricula. When evaluating phlebotomy technician programs it is important that the institution be nationally accredited. Institutional and program accreditation ensures that the school has been evaluated and has met the minimum required educational and/or program standards. In addition, quality programs will seek program approval through one of the certification agencies. The National Accrediting Agency for Clinical Laboratory Sciences (NAACLS) and The National Committee for Clinical Laboratory Standards (NCCLS) have set guidelines and standards for phlebotomy curriculum. Quality programs will meet or exceed these standards. Most certification agencies base their certification standards on these guidelines.

The College of American Pathologists (CAP) also influences the standards of phlebotomy. This organization is composed entirely of board-certified pathologists. It functions as a laboratory review committee. A CAP-certified laboratory undergoes laboratory inspections routinely and works in conjunction with the Joint Commission on Accreditation of Health Care Organizations (JCAHO) in a hospital setting.

PHLEBOTOMIST'S RESPONSIBILITIES

The phlebotomist is a vital part of the medical laboratory team. The phlebotomist's primary responsibility is the collection of blood samples from patients using venipuncture or microcollection techniques. The phlebotomist also facilitates the expedient collection and transport of specimens to the laboratory and is often the patient's only contact with the medical lab. Furthermore, the phlebotomist ensures that the integrity of the draw and the patient's comfort and safety are maintained. With the ever-increasing number and complexity of laboratory testing, as well as the need to contain costs and efficiently control quality, the phlebotomist has become a highly trained specialist in the clinical laboratory. With the increased demands of the profession, phlebotomists must obtain specialized training in a formal educational setting and seek certification.

The role of the phlebotomist has increased over the past several years to include more and more patient care. Phlebotomists in most laboratories are now required to know how to perform vital signs, electrocardiograms, and point-of-care testing. Most laboratories require that the phlebotomist is current in cardiopulmonary resuscitation (CPR) certification and automated external defibrillation (AED). The phlebotomist must also be trained in laboratory computer software and medical record documentation.

Clinical skills are but one area in which the phlebotomist must excel. The phlebotomist must be highly motivated, have a pleasant personality, work well under pressure, and be detail oriented, as well as compassionate and empathetic.

The following list identifies the primary skills required of entry-level phlebotomists:

● Obtaining blood samples
● Specimen collection and processing
● Performing vital signs
● Professional communication and appropriate client/patient interaction
● Performing point-of-care testing
● Laboratory computer skills
● Medical terminology
● Anatomy and physiology
● Medicolegal awareness
● Knowledge and compliance of safety standards—Standard Precautions
● CPR- and AED-certified
● Accurate tube identification and correct sequence of draw
● Knowledge of frequently ordered laboratory tests
● Electrocardiography (ECG)
● Time management and task prioritization
● Understanding of compliance with Quality Assurance and Quality Control
● Preparation of blood film slides
● Clerical skills

THE PHLEBOTOMIST AS PART OF THE HEALTH CARE TEAM

Hospitals and independent laboratories are often very large organizations, with multiple departments subdivided by specialties. The phlebotomist is an integral part of the health care team and as such must be familiar with all departments and specialties. The phlebotomist may be required to perform blood collections or point-of-care testing before, during, or after procedures in any department. Table 1-2 describes major departments within a hospital.

Table 1-2: Hospital Departments	
DEPARTMENT	**DESCRIPTION**
Anesthesiology	Administers anesthesia to provide partial or complete loss of sensation. Generally performed prior to surgical procedures.
Cardiology	Subspecialty of Internal Medicine dealing with the blood vessels and the heart. Cardiovascular surgery.

(continues)

DEPARTMENT	DESCRIPTION
Emergency Room	Specializes in emergency care of the acutely ill and injured.
Intensive Care Unit	Unit of the hospital for patients who require continuous monitoring by specially trained personnel. Types of ICUs include CCU, PCU, PICU, NICU.
Internal Medicine	Treats diseases of the internal organs by other than surgical procedures.
Obstetrics/Gynecology	Concerned with management of women's health, during pregnancy, childbirth, puerperium, gynecologic surgery, and menopausal disorders.
Oncology	Diagnosis and treatment of malignant tumors and blood disorders.
Orthopedics	Deals with disorders of the musculoskeletal system.
Pathology/Laboratory	Study of the nature and cause of disease through clinical laboratory test results.
Pediatrics	Treatment and care of children from birth to adolescence, including diagnosis and management of disease, wellness checks, and vaccinations.
Physical Medicine	Diagnosis and treatment of diseases and disorders of the neuromuscular systems, to include physical therapy and occupational therapy.
Psychiatry/Neurology	Diagnosis, treatment, and prevention of mental illness and disorders of the brain.
Radiology/Medical Imaging	Diagnosis, treatment, and prevention of disease through the use of X-rays, radioactive isotopes, ionizing radiations, ultrasonography, and magnetic resonance imaging.
Surgery	Branch of medicine dealing with manual and operative procedures for correction of deformities and defects, repair of injuries, and diagnosis and cure of certain diseases.

Table 1-2: Hospital Departments *(continued)*

It is also important for the phlebotomist to identify and know the various personnel affiliated with hospitals and independent laboratories.

Hospital Personnel

● Physician: A doctor; a person who has been educated, trained, and state licensed to practice the art and science of medicine.
● Physician's assistant (PA): A health care professional who provides patient services ranging from physical examinations to surgical procedures. The physician's assistant works under the supervision of a physician. A PA receives two years of post-college training and is licensed by the state where he or she works.

- Nurse practitioner (NP or ANP): A registered nurse with a minimum of a master's degree in nursing and advanced education in a particular primary care (e.g., OB/gyn, pediatrics, oncology, etc.). A nurse practitioner is capable of independent practice in a variety of settings.
- Registered nurse (RN): A nurse who graduated from an accredited nursing program, passed the state exam for licensure, and is registered and licensed to practice by state authority.
- Licensed practical nurse (LPN): A nurse who graduated from an accredited school of practical (vocational) nursing, passed the state examination for licensure, and is licensed to practice by a state authority. A LPN program is generally one year in length.
- Certified nursing assistant (NA or CNA): An unlicensed nursing staff member who assists with basic patient care such as giving baths, checking vital signs, bed making, and postioning. Nursing assistants usually must complete a training course, including classroom instruction and clinical practice under supervision. Each state regulates nursing assistant practice. Upon completion of training the nursing assistant may take a certification examination and upon successful completion of the examination become a certified nursing assistant. (Some states require state licensure of nursing assistants.)
- Anesthesiologist: A physician specializing solely in anesthesiology and related areas. An individual with a medical degree who is board-certified and state-licensed to administer anesthetics and related techniques.
- Pharmacist: A pharmacist is a specialist in formulating and dispensing medications. They are licensed by individual states to practice pharmacy, which is the study of preparing and dispensing drugs. Training consists of two years of postgraduate study in pharmacology.
- Respiratory therapist (RT): A licensed allied health professional trained to provide respiratory care. A respiratory therapist works under the direction of a physician, educating patients, treating and assessing patient response to therapy, and managing and monitoring patients with deficiencies and abnormalities of cardiopulmonary function.
- Physical therapist (PT): A medical practitioner with either a bachelor's or master's degree in physical therapy. The PT treats patients with the restoration of physical strength and endurance, coordination, and range of motion through exercises, heat or cold therapy, and massage.

● Occupational therapist (OT): A medical practitioner with either a bachelor's or master's degree in occupational therapy. Following training an OT must pass an examination administered by the National Board for the Certification of Occupational Therapists. Upon successfully passing this examination, the OT is registered and uses the credentials OTR. Occupational therapists help people with physical or mental disabilities use the activities of everyday living to achieve maximum functioning and independence at home and in the workplace.

● Radiologist: A physician trained in the diagnostic and/or therapeutic use of X-rays and radionuclides, radiation physics, and biology. A diagnostic radiologist is also trained in diagnostic ultrasound and magnetic resonance imaging and applicable physics.

Laboratory Personnel (May be employed by hospitals or independent laboratories)

● Laboratory director/pathologist: A physician who practices, evaluates, or supervises diagnostic tests, using materials removed from living or dead patients. The laboratory director/pathologist functions as a laboratory consultant to clinicians, and may conduct experiments or other investigations to determine the causes of diseases or nature of their changes.

● Laboratory manager: Position typically requires a bachelor's degree in health science, plus additional years of clinical laboratory experience or the equivalent combination of education and experience, including a minimum of three years' prior supervisory experience, for example, a medical technologist with an advanced degree in management or business with many years of experience. The responsibilities of a laboratory manager include overseeing all business operations of the laboratory, such as developing and maintaining the clinical laboratory budget, hiring laboratory personnel, setting goals and objectives, and providing continuing education. Some states require the laboratory manager to be a bioanalyst, which is a licensed position requiring extensive postgraduate work.

● Medical technologist/Clinical laboratory scientist: A medical technologist (MT) or clinical laboratory scientist (CLT) has a four-year bachelor's degree in medical technology, which includes one year of study in an MT program. Some states require licensure for MTs, but will grant reciprocity to those MTs who are nationally certified. MTs are often employed as laboratory supervisors of one or more departments in large clinical laboratories and are ultimately responsible for all test results in their department(s). MTs are authorized to perform any and all clinical laboratory tests.

- Medical laboratory technicians: Medical laboratory technicians have graduated from a two-year associate degree program and have completed several semesters of hands-on clinical training as part of their degree. MLTs can perform clinical laboratory testing under the direction of a medical technologist (MT)
- Phlebotomist: A clinical laboratory employee whose responsibilities have been described previously in this chapter. Generally, a phlebotomy technician graduates from an accredited phlebotomy technician program or has been cross-trained from another medical profession.
- Clinical laboratory clerical staff: A clerical staff employee is generally required to have a high school diploma and some prior clinical training. The clerical person may answer telephones, take messages, perform data entry of test results on the laboratory computer, retrieve test results for the physician, file laboratory reports, and distribute reports to physicians or the medical records department.

LAW AND ETHICS

Every health care practitioner from physician to phlebotomist is governed by the same legal and ethical standards. Knowing and understanding these standards not only protect the phlebotomist, laboratory, hospital, and physician from possible lawsuit, but protect the patient from harm as well.

The phlebotomist must respect the rights and privileges of every patient while in a health care facility or hospital including the clinical laboratory. The patient is protected by a document called The Patient Care Partnership. The Patient Care Partnership was adopted in April of 2003 as a replacement for the Patient's Bill of Rights, originally developed in 1973 by the American Hospital Association.

Although it is not legally binding, this document is accepted throughout medical health care as the standard to which all patients have the right to be treated. It declares that all health care professionals have a duty to provide quality health care to their patients.

There are two broad divisions of law that affect the health care provider: civil law and criminal law.

Civil Law

Civil law is defined as the law of private rights between persons or parties. Civil law actions comprise the majority of all health care cases. Civil law is based on tort law. Tort law is a civil wrong and is based on an act that is committed without just cause. The act

TORT

A private wrong or injury, other than breach of contract, for which the court will provide a remedy.

Box 1-3: Patient Care Partnership

The Patient Care Pertnership:
Understanding Expectations, Rights, and Responsibilities

When you need hospital care, your doctor and the nurses and other professionals at our hospital are committed to working with you and your family to meet your health care needs. Our dedicated doctors and staff serve the community in all its ethnic, religious, and economic diversity. Our goal is for you and your family to have the same care and attention we would want for our families and ourselves.

The sections below explain some of the basics about how you can expect to be treated during your hospital stay. They also cover what we will need from you to care for you better. If you have questions at any time, please ask them. Unasked or unanswered questions can add to the stress of being in the hospital. Your comfort and confidence in your care are very important to us.

What to Expect During Your Hospital Stay

- **High quality hospital care.** Our first priority is to provide you the care you need, when you need it, with skill, compassion, and respect. Tell your caregivers if you have concerns about your care or if you have pain. You have the right to know the identity of doctors, nurses, and others involved in your care, as well as students, residents, or other trainees.

- **A clean and safe environment.** Our hospital works hard to keep you safe. We use special policies and procedures to avoid mistakes in your care and keep you free from abuse or neglect. If anything unexpected and significant happens during your hospital stay, you will be told what happened and any resulting changes in your care will be discussed with you.

- **Involvement in your care.** You and your doctor often make decisions about your care before you go to the hospital. Other times, especially in emergencies, those decisions are made during your hospital stay. When they take place, making decisions should include:

  ➤ *Discussing your medical condition and information about medically appropriate treatment choices.* To make informed decisions with you doctor, you need to understand several things:
    - The benefits and risks of each treatment.
    - Whether it is experimental or part of a research study.
    - What you can reasonably expect from your treatment and any long-term effects it might have on your quality of life.
    - What you and your family will need to do after you leave the hospital.
    - The financial consequences of using uncovered services or out-of-network providers.
  Please tell your caregivers if you need more information about treatment choices.

  ➤ *Discussing your treatment plan.* When you enter the hospital, you sign a general consent to treatment. In some cases, such as surgery or experimental treatment, you may be asked to confirm in writing that you understand what is planned and agree to it. This process protects your right to consent to or refuse a treatment. Your doctor will explain the medical consequences of refusing recommended treatment. It also protects your right to decide if you want to participate in a research study.

➤ *Getting information from you.* Your caregivers need complete and correct information about your health coverage so that they can make good decisions about your care. That includes:
  – Past illnesses, surgeris, or hospital stays.
  – Past allergic reactions.
  – Any medicines or diet supplements (such as vitamins and herbs) that you are taking.
  – Any network or admission requirements under your health plan.

➤ *Understanding your health care goals and values.* You may have health care goals and values or spiritual beliefs that are important to your well-being. They will be taken into account as much as possible throughout your hospital stay. Make sure your doctor, your family, and your care team know your wishes.

➤ *Understanding who should make decisions when you cannot.* If you have signed a health care power of attorney stating who should speak for you if you become unable to make health care decisions for yourself, or a "living will" or "advance directive" that states your wishes about end-of-life care, give copies to your doctor, your family and your care team. If you or your family need help making difficult decisions, counselors, chaplains and others are available to help.

- **Protection of your privacy.** We respect the confidentiality of your relationship with your doctor and other caregivers, and the sensitive information about your health and health care that are part of that relationship. State and federal laws and hospital operating policies protect the privacy of your medical information. You will receive a Notice of Privacy Practices that describes the wasy that we use, disclose, and safeguard patient information and that explains how you can obtain a copy of information from our records about your care.

- **Help preparing you and your family for when you leave the hospital.** Your doctor works with hospital staff and professionals in your community. You and your family also play an important role. The success of your treatment often depends on your efforts to follow medication, diet and therapy plans. Your family may need to help care for you at home.

You can expect us to help you identify sources of follow-up care and to let you know if our hospital has a financial interest in any referrals. As long as you agree that we can share information about your care with them, we will coordinate our activities with your caregivers outside the hospital. You can also expect to receive information and, where possible, training about the self-care you will need when you go home.

- **Help with your bill and filing insurance claims.** Our staff will file claims for you with health care insurers or other programs such as Medicare or Medicaid. They will also help your doctor with needed documentation. Hospital bills and insurance coverage are often confusing. If you have questions about your bill, contact our business office. If you need help understanding your insurance coverage or health plan, start with your insurance company or health benefits manager. If you do not have health coverage, we will try to help you and your family find financial help or make other arrangements. We need your help with collecting needed information and other requirements to obtain coverage or assistance.

While you are here, you will receive more detailed notices about some of the rights you have as a hospital patient and how to exercise them. We are always interested in improving. If you have questions, comments, or concerns, please contact _____.

ABANDONMENT

A premature termination of the professional treatment relationship by the health care provider without adequate notice of the patient's consent.

ASSAULT

The act of intentionally causing someone to fear that he or she is about to become the victim of battery, or incomplete battery.

BATTERY

The act of intentionally touching someone in a harmful or offensive manner without the person's consent.

DUTY OF CARE

The responsibility not to infringe on another's rights by either intentionally or carelessly causing him or her harm.

FALSE IMPRISONMENT

The intentional and unjustifiable act of preventing someone from moving about.

FRAUD

An intentional misrepresentation. A deliberate deception intended to produce unlawful gain.

INTENTIONAL INFLICTION OF EMOTIONAL DISTRESS

The willful infliction of emotions or actions causing the patient to suffer duress.

may be intentional or unintentional. There are three basic types of torts: intentional torts, negligence torts, and strict liability torts.

Intentional Tort

Intentional torts arise out of an intentional act or willful breach of duty. For example, a patient is scheduled for lab work in an outpatient lab. When the patient arrives for the scheduled appointment, the phlebotomy technician begins the blood draw. During the draw the phlebotomy technician receives a phone call and leaves the patient sitting in the chair with the needle still in his arm to answer the call. After waiting a few minutes for the phlebotomy technician to return, the patient removes the needle from his own arm and files a complaint of **abandonment**. Other examples of intentional torts include: **assault**, **battery**, **duty of care**, **false imprisonment**, **fraud**, **intentional infliction of emotional distress**, **invasion of privacy**, **libel**, and **slander**.

Negligence

Negligence torts occur when a duty of care is breached unintentionally, causing harm. The law states that everyone has the duty to act with reasonable care to avoid creating undue risk of harm to others. Health care providers are responsible to take the precautions that a reasonably prudent person would take to prevent bringing about foreseeable harm to another. If a health care provider fails to observe such care and a patient suffers harm as a result, negligence can be charged.

For negligence to occur there must be:

1. a legal obligation owed by one person to another

2. a breach of duty

3. harm done as a direct result of the action.

Negligence does not require intent. If the harm is caused with intent it is covered by one of the intentional torts, that is, assault, battery, or slander. By definition, negligence is done unintentionally. The following is an example of negligence: A patient informs the phlebotomy technician prior to a venipuncture that she faints every time her blood is drawn. The phlebotomy technician disregards the warning and continues with the draw. The patient faints, falls out of the chair, and hits her head on the corner of the counter. The patient is seen in the emergency room with a slight concussion, and requires 14 sutures to repair the laceration. The patient misses four days of work and sues the phlebotomy technician for negligence. Examining this scenario we find: 1) A legal duty was es-

INVASION OF PRIVACY

A tort involving one or more of the following four categories: illegal appropriation of another's name for commercial use, intrusion into a person's privacy, placing a person in false light, or disclosure of private facts.

LIBEL

A written statement falsifying facts about someone that causes harm to that person's reputation.

SLANDER

The act of falsifying of facts which causes harm to a person's reputation. Slander is spoken as opposed to libel, which is written.

NEGLIGENCE

The failure to act with reasonable care, resulting in the harming of others.

RESPONDEAT SUPERIOR

A Latin phrase which means "let the master answer." In more common language, employers must answer for damage their employees cause within the scope of the employee's position.

MALPRACTICE

The misconduct or unprofessional treatment by someone in a professional or official position.

tablished. The patient came to the laboratory for blood testing. The phlebotomy technician had the legal duty as a laboratory employee to perform the blood collection. 2) There was a breach of duty. The patient warned the phlebotomist that she fainted every time her blood was drawn. A reasonable phlebotomist would have asked the patient to lie down, so she would not fall if she fainted. 3) Harm was done. The patient fell and required emergency medical treatment, 14 sutures, and missed time from work. If negligence is established, the plaintiff (patient) is entitled to damages that will compensate for her loss. In this case the plaintiff is entitled to the reimbursement of all medical bills, any lost wages caused by her inability to work after the incident, and a reasonable award to compensate her for her "pain and suffering," plus any loss of future income resulting directly from the injury.

Due care is the responsibility of health care providers to protect others from harm. Due care also implies that the person performing the procedure or care possesses the qualifications and training to provide the necessary level of care. In one negligence case a health care worker who had not received the proper training performed a venipuncture by inserting the needle approximately two inches above the antecubital space. The needle went through the vein, through the muscle, and into a nerve, causing severe damage to the patient's arm. The damage remained permanent even after three corrective surgeries. Not only was the health care worker held responsible, but the laboratory was named in the suit as well. Due care requires the physician, laboratory, or hospital to hire competent personnel. The term **respondeat superior** is a Latin phrase that means "let the master answer." This term means that the employer is ultimately responsible and accountable and must answer for any improprieties or damages caused by an employee, committed within the scope of employment. If the employee acts outside the scope of duties or training, the employee may be held solely responsible.

Malpractice is a claim of improper treatment or negligence brought against a professional person and/or institution by means of a civil lawsuit. Generally, medical malpractice lawsuits are brought against a hospital or physician. However, a phlebotomy technician can be named in a malpractice lawsuit. Malpractice or liability insurance is usually obtained by the physician or laboratory and covers all employees. Phlebotomy technicians may also purchase their own malpractice insurance for a nominal fee each year.

Strict Liability

There are very few instances when a health care provider can be found guilty of a tort even though the health care provider neither intentionally nor unintentionally committed a tort. When this occurs it is called strict liability. In medicine this generally occurs with product liability. Manufacturers and retailers of commercial products can be held strictly liable for damages caused by products they manufacture or sell. Collecting blood specimens involves many types of equipment and supplies. Both patients and phlebotomists have been injured as the result of malfunctioning equipment. In 1990, the federal government issued the Safe Medical Devices Act. This law was enacted to protect health care workers and patients from injuries caused by health care devices.

Criminal Law

Criminal law is the division of law concerned with violations of laws established by local, state, or federal government agencies. Criminal laws are imposed to protect the public. Violations of these laws are called crimes. There is a strong relationship between tort law and criminal law. In fact, many torts are considered crimes. What distinguishes the two from each other is the nature of the offense. A tort is a wrong against an individual and a crime is a wrong against a society. Criminal laws are divided into two classifications: **felonies** and **misdemeanors**. Misdemeanors are the lesser of the two crimes and are punishable by fines and/or up to one year in jail. Some common misdemeanors are petty larceny, simple assault, reckless endangerment, and disorderly conduct. Felonies are the most serious types of crimes and include murder, rape, arson, burglary, embezzlement, grand larceny, and aggravated assault. Felonies are punishable by fines and more than one year in state or federal prison.

Preventive Law

The avoidance of legal conflicts through education and planning is called preventive law. The phlebotomist follows these basic guidelines to prevent a lawsuit:

- Accurately and legibly document all information.
- Acquire **informed consent** prior to specimen collection.
- Document all incidents immediately.
- Participate in continuing education.
- Perform at the accepted standard of care.
- Strictly adhere to all laboratory policies and procedures.
- Use proper safety measures.

FELONY

A crime more serious than a misdemeanor, punishable by a sentence of more than one year in prison or death.

MISDEMEANOR

A crime less serious than a felony, punishable by a fine or imprisonment of up to one year in jail.

INFORMED CONSENT

Agreement by the patient to a medical procedure or treatment after receiving adequate information about the procedure or treatment, risks, and/or consequences.

BURDEN OF PROOF

A legal term used in conjunction with the terms malpractice and negligence. Must be proved by the client when an accusation of malpractice or negligence is claimed, rather than the health care provider proving that none existed.

CHAIN OF CUSTODY

The procedure for ensuring that material obtained for diagnosis has been taken from the named patient, is properly labeled, and has not been tampered with en route to the laboratory.

The **burden of proof** in proving malpractice or negligence is the responsibility of the plaintiff. Although most cases or situations are very difficult to prove, it has not prevented lawsuits to increase in number, including cases against phlebotomists.

Most cases against phlebotomists involve malpractice or negligence, and include practices such as mislabeling specimens; failure to properly identify the patient; failure to use sterile techniques, causing infection; reuse of needles; failure to properly perform a test, resulting in misdiagnosis; injury to a vein, injury to a nerve, and/or scarring; failure to properly inform a patient of the risks, such as fainting; drawing blood without the patient's consent; breech of confidentiality; breakage of equipment causing injury to the patient; and failure to control the **chain of custody**.

In order for a patient to prove negligence, four conditions must exist:

● A standard of care must exist.
● The standard of care must be breached.
● An injury must be sustained.
● The injury must be proven to be caused by acts that resulted from a breach of the standard of care.

Ethics

Ethics is the area of philosophical study that examines society's values, actions, and choices to determine right and wrong. The term ethics is derived from the Greek word *ethos,* which means custom or practice. From the beginning of time, the human race has grouped together to share a common goal. In order to accomplish the goal, rules were established. The degree to which the rules were followed dictated the fate of the group. The rules were decided upon by what the group accepted as ethical; in other words, what the group accepted as right and wrong. Today's society has established rules of right and wrong. The medical profession's rules of right and wrong are called the medical code of ethics. It outlines acceptable and unacceptable acts and behaviors in order to avoid harming the life, well-being, and privacy of medical employers, workers, and patients. For example, a phlebotomy technician would not disclose the results of a laboratory test to any one other than an authorized person, such as a physician. To do so would violate the principle of good conduct or ethics. The following is an example of a code of ethics used by the associate membership of the American Society of Clinical Pathologists (ASCP).

Recognizing that my integrity and that of my profession must be pledged to the best possible care of patients based the reliability of my work, I will:

- Treat patients and colleagues with respect, care, and thoughtfulness.
- Perform my duties in an accurate, precise, timely, and responsible manner.
- Safeguard patient information as confidential within the limits of the law.
- Prudently use laboratory resources.
- Advocate the delivery of quality laboratory services in a cost-effective manner.
- Work within the boundaries of the laws and regulations and strive to disclose illegal or improper behavior to the appropriate authorities.
- Continue to study, apply, and advance medical laboratory knowledge and skills and share such with my colleagues, other members of the health care community, and the public.

OSHA AND CLIA

Occupational Safety and Health Administration (OSHA)

OSHA is a division of the U.S. Department of Labor and is responsible for enforcing OSHA standards. The Occupational Safety and Health Act was passed into law by the federal government in 1970, establishing the original OSHA standards. With the passing of this law, it became mandatory for every employer with 10 or more employees to maintain a workplace free of recognized hazards. OSHA has the authority to impose fines for noncompliance of standards. Several areas of these standards directly affect the health care industry. These are standards regarding:

- **Blood-borne pathogens**
- Personal protective equipment
- Formaldehyde (standard)
- Eye wash protection
- Respirator (standard)
- Maintenance of the Log for Injuries and Illnesses
- Electrical systems

In December 1991, OSHA standards for the Occupational Exposure to Blood-borne Pathogens, and the recommendations regarding Universal Precautions, were published. These standards were put into place to minimize the risk of exposure to the hepatitis B and HIV viruses, as well as all other blood-borne pathogens. The standards mandate the availability and use of **personal protective equipment** (PPE), specific training, availability of the hepatitis B vaccination for all employees who have contact with

BLOOD-BORNE PATHOGEN

A term applied to any infectious microorganism present in the blood and/or other body fluids and tissues.

PERSONAL PROTECTIVE EQUIPMENT

le gloves, lab ons, protective as masks side hy

BIOHAZARDOUS WASTE

Any waste material that is harmful or potentially harmful to humans, or other species, or the environment.

blood-borne pathogens, and disposal of **biohazardous waste**. Specific OSHA standards will be addressed in Chapter 4.

Clinical Laboratory Improvement Amendments (CLIA)

The Clinical Laboratory Improvement Amendments were signed into federal law on October 31, 1988, stipulating that all clinical laboratories use the same standards, regardless of their location, type, or size.

The Clinical Laboratory Improvement Amendment law states that every facility in the country with a clinical laboratory must obtain a certificate from the federal government. This certificate assures the clients that all laboratory testing done in the facility meets federal standards. The laboratory must agree to routine site inspections in order to maintain certification.

CLIA also establishes levels of laboratory testing certification. This certification is based on the complexity of the test. A Physician Office Laboratory (POL) that performs tests such as pregnancy testing, microhematocrits, dipstick urinalysis, or blood-glucose determinations is considered "waived" from inspection. Waived tests, also known as low-complexity tests, are simple to perform, require minimum judgment, and are easily interpreted. Properly trained phlebotomy technicians are authorized to perform CLIA waived tests. Most "waived" test kits will say either on their packaging or within the kit's literature if they are CLIA waived. As technology continues to improve, laboratory tests can be reclassified, and a higher complexity test may become a lower complexity test. This is one reason why continuing education and keeping current with industry changes are so important to the phlebotomist.

Box 1-4: CLIA Certification Levels

Three level of tests are defined by CLIA and are categorized according to their complexity.

● Waived Tests: The general types of test that are listed as waived are simple to perform, require a minimum of quality control, and have an insignificant risk of harm to the patient. Tests on the waived list may be billed to Medicare and Medicaid. Certificate of Waiver must be renewed every two years. The following is a list of some CLIA waived tests.
  ▪ Urinalysis by reagent strip
  ▪ Microscopic urine sediment
  ▪ Urine pregnancy tests
  ▪ Occult blood/Guaiac tests

(continues)

Box 1-4: CLIA Certification Levels *(continued)*

- Microscopic examination of:
  - Pinworm preparation
  - Vaginal wet mount preparation
  - KOH preparation of cutaneous scrapings
  - Semen analysis
  - Gram stain (of discharge and exudate)
- Screen-slide card agglutination test for:
  - ASO (antistreptolysin O)
  - CRP (C-reactive protein)
  - Infectious mononucleosis screening
  - Rheumatoid factor screening
  - Sickle cell screening
- Ovulation tests (visual color test for human luteinizing hormone)
- Whole blood clotting time
- Glucose reagent strip screening
- Spun microhematocrit
- Erythrocyte sedimentation rate
- Level 1—Moderate Complexity Tests: More complicated to perform than waived tests; require an understanding of methodology, quality control, reagent stability, and instrument calibration. Any abnormal test results that apply to previously undiagnosed conditions of a patient must be referred to a Level 2 lab for verification. Must have a Quality Assurance program. Approximately 7,500 tests fall within this category. Some examples follow:
  - Urine cultures for colony counts (excluding identification and susceptibility)
  - Red and white blood cell counts
  - Hematocrit
  - BUN (blood urea nitrogen) uric acid
  - Glucose
  - Creatinine
  - Direct strep-antigen test
- Level 2—High Complexity Tests: Include sophisticated testing methodology, and often require independent judgment for interpretation. Examples of high complexity tests are:
  - Automated multichannel chemical profiles
  - Radioimmunoassay procedures
  - Drug and toxicology procedures
  - Coagulation studies

QUALITY ASSURANCE—QUALITY CONTROL

Quality Assurance (QA) is a group of activities and programs designed to guarantee the highest level of quality patient care. QA is accomplished by tracking outcomes through scheduled evaluations in which the hospital/laboratory looks at the suitability, adequacy, and timeliness of patient care. The Quality Assurance program must have evaluations and educational components to identify and correct problems. QA programs are required by hospitals and laboratories to receive funding by the Public Health Act.

The Joint Commission on Accreditation of Healthcare Organizations (JCAHO) is the leading national accreditation body for hospitals. In 1994, JCAHO required all hospitals to implement Quality Assurance programs. Quality Assurance programs are a subset of larger and more comprehensive programs called Total Quality Management (TQM). TQM is a combination of concepts based on continuously improving services and client care through the involvement of all employees. Because health care is very expensive and clients/patients can make educated choices regarding their care, TQM is directed at customer satisfaction.

It is a phlebotomy technician's responsibility to work effectively within the parameters of your health care facility's Quality Assurance program. What this means specifically is that the phlebotomy technician is to provide accurate, reproducible, and reliable "waived" test results and quality specimens, so that reliable and accurate client diagnoses can be made. As part of the health care team you must be continuously thinking quality, and constantly ask yourself, "Where are the possible sources of error?" and "How can I make the analysis most accurate?"

Quality Control (QC) is a component of Quality Assurance and is built on specific procedural steps to obtain accurate and reliable client test results. Examples of QC are collecting timed specimens such as Glucose Tolerance Tests (GTT) on schedule and ensuring that evacuated collection tubes have not expired.

QA/QC begins before every specimen is collected and every test is performed. The process begins with proper identification of the patient, proper selection of equipment, and proper positioning of the patient. Every specimen should be collected so that the integrity of the specimen is maintained. **Hemolysis** of the blood should not occur; the correct amount of blood should be drawn into the tube or syringe. Specimens requiring that the serum be tested should be allowed to clot for the correct amount of time and the serum must be drawn off using the appropriate procedures, which will be described

HEMOLYSIS

The destruction of the membrane of red blood cells and the liberation of hemoglobin, which diffuses into the surrounding fluid.

in Chapter 10. QA/QC affects how the patient is treated, and the patient's comfort and safety are the main objectives.

Procedure manuals must be made available to every health care worker who collects blood specimens and performs laboratory tests. Procedure manuals are a necessary part of a good TQM program. Procedure manuals outline the correct steps to be taken for every procedure performed in the facility. They must meet JCAHO, CLIA, CAP, and OSHA guidelines. The procedures must be clearly described in a detailed manner, ensuring every laboratory employee can understand the procedure and perform job duties with a high level of professionalism and accuracy.

RISK MANAGEMENT

Risk Management is a program used in conjunction with QA/QC. It is designed to minimize the exposure to the risk of loss or injury, for both the health care provider and the patient. Risk management encompasses organizational policies and procedures developed to protect the employees, employer, and the clients. There are two main areas of concern to the phlebotomist: 1) practices that create a high risk of injury, particularly in the area of blood-borne pathogen exposure, and 2) practices that might place the health care worker at risk for litigation. The specific guidelines to minimize the risk of exposure are further discussed in Chapter 4.

SUMMARY

The art of phlebotomy has been a medical practice for generations. It has evolved into the diagnostic practice used in medicine today. The phlebotomy technician is an integral part of the health care team and as such is held to a specific standard of care and must work within the legal and ethical boundaries of the health care industry. Formal education and certification are encouraged and often required to become employed as a phlebotomy technician. National certifying organizations provide an avenue for phlebotomy technicians to become certified, and most certifying agencies require continuing education to maintain certification. Successful phlebotomy technicians are highly motivated, detail oriented, compassionate, and empathetic health care workers with an ongoing commitment to the profession. They understand and comply with the professional guidelines and standards set by regulatory agencies such as OSHA, CLIA, and JCAHO.

STUDY AND REVIEW EXERCISES
Defining Key Terms
Write the definition for each of the following key terms.

1) abandonment _____

2) antisepsis _____

3) assault _____

4) battery _____

5) biohazardous waste _____

6) blood-borne pathogens_____

7) burden of proof _____

8) chain of custody _____

9) duty of care _____

10) false imprisonment _____

11) felony_____

12) fraud_____

13) hemochromatosis _____

14) hemolysis_____

15) informed consent _____

16) intentional infliction of emotional distress _____

_____

17) invasion of privacy_____

18) libel_____

19) malpractice _____

20) misdemeanor _____

21) negligence _____

22) personal protective equipment_____

23) polycythemia _____

24) respondeat superior_____

25) slander_____

26) tort _____

Reviewing Key Points

1) Briefly describe the advancement of phlebotomy as a profession.

2) List the basic responsibilities of a phlebotomy technician.

3) List the personal characteristics of a phlebotomy technician that employers find valuable.

4) Contrast the two main divisions of law as they affect the health care professional.

5) Identify the regulatory agencies involved with health care.

Sentence Completion

1) _____ provided the first written documentation of the practice of bloodletting.

2) Even today bloodletting is a valuable tool in treating _____ and _____.

3) _____ is evidence that an individual has mastered the skills required to perform in a specific technical area.

4) The _____, although not a legally binding document, is the standard to which all patients have the right to be treated.

5) _____ occurs when a duty of care is breached unintentionally, causing harm to the patient.

6) The _____ in proving malpractice or negligence is the responsibility of the client/patient.

7) _____ is a division of the U.S. Department of Labor and is responsible for enforcing the Occupational Safety and Health Act.

8) _____ is a group of activities and programs designed to guarantee the highest level of quality patient care.

9) _____ is a program used in conjunction with QA/QC and is designed to minimize the exposure to the risk of loss or injury to both the health care provider and the patient.

10) _____ is a combination of concepts based on continuously improving services and client care through the involvement of all employees and is directed at customer satisfaction.

Multiple Choice

1) A device that consisted of a small box that contained 12 small spring-driven rotary blades.
   A. Fleam
   B. Scarificator
   C. Flint cup
   D. Lancet

2) The medicinal leech is typically _____ to _____ inches in length and when full, contains from _____ to _____ ounce of blood.
   A. 3–6; $\frac{1}{2}$–1
   B. 2–4; $\frac{1}{2}$–1
   C. 5–7; 1–2
   D. 2–4; 1–2

3) The agency that has set guidelines and standards for phlebotomy curriculum is:
   A. OSHA
   B. NCCLS
   C. CLIA
   D. CAP

4) A health care professional with a minimum of a master's degree in nursing and advanced education in a particular primary care group such as Pediatrics, and who can practice independently.
   A. Physician's assistant
   B. Licensed practical nurse
   C. Registered nurse
   D. Nurse practitioner

5) A health care professional who treats patients with the restoration of physical strength and endurance, coordination, and range of motion through exercises, heat and cold therapy, and massage.
   A. Massage therapist
   B. Physician's assistant
   C. Occupational therapist
   D. Physical therapist

6) A technologist with an advanced degree in management who is responsible for overseeing all business operations of the laboratory.
   A. Physician
   B. Pathologist
   C. Laboratory manager
   D. Clinical laboratory scientist

7) A civil wrong, that is based on an act that is committed without just cause such as negligence.
   A. Tort
   B. Due care
   C. Respondeat superior
   D. Criminal law

8) Assault, battery, and invasion of privacy are examples of:
   A. negligence
   B. intentional tort
   C. strict liability
   D. respondeat superior

9) _____ is a claim of improper treatment or negligence brought against a professional person and/or entity by means of a civil lawsuit.
   A. Malfeasance
   B. Misdemeanor
   C. Malpractice
   D. Misfeasance

10) OSHA mandates all of the following except:
   A. Proper disposal of hazardous waste
   B. Personal protective equipment
   C. Availability of hepatitis B vaccination
   D. All of the above are mandated by OSHA

Critical Thinking

1) The patient in the emergency room you have orders to draw blood on is being uncooperative; she is yelling and screaming at you to leave her alone. She seems to be coherent and logical except for the fact that she does not want you to draw her blood. What would you do?

2) The patient in Room 112, Mrs. Henderson, has been hospitalized for the past two days. Your coworker has been assigned to draw her labs both days. Today at lunch your coworker tells you that the "mean old lady" in 112 has been so verbally abusive that he has not drawn her blood either day, but has "pulled" an extra tube from another patient and sent in down as Mrs. Henderson's. Could Mrs. Henderson or her family sue your coworker? If so, what would the charges be? Explain. Could your coworker sue Mrs. Henderson? If so, what would the charges be? Explain.

Medical Terminology

CHAPTER 2

KEY TERMS

All medical terms throughout this chapter should be considered key terms.

OBJECTIVES

Upon completion of this chapter the student should be able to:

- Define the terms word root, prefix, suffix, combining form, and combining vowel.
- Describe how word parts fit together to create a variety of medical terms.
- Correctly form, define, and use in a sentence medical terms created from combining forms, prefixes, and suffixes.
- State the meaning of a variety of commonly used combining forms, prefixes, and suffixes.
- Appropriately use common medical abbreviations.

OUTLINE

- Introduction: The Language of Medicine
- Word Roots
- Combining Forms
- Prefixes
- Suffixes
- Abbreviations—Medical Laboratory

❶ INTRODUCTION: THE LANGUAGE OF MEDICINE

The medical profession has a language all its own. Every medical professional needs to master the basics of this language to properly function as a member of the health care team.

Medical terminology was primarily derived from the Latin and Greek languages. Understanding how medical terms originate and how they can be broken down into word roots, suffixes, and prefixes, using combining forms, will help to simplify this process.

What once was a matter of rote memorization is now a matter of learning some basics. By learning how to combine word parts and exchanging suffixes and prefixes, you can build quite an extensive medical vocabulary. For an example, see Figure 2-1.

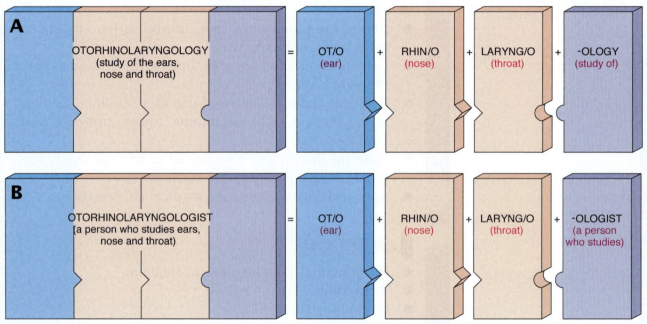

FIGURE 2-1: (A) A medical term may be taken apart to determine its meaning. (B) Change the ending (suffix) and a new term is made.

At first glance "otorhinolaryngology" is a 19-letter word that seems to have no rhyme or reason. However, when broken down into manageable parts, the term starts to make sense.

❶ WORD ROOTS

Word roots are the basis from which all medical terms are derived. The word root establishes the meaning of the term, and generally pertains to a tissue, organ, or body system. Word roots are also used to indicate colors. They are used with prefixes, suffixes, and other word roots to create new words.

● COMBINING FORMS

The combining form aids in the ease of pronunciation of medical terms. It is an extension of the word root and may be used to modify the spelling of a term generally by using the letters **o** or **i**. These are called combining vowels. The following basic rules are used to determine when the vowel is used or not used.

The combining vowel is not used when the suffix begins with a vowel. For example, when the combining form **cardi/o** is used with **-itis** the term would be **carditis**, because -itis starts with a vowel. ("Carditis" means inflammation of the heart; "cardi/o" meaning heart and "itis" meaning inflammation of).

The combining vowel is used when the suffix begins with a consonant. For example, when "cardi/o" is combined with **-pathy**, they form the term **cardiopathy**. The suffix -"pathy" starts with a consonant (-"pathy" means disease). Cardiopathy means any disease of the heart.

Table 2-1 lists some of the combining forms that are commonly used in the phlebotomy profession. Additional terms are presented in subsequent chapters as introduced by the chapter topics. For additional references, refer to any of the several medical terminology textbooks available on today's market.

Table 2-1: Commonly Used Combining Forms	
abdomin/o	abdomen
abrupt/o	broken away from
abscess/o	going away, collection of pus
aer/o	air, gas
agglutin/o	clumping, stick together
aneurysm/o	aneurysm
angin/o	choking, strangling
aort/o	aorta
appendic/o	appendix
arteri/o	artery

(continues)

Table 2-1: Commonly Used Combining Forms *(continued)*

articul/o	joint
arthr/o	joint
asphyxi/o	absence of a pulse
aspirat/o	to breathe in
ather/o	plaque, fatty substance
atri/o	atrium
attenuat/o	diluted, weakened
bacill/o	little stick or rod
bacteri/o	bacteria, rod or staff
bilirubin/o	bilirubin
brachi/o	arm
bronc/i,	bronchial tube, windpipe
broncho/o	bronchial tube, windpipe
calc/o	calcium
carcin/o	cancerous
cardi/o	heart
caud/o	tail
cauter/o	burn, burning
cephal/o	relating to a head
cerebell/o	cerebellum
cerebr/o	brain, cerebrum
cholesterol/o	cholesterol
coagulat/o	congeal, curdle, fix together
cocc/i, cocc/o	berry-shaped bacterium
constrict/o	draw tightly together
contagi/o	unclean, infection
contaminat/o	pollute, render unclean by contact
corpuscul/o	little body
crani/o	skull
cry/o	cold
cyst/o	urinary bladder, cyst, sac of fluid
cyt/o	cell

Table 2-1: Commonly Used Combining Forms *(continued)*

derm/o	skin
diastol/o	standing apart, expansion
dilat/o	spread out, expand
ecchym/o	pouring out of juice
electr/o	electric, electricity
encephal/o	brain
endocrin/o	secrete within
eosin/o	red, rosy, dawn-colored
erythem/o	flushed, redness
erythr/o	red
fibrin/o	fibrin, fibers, threads of a clot
gastr/o	stomach, belly
glyc/o	glucose, sugar
hem/o	blood, relating to the blood
hemat/o	blood, relating to the blood
hemangi/o	blood vessel
hepat/o	liver
immun/o	immune,
jugul/o	throat
lip/o	fat, lipid
lymph/o	lymph, lymphatic tissue
micr/o	small
morph/o	shape, form
my/o	muscle
myocardi/o	myocardium, heart muscle
nephro/o	kidney
nerv/o	nerve, nerve tissue
neur/o, neur/i	pertaining to the nerves, nervous tissue
nucle/o	nucleus
nucleol/o	little nucleus, nucleolus
occlud/o	shut, close up
occult/o	hidden, concealed

(continues)

Table 2-1: Commonly Used Combining Forms *(continued)*

onc/o	tumor
oste/o	bone
path/o	disease, suffering
phleb/o	vein
plasm/o	something molded or formed
pulm/o	lung
pulmon/o	lung
py/o	pus
ren/o	kidney
resuscit/o	revive
retr/o	behind, backward
scler/o	sclera, white of eye
sphincter/o	tight band
staphyl/o	cluster, bunch of grapes
strept/o	twisted chain
syring/o	tube
systol/o	contraction
thorac/o	chest
thromb/o	clot
tox/o, toxic/o	poison
trache/o	trachea, windpipe
tunic/o	covering, cloak, sheath
tympan/o	tympanic membrane, eardrum
varic/o	swollen or dilated vein
vascul/o	little vessel
ven/o	vein
ventr/o	in front, belly side of body
ventricul/o	ventricle of brain or heart
venul/o	venule, small vein

● PREFIXES

Prefixes are often added to the beginning of a word root to change the meaning of the word. They often indicate an amount, location, or time. A prefix never stands alone. Many prefixes are paired with another prefix with the opposite meaning. It is important to pay special attention when studying these prefixes until you have them committed to memory. Learn the prefixes listed in Table 2-2.

Table 2-2: Prefixes	
a-, an-	away from, negative, no, not without
ab-	away from
ac-, ad-, af-, as-, at-	toward, to
al-	like, similar
ante-	before, forward
anti-	against, counter
bi-	twice, double, two
brachy-	short
brady-	slow
cent-	hundred
circum-	around, about
co-, com-, con-	together, with
contra-	against, counter, opposite
cort-	covering
cyst-	bag, bladder
de-	from, not, down, lack of
demi-	half
di-	twice, twofold, double
dia-	through, between, apart, complete
dis-	negative, apart, absence
dys-	difficult, painful, bad
ecto-	out, outside
em-	in
en-	in, into, within
endo-	within, in, inside

(continues)

Table 2-2: Prefixes *(continued)*

epi-	upon, above, on, upper
eu-	well, easy, good
ex-, exo-	out of, outside, away from
extra-	on the outside, beyond, outside
fore-	before, in front of
hem-	relating to the blood
hemi-	half
hydra-	relating to water
hyper-	over, above, increased, excessive
hypo-	under, decreased, deficient, below
in-	in, into, not, without
infra-	beneath, below, inferior to
inter-	between, among
intra-, intro-	within, into, inside
mal-	bad, poor, evil
med-, mes-	middle
mega-	large, great
meta-	change, transformation, subsequent to, behind, hindmost, after or next
multi-	many, much
neo-	new, strange
nitro-	nitrogen
non-	no
nuli-	none
ortho-	straight, normal, correct
os-	mouth, bone
pan-	all, entire, every
para-	apart from, beside, near, abnormal
per-	excessive, through
peri-	around, surrounding
poly-	many
post-	after, behind
pre-	before, in front of

Table 2-2: Prefixes *(continued)*	
pro-	before, in behalf of
re-	back, again
retro-	behind, backward, back of
semi-	half
sub-	under, less, below
super-	above, excessive, higher than
sym-	with, together
syn-	union, association
tachy-	fast, rapid
tetra-	four
trans-	across, through
tri-	three
ultra-	beyond, excess
un-	not
uni-	one
venter-	the abdomen

● SUFFIXES

Suffixes are added to the end of a combining form to add to or change its meaning. They usually indicate a procedure, condition, disorder, or disease. As with prefixes, suffixes cannot stand alone. There are several suffixes that mean "pertaining to" or "relating to"; be sure to pay particular attention to these. Learn the suffixes listed in Table 2-3.

Table 2-3: Suffixes	
-able	capable of, able to
-ac	pertaining to
-ago	attack, diseased state or condition
-agra	excessive pain, seizure, attack of severe pain
-aise	comfort, ease
-al	pertaining to

(continues)

Table 2-3: Suffixes *(continued)*

-algesic	painful
-ar	pertaining to
-arche	beginning
-ary	pertaining to
-ase	enzyme
-blast	embryonic, immature
-cele	tumor, cyst, hernia
-centesis	surgical puncture to remove fluid
-cidal	pertaining to death
-cide	causing death
-clasis, -clast	break
-clysis	irrigation, washing
-crasia	a mixture or blending
-crit	separate
-cytic	pertaining to a cell
-cytosis	condition of cells
-dema	swelling (fluid)
-desis	bind, tie together, surgical fixation of bone or joint
-duct	opening
-dynia	pain
-eal	pertaining to
-ectasia, -ectasis	stretching, dilation, enlargement
-ectomy	surgical removal, cutting out, excision
-emesis	vomiting
-emia	blood, blood condition
-esis	state or abnormal condition
-esthesia	sensation, feeling
-exia, -exis	condition
-ferent	carrying
-form	form, figure, shape
-fuge	to drive away
-gene	production, origin, formation

Table 2-3: Suffixes (continued)

-genesis, -genic	producing, forming
-genous	producing
-grade	go
-gram	tracing, picture, record
-graph	instrument for recording, picture
-graphy	process of recording a picture or record
-ia	state or condition
-iac	pertaining to
-iasis	condition, pathologic state, abnormal condition
-ible	able to be, capable of being
-ic	pertaining to
-ific	making, producing
-iform	shaped or formed like, resembling
-igo	attack, diseased condition
-ile	capable of (being), able to, pertaining to
-ism	state of, condition
-istis, -itis	inflammation
-ium	structure, tissue
-kinesis	motion
-lith	stone, calculus
-lithiasis	presence of stones
-lysis	setting free, break down, separation, destruction
-lyst	agent that causes lysis or loosening
-lytic	reduce, destroy
-mania	obsessive, preoccupation
-megaly	large, great, extreme, enlargement
-meter	measure
-necrosis	death of tissue
-oid	like, resembling
-ologist	specialist
-ology	the science or study of

(continues)

Table 2-3: Suffixes *(continued)*

-oma	tumor, neoplasm
-osis	disease, an abnormal condition
-ostomosis, -ostomy	surgically creating a mouth or opening
-otomy	cutting, surgical incision
-ous	pertaining to
-paresis	partial or incomplete paralysis
-pathic	pertaining to, affected by disease
-penia	lack, deficiency, too few
-pexy	surgical fixation, to put in place
-phage	one that eats, a cell that destroys
-phagia	eating, swallowing
-phasia	speak or speech
-pheresis	removal
-phoresis	carrying, transmission
-phoria	to bear, carry, feeling, mental state
-phylactic	protective, preventive
-phylaxis	protection
-physis	to grow
-plasia	formation, development, growth
-plasm	formative material of cells
-plasty	surgical repair
-plegia	stroke, paralysis, palsy
-plegic	paralysis, one affected with paralysis
-pnea	breathing
-poiesis	formation
-porosis	passage, porous condition
-praxia	action, condition concerning the performance of movements
-ptosis	drooping, sagging, prolapse, dropping down
-ptysis	spitting
-rrhage, -rrhagia	bursting forth
-rrhaphy	suturing, stitching
-rrhea	flow, discharge

Table 2-3: Suffixes *(continued)*	
-rrhexis	rupture
-sarcoma	tumor, cancer
-scope	instrument for visual examination
-scopic	pertaining to visual examination
-scopy	see, visual examination
-stalsis	contraction
-statis	stopping, controlling
-stenosis	narrowing, tightening, stricture of a duct or canal
-stomosis, - stomy	furnish with a mouth or outlet, new opening
-tic	pertaining to
-tome	instrument to cut
-tomy	cutting, incision
-tripsy	crushing stone
-tropic	having an affinity for, turning toward
-uresis	urination
-uria	urination, urine
-us	thing
-version	to turn

ABBREVIATIONS—MEDICAL LABORATORY

Abbreviations are frequently used to shorten medical terms, laboratory tests, and medical phrases. It is very important to use abbreviations correctly. Some abbreviations have more than one meaning. For example, **be** can mean "below elbow" or "barium enema." Some terms and phrases have more than one abbreviation; for example, subcutaneous can be abbreviated as **sc**, **sub-Q**, and **subcu**. It is also very important to pay particular attention to the capitalization use of abbreviations; for example, **Ca** stands for calcium, **CA** means cancer. *Remember: when in doubt spell it out.* Some of the most common medical abbreviations are listed in Table 2-4.

Table 2-4: Common Medical Abbreviations

abd	abdomen	bil	bilateral
AB	abnormal	Bld	blood
ABG	arterial blood gas	B/P, BP	blood pressure
AC, ac	before meals	BT	bleeding time
ACLS	advanced cardiac life support	BUN	blood, urea, nitrogen
ACTH	adrenocorticotropic hormone	bx	biopsy
ADH	antidiuretic hormone	C	Celsius; centigrade
ad lib	as desired	c̄	with
adm	admission	Ca	calcium
AIDS	acquired immune deficiency syndrome	CA	cancer
		CAD	coronary artery disease
AKA	also known as	CAT	computed axial tomography
alb	albumin	cath	catheter; catheterize
alk	alkaline	CBC	complete blood count
ALL	acute lymphocytic leukemia	CC	chief complaint
alt hor	alternate hours	cc	cubic centimeter
alt noct	alternate nights	CCU	coronary care unit
am, a.m.	morning	CDC	Centers for Disease Control
AMA	against medical advice; American Medical Association	Ch, chol	cholesterol
		CHF	congestive heart failure
AMI	acute myocardial infarction	CK	creatinine kinase
AML	acute myelocytic leukemia	cm	centimeter
AMS	amylase	CML	chronic myelocytic leukemia
amt	amount	CNS	central nervous system
ANS	autonomic nervous system	c/o	complains of
ant	anterior	CO2	carbon dioxide
A&P	anterior and posterior	contra	against
aq	aqueous	COPD	chronic obstructive pulmonary disease
ASA	aspirin		
ASAP	as soon as possible	CPK	creatinine phosphokinase
AST	aspartate aminotransferase	CPR	cardiopulmonary resuscitation
AZT	azidothymindine	creat	creatinine
BID, bid, b.i.d.	twice a day	C&S	culture and sensitivity

Table 2-4: Common Medical Abbreviations *(continued)*

CSF	cerebrospinal fluid		ETOH	ethyl alcohol
CT, C-T	computerized tomography		ex	excision
CVA	cardiovascular accident; cerebrovascular accident		exam	examination
			exp	expiration
CXR	chest X-ray film		F	Fahrenheit
d	day		FAS	fetal alcohol syndrome
DC	discontinue		FBS	fasting blood sugar
diag	diagnosis		FH	family history
DIC	diffuse intravascular coagulation		FOB	fecal occult blood
diff	differential		FTT	failure to thrive
disch	discharge		FU, F/U	follow-up
DNA	deoxyribonucleic acid		FUO	fever of unknown origin
DNR	do not resuscitate		FX, Fx, fx	fracture
DOA	dead on arrival		g	gram
DOB	date of birth		GI	gastrointestinal
Dx	diagnosis		gm	gram
EBV	Epstein-Barr virus		gr	grain
ECG	electrocardiogram; electrocardiograph		GSW	gunshot wound
			GTT	glucose tolerance test
ECHO	echocardiogram		gtt	drops
E. coli	Escherichia coli		GU	genitourinary
EEG	electroencephalogram		GYN, Gyn, gyn	gynecology
EENT	eye, ear, nose, and throat		h	hour
EIA	enzyme immunoassay		H2O	water
EKG	electrocardiogram; electrocardiograph		H&H	hemoglobin and hematocrit
ELISA	enzyme-linked immunoassay; enzyme-linked immunosorbent assay		Hb, hgb	hemoglobin
			HbF	fetal hemoglobin
			HBV	hepatitis B virus
eos, eosins	eosinophils		HCFA	Health Care Financing Administration
ER	emergency room			
ESR	erythrocyte sedimentation rate		hct	hematocrit
et	and		hdk, H/A	headache

(continues)

Table 2-4: Common Medical Abbreviations *(continued)*

HDL	high-density lipoprotein	liq	liquid
HIV	human immunodeficiency virus	LLQ	left lower quadrant
H&P	history and physical	LMP	last menstrual period
hr	hour	LOC	level of consciousness
Hs, h.s.	at bedtime; hour of sleep	LTC	long-tem care
ht	height; hematocrit	LUQ	left upper quadrant
Hx	history	lymphs	lymphocytes
ICU	intensive care unit	lytes	electrolytes
Ig	immunoglobulin	m	minim
IgA	immunoglobulin A	mcg	microgram
IgD	immunoglobulin D	MCH	mean corpuscular hemoglobin
IgG	immunoglobulin G	MCHC	mean corpuscular hemoglobin concentration
IgM	immunoglobulin M		
IM	infectious mononucleosis; intramuscular	MCV	mean corpuscular volume
		mEq	milliequivalent
inf	inferior; infusion	mg	milligram
I&O	intake and output	MI	myocardial infarction
irrig	irrigation	mL	milliliter
isol	isolation	mm	millimeter
IV	intravenous; intravenously	mono	monocytes
IVP	intravenous pyelogram	MRI	magnetic resonance imaging
K	potassium	MS	mitral stenosis; multiple sclerosis
kg	kilogram		
KO	keep open	Na	sodium
KVO	keep vein open	NaCL	sodium chloride
L	liter	NEG, neg	negative
lab	laboratory	NG	nasogastric
lac	laceration	NKA	no known allergies
lat	lateral	NKDA	No known drug allergies
lb	pound	No, #	number
LD	lactic dehydrogenase	noct	night
LDL	low-density lipoprotein	NPO	nothing by mouth
lg	large	N/S	normal saline

Table 2-4: Common Medical Abbreviations *(continued)*

O2	oxygen	preop	preoperative
OB	obstetrics	prep	prepare
OB-GYN	obstetrics and gynecology	prn, PRN	as needed
OCC	occasional	prog	prognosis
OD	overdose	pro time	prothrombin time
od	once a day, also right eye	psych	psychiatry
O&P	ova and parasites	pt	patient; pint
OR	operating room	PPT	partial prothrombin time
oz	ounce	PTT	partial thromboplastin time; prothrombin time
p̄	after; phosphorus	PVD	peripheral vascular disease
P	pulse	Px	prognosis
Pap	Papanicolaou	q	every
Path	pathology	qd, q.d.	every day
pc	after meals	qh, q.h.	every hour
PCO2	pressure of carbon dioxide in the blood	q2h	every 2 hours
PCV	packed cell volume	qid, q.i.d.	four times a day
PE	physical examination	qm	every morning
Peds	pediatrics	qns	quantity not sufficient
pH	acidity; hydrogen ion concentration	qod	every other day
PI	present illness	qoh	every other hour
PKU	phenylketonuria	qt	quart; quiet
PLTS	platelets	q.q	each
PM, p.m.	evening or afternoon	quad	quadrant
PMNS	polymorphonuclear leukocytes	RBC	red blood cell; red blood count
PNS	peripheral nervous system	RBCV	red blood cell volume
PO, p.o.	by mouth; orally; postoperative	Rh neg, Rh–	Rhesus factor negative
Polys	polymorphonuclear leukocytes	Rh pos, Rh+	Rhesus factor positive
pos	positive	RIA	radioimmunoassay
post-op	postoperatively	RLQ	right lower quadrant
PP	postpartum; postprandial (after meals)	RNA	ribonucleic acid
		R.O, R/O	rule out

(continues)

Table 2-4: Common Medical Abbreviations *(continued)*

RPR	rapid plasma reagin		strep	streptococcus
RR	recovery room; respiratory rate		subcu	subcutaneous
rt	right; routine		sub-Q	subcutaneous
RT	radiation therapy; respiratory therapy		Sx	symptoms
RUQ	right upper quadrant		T	temperature
Rx	prescription; take; therapy; treatment		T3	triiodothyronine (thyroid hormone)
s̄	without		T4	thyroxine (thyroid hormone)
sc	subcutaneous		TB	tuberculosis
SCA	sickle cell anemia		T&C	type and crossmatch
SCPK	serum creatinine phosphokinase		temp	temperature
SCT	sickle cell trait		TIA	transient ischemic attack
sed rate	sedimentation rate		TIBC	total iron binding capacity
seg	segmented neutrophils		TID, t.i.d.	times interval difference; three times a day
semi	half		TKO	to keep open
SGOT	serum glutamic oxaloacetic transaminase		TPN	total parenteral nutrition
SGPT	serum glutamic pyruvic transaminase		TPR	temperature, pulse, respiration
SIDS	sudden infant death syndrome		Trig	triglycerides
SLE	St. Louis encephalitis; systemic lupus erythematosus		TSH	thyroid-stimulating hormone
			Tx	traction; treatment
SSMA	sequential multiple analysis		U	units
SMAC	sequential multiple analysis computer		UA	urinalysis
			UK	unknown
SOAP	symptoms, observations, assessments, plan		URI	upper respiratory infection
			UTI	urinary tract infection
SOB	shortness of breath		UV	ultraviolet
sp gr	specific gravity		VCUG	voiding cystourethrogram
SR	sedimentation rate		VD	venereal disease
ss	half		VDRL	Venereal Disease Research Laboratory
staph	staphylococcus			
stat	immediately		VP	venipuncture; venous pressure
STD	sexually transmitted disease		VS	vital signs

Table 2-4: **Common Medical Abbreviations** *(continued)*			
W	water	X	multiplied by; times
WBC	white blood cell; white blood count	XR	X-ray
wd	wound	y/o	year(s) old
WNL	within normal limits	YOB	year of birth
w/o	without	yr	year
wt	weight		

STUDY AND REVIEW EXERCISES
Defining Key Terms

Word Parts: Write the definition for each of the following terms:

1) word root _____

2) prefix _____

3) suffix _____

4) combining form _____

5) combining vowel _____

Combining Forms: Define each of the combining form:

1) aort/o _____

2) oste/o _____

3) cardi/o _____

4) thromb/o _____

5) strept/o _____

6) hem/o _____

7) venul/o _____

8) angin/o _____

9) cyt/o _____

10) plasm/o _____

11) erythem/o _____

12) hemangi/o _____

Combining Forms: Write the correct combining form for each of the following definitions:

1) small _____

2) little vessel _____

3) skin _____

4) clumping together _____

5) brain _____

6) heart _____

7) tumor _____

8) contraction _____

9) vein _____

10) kidney _____

11) little body _____

12) stomach, belly _____

Prefixes: Define each of the prefixes:

1) demi- _____

2) tachy- _____

3) neo- _____

4) endo- _____

5) a- _____

6) pre- _____

7) trans- _____

8) epi- _____

9) peri- _____

10) dys- _____

11) hypo- _____

12) poly- _____

Prefixes: Write the correct prefix for each of the following definitions.

1) three _____

2) against, counter _____

3) relating to blood _____

4) around, about _____

5) bad, poor, evil_____

6) beyond, excess_____

7) none _____

8) half _____

9) all, entire, every_____

10) after, behind _____

11) not_____

12) under, less, below _____

Suffixes: Define each of the following suffixes.

1) -dynia_____

2) -pnea_____

3) -lysis _____

4) -pathic _____

5) -rrhage _____

6) -otomy _____

7) -plasm _____

8) -lytic _____

9) -ism_____

10) -emia_____

11) -ary _____

12) -crit _____

Suffixes: Write the correct suffix for each of the following definitions.

1) large _____

2) surgical repair _____

3) one that eats, a cell that destroys _____

4) the science or study of _____

5) embryonic, immature _____

6) pertaining to _____

7) narrowing, tightening _____

8) removal _____

9) condition _____

10) surgical puncture to remove fluid _____

11) painful _____

12) like, resembling _____

Creating Medical Terms: Create 12 medical terms, define each term, and correctly use each in a sentence. Each of the 12 terms must contain at least one word part from the list below.

angi/o	-graphy	-itis	-otomy	multi-
hemat/o	-osis	aort/o	cardi/o	-ectomy
phleb/o	brady-	peri-	my/o	intra-
-ologist	-oma	thromb/o		

1) _____
_____

2) _____
_____

3) _____
_____

4) _____
_____

5) _____
_____

6) _____
_____

7) _____
_____

8) _____
_____

9) _____
_____

10) _____

_____

11) _____

_____

12) _____

_____

Medical Terms: Write the definition for each of the following medical terms.

1) cardiopathy _____

2) angiography_____

3) hemolysis _____

4) cardiac _____

5) venules _____

6) ventricular _____

7) ecchymosis _____

8) hemangioma _____

9) dysphagia_____

10) glycosuria_____

11) phlebotomy _____

12) diaphoresis _____

Medical Abbreviations: Write the definition for each of the following medical abbreviations.

1) TPR _____

2) ECG _____

3) gm _____

4) CAD_____

5) FBS_____

6) alt noct _____

7) SMAC _____

8) I&O _____

9) HDL_____

10) T$_3$ _____

11) ABG _____

12) ASAP _____

Medical Abbreviations: Write the correct medical abbreviation for each of the following definitions.

1) sedimentation rate _____

2) every day _____

3) fecal occult blood _____

4) with _____

5) hematocrit _____

6) complete blood count _____

7) lymphocytes _____

8) white blood cell _____

9) mean corpuscular _____

10) volume _____

11) serum glutamic oxaloacetic transaminase _____

_____

12) packed cell volume _____

13) within normal limits _____

Medical Abbreviations: In the following paragraph define the highlighted medical abbreviations.

A 16 **y/o** female **pt** was brought by ambulance to the **ER**, **c/o** of **SOB**, **hdk**, and blurred vision. Upon further questioning it was found that the pt was **HIV** positive. Examination revealed the **VS** were **WNL**. A **stat CBC** and **chem** panel were ordered and the phlebotomist performed a **VP** successfully. After review of the results an **ABG** was also ordered. During the draw the pt's **LOC** deteriorated. **CPR** was initiated. 10 **mg.** of Epinephrine was administered, the patient was defibrillated **X** 3, but after 40 minutes s̄ resuscitation, CPR was **DC**. The time of death was 4:32 **a.m.**

1) _____

2) _____

3) _____

4) _____

5) _____

6) _____

7) _____

8) _____

9) _____

10) _____

11) _____

12) _____

13) _____

14) _____

15) _____

16) _____

17) _____

18) _____

19) _____

20) _____

21) _____

Anatomy and Physiology

KEY TERMS

afferent (**AF**-er-ent)
agranulocytes
   (a-**GRAN**-u-lo-site)
albinism (**AL**-bye-nizm)
alveoli (al-**VE**-o-lye)
anatomy (a-**NAT**-o-me)
antecubital fossa
   (**an**-tee-**KU**-bi-tal)
anterior
antigen (**AN**-tih-jen)
anuria (ah-**NEW**-ree-ah)
aortic semilunar valve
   (aye-**OR**-tik **sem**-ee-**LOO**-
   nur valv)
arteriole (ahr-**TEER**-ee-ole)
arteriosclerosis
   (ahr-**teer**-ee-o-skleh-
   ROH-sis)
atherosclerosis
   (**ath**-er-o-scle-**ROH**-sis)
atrium (**AY**-tree-um)
axon (**AK**-son)
basophil (**BAY**-suh-fil)
bicuspid valve (bye-**KUS**-pid
   valve)
bilateral symmetry
   (bye-**LAT**-ur-al **SIM**-eh-tree)
bolus (**BOH**-lus)
cerebrospinal fluid
   (seh-**ree**-bro-**SPY**-nuyl
   FLEW-id) (Abbr. CSF)
chyme (kime)
contractility
   (kon-trak-**TIL**-ih-tee)

(continues)

OBJECTIVES

Upon completion of this chapter the student should be able to:

- Define the terms anatomy and physiology.
- Describe the correct anatomic position and the supine and prone body positions.
- Identify the body's planes, cavities, and regions, using the correct directional terms to describe the relationships between areas of the body with respect to other areas of the body.
- Define homeostasis and the process of metabolism.
- Describe the organization of the body, identifying the structural components of cells, body tissues, and organs.
- Describe the functions, structures, disorders, and diagnostic tests relating to the skeletal, muscular, nervous, integumentary, digestive, endocrine, urinary, lymphatic, reproductive, and respiratory systems.
- Describe the functions, structures, disorders, and diagnostic tests relating to the cardiovascular system, including the blood and vessels.
- Identify the layers of the heart.
- Describe the various types of circulation in the human body.
- Trace a drop of blood from the right atrium back to the right atrium of the heart.
- Differentiate between and describe the structure and function of the blood vessels of the human body.
- Name and locate the veins of the arm and discuss their suitability.

(continues)

KEY TERMS
(continued)

cranial cavity
(**KRAY**-nee-al **KAV**-eh-tee)

cytoplasm
(**SIGH**-toh-plazm)

deep

dendrite (**DEN**-drite)

deoxygenated
(dee-**OCK**-si-jen-ate-ted)

dermis (**DUR**-mis)

distal (**DIS**-tul)

dorsal cavity
(**DOR**-sul **KAV**-eh-tee)

duodenum
(dew-o-**DEE**-num)

efferent

elasticity (**e**-las-**TIS**-ih-tee)

electrolytes
(ee-**LEK**-tro-lites)

endocardium
(**en**-do-**KAR**-dee-um)

endocrine gland
(**EN**-doh-crin gland)

eosinophil (**ee**-o-**SIN**-uh-fil)

epidermis (**ep**-ih-**DUR**-mis)

epiglottis (**ep**-ih-**GLOT**-is)

erythrocytes
(e-**RITH**-ro-sites)

excitability
(ek-**sye**-tah-**BIL**-eh-tee)

exocrine gland
(**EX**-o-crin gland)

extensibility
(**ek**-**STEN**-sih-bil-eh-tee)

fimbria (**FIM**-bree-ah)

frontal plane

gamete (**GAM**-eet)

glomerulus
(gloh-**MER**-yah-lus)

granulocyte
(**GRAN**-yu-loh-site)

hematuria
(**he**-mah-**TOOR**-ee-ah)

hemoglobin
(**HE**-muh-gloh-bin)

hemolysis (he-**MOL**-ih-sis)

hemopoiesis
(**he**-mo-poy-**EE**-sis)
(hematopoiesis)

hemostasis
(**he**-moh-**STAY**-sis)

- List the major components of blood, differentiate between serum and plasma, and describe the formed elements and their functions.
- Describe how ABO and Rh blood types are determined and the importance of type and crossmatch testing.
- Define hemostasis and describe the basic coagulation process.

● OUTLINE
- Introduction to the Human Body
- Anatomic Terminology
- Body Functions
- Body Organization
- Skeletal System
- Muscular System
- Nervous System
- Integumentary System
- Digestive System
- Endocrine System
- Urinary System
- Lymphatic System—Immune System
- Reproductive System
- Respiratory System
- Cardiovascular System

homeostasis (**ho**-me-oh-**STAY**-sis)

hormone (**HOR**-mone)

ileum (**IL**-ee-um)

inferior (in-**FEH**-re-or)

interstitial fluid
(**in**-tur-**STISH**-ul **FLEW**-id)

jejunum (je-**JOO**-num)

lateral (**LAT**-ur-ul)

leukocyte (**LOO**-ko-site)

lumen (**LEW**-min)

lymph (limf)

lymphocyte (**LIM**-foh-site)

mastication (**mas**-ti-**KAY**-shun)

medial (**MEE**-dee-ul)

mediastinum
(**mee**-dee-as-**TIH**-num)

melanocyte (**MEL**-an-o-sit)

meninges (men-**IN**-jeez)

metabolism (meh-**TAB**-oh-**lizm**)

midsagittal plane
(**mid**-**SAJ**-eh-tel plane)

monocyte (**MON**-oh-site)

myelin sheath
(**MY**-eh-lin)

myocardium
(**MY**-oh-**kar**-dee-um)

nephron (**NEF**-ron)

neuron (**NEW**-ron)

neutrophil (**NOO**-trah-fil)

oliguria (**ol**-ih-**GOO**-ree-ah)

ova (**O**-va)

papilla (pa-**PIL**-uh)

paresthesia
(**par**-es-**THEE**-zee-ah)

pericardium
(**per**-ih-**KAR**-dee-um)

periosteum (**per**-ee-os-**TEE**-um)

peristalsis (**per**-ih-**STAL**-sis)

phagocytosis
(**fag**-oh-sigh-**TOH**-sis)

phospholipids (**fos**-foh-**LIP**-ids)

physiology (**fiz**-ee-**OL**-oh-jee)

posterior (pos-**TEER**-ee-ur)
prone
proximal (**PROK**-sih-mul)
pulmonary semilunar
valve (**PUL**-mo-neh-ree
sem-ee-**LOO**-nar valv)
sagittal plane
(**SAJ**-ih-tel plane)
Schwann cell (shwon cell)
sebaceous gland
(seh-**BAY**-shus)
sebum (**SE**-bum)
solute (**SOL**-yoot)
spermatozoa
(sper-**mat**-oh-**ZOH**-ah)
spinal cavity
(**SPY**-nel **CAV**-eh-tee)

stratum corneum
(**STRAH**-tum **KOR**-nee-um)
stratum germinativum
(**strah**-tum
jer-mi-nah-**TIVE**-um)
subcutaneous (**sub**-ku-**TAY**-nee-us)
superficial (**soo**-per-**FISH**-al)
superior (soo-**PEER**-ee-ur)
supine (soo-**PINE**)
surfactant (sur-**FAK**-tent)
synapse (**SIN**-aps)
thrombocyte (**THROM**-boh-site)
thromboplastin
(**throm**-boh-**PLAS**-tin)
transverse plane
tricuspid valve
(tri-**KUS**-pid valv)

tunica adventitia
(**TOON**-ih-kah ad-ven-**TISH**-uh)
tunica intima
(**TOON**-ih-kah **IN**-tih-ma)
tunica media
(**TOON**-ih-kah **ME**-dyuh)
universal donor
universal recipient
uremia (**yoo**-**REE**-mee-ah)
urethra (yoo-**REE**-thra)
uvula (**YOO**-vew-luh)
vasoconstriction
(**vas**-oh-kon-**STRIK**-shun)
ventral cavity
ventricle (**VEN**-trik-ul)
villi (**VIL**-eye)

INTRODUCTION TO THE HUMAN BODY

The human body is an amazing organism. Each body system is unique, its structure and function specific, and even though each system performs a specialized activity, the body's systems work together to create a well-organized and structured unit—the human body.

ANATOMY

The study of the structure of an organism.

The study of the structure of an organ and the relationship of that organ to other parts of the body is the study of **anatomy**. The word anatomy is derived from two Greek words, *ana,* meaning apart, and *temuein,* to cut. Human anatomy was discovered and labeled when scientists and physicians dissected the human body. **Physiology** is the study of the function of living organisms and their structures. By studying and understanding the anatomy and physiology of the human body the phlebotomist is better equipped to understand the reasoning behind why specific laboratory tests are ordered and how the patient's body may be responding to diseases, disorders, and conditions.

PHYSIOLOGY

The study of the functions of the living organism and its components.

BILATERAL SYMMETRY

Relating to both sides of the body equally.

The human body is a very complex and intricate organism. It has very distinct characteristics. For example, the human body exhibits **bilateral symmetry** (is bisymmetric), is divided into nine regions with five levels of organization, and has eleven major body systems (Figure 3-1). Understanding the five levels of organization of the human body, from the basis of life in the chemical form (atoms and molecules) to the most complex stage of life (the body), sets the stage for understanding the complexities of diseases, disorders, and conditions.

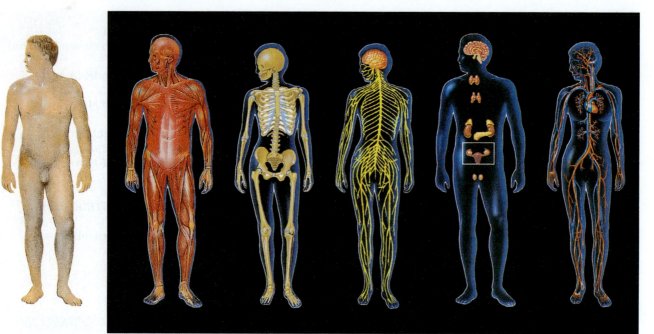

INTEGUMENTARY SYSTEM	MUSCULAR SYSTEM	SKELETAL SYSTEM	NERVOUS SYSTEM	ENDOCRINE SYSTEM	CIRCULATORY SYSTEM
Protection from injury and dehydration; body temperature control; excretion of some wastes; reception of external stimuli; defense against microbes.	Movement of internal body parts; movement of whole body; maintenance of posture; heat production.	Support, protection of body parts; sites for muscle attachment, blood cell production, and calcium and phosphate storage.	Detection of external and internal stimuli; control and coordination of responses to stimuli; integration of activities of all organ systems.	Hormonal control of body functioning; works with nervous system in integrative tasks.	Rapid internal transport of many materials to and from cells; helps stabilize internal temperature and pH.

FIGURE 3-1: The body systems (from *Biology: The Unity and Diversity of Life*, 5th ed., Starr, and Taggart, copyright 1989, Wadsworth).

In order, beginning with the simplest and proceeding to the most complex, the body's five levels of organization are:

● Cells: The smallest living units of structure and function in the body. Although the smallest units, cells are far from being the simplest. Greater explanation of cells continues later in this chapter.

● Tissues: An organization of many similar cells working together to perform a specific function. For example, the cardiac cells of the heart together create cardiac muscle tissue, which contracts and relaxes, thereby pumping blood to all parts of the body.

● Organs: More complex than cells or tissues. Made of like tissues arranged to perform a specific function. For example, the lungs are organs of the respiratory system which perform the function of supplying the body with oxygen through respiration.

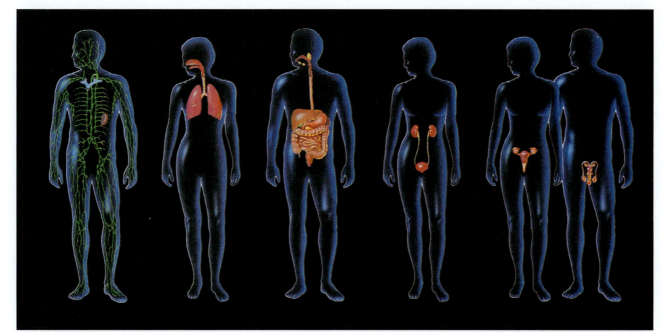

LYMPHATIC SYSTEM
Return of some tissue fluid to blood; role in immunity (defense against specific invaders of the body).

RESPIRATORY SYSTEM
Provisioning of cells with oxygen; removal of carbon dioxide wastes produced by cells; pH regulation.

DIGESTIVE SYSTEM
Ingestion of food, water; preparation of food molecules for absorption; elimination of food residues from the body.

URINARY SYSTEM
Maintenance of the volume and composition of extracellular fluid. Excretion of blood-borne wastes.

REPRODUCTIVE SYSTEM
Male: production and transfer of sperm to the female. Female: production of eggs; provision of a protected, nutritive environment for developing embryo and fetus. Both systems have hormonal influences on other organ systems.

- Systems: The most complex units functioning together, making a human body. A system is an organization of different organs functioning together to perform a specific task. For example, the organs of the circulatory system are the heart and blood vessels. They work together to provide the body with blood.
- The body as a whole: All the body's systems working together efficiently and effectively to sustain life.

Before exploring each of the organizational levels in detail it is important to understand the anatomic terminology used to describe the location of the organs in relationship to the position and structure of other organs.

Anatomic Position

When discussing the specific location of a body structure, or the relationship of one body structure to another, it is assumed the body is in a specific position called the anatomic position

SUPINE

The position of lying on the back with the face upward.

PRONE

A position which is horizontal with the face downward.

ANTERIOR

Before or in front of; refers to the ventral or abdominal side of the body.

POSTERIOR

A location behind or at the back; opposite to anterior.

SUPERIOR

In anatomy, higher; denoting upper of two parts, toward vertex.

INFERIOR

Beneath, lower; referring to the underside of an organ or indicating a structure below another.

MEDIAL

Toward the midline of the body.

LATERAL

Toward the side.

PROXIMAL

A location nearest the point of attachment, center of the body, or point of reference.

(Figure 3-2). The correct anatomic position is when the body is standing erect with the arms at the sides and palms turned forward. The head and feet are also facing forward. All references to anatomic directional terms or the location of a given structure of the body are identified or referred to as if the patient were in this position, regardless of the actual body position.

The terms **supine** and **prone** are used to describe two other patient positions that are of particular importance to the phlebotomist. In the supine position, the patient is lying face up on his/her back. When the patient is lying face down on the stomach it is the prone position. Prone can also refer to the patient's hand when the palm is face down, as, for example, when drawing blood from the back of the hand.

Directional Terms

Directional terms are helpful when describing a particular body structure location in relationship to another body structure location (Figure 3-3).

- **Anterior** (ventral) and **posterior** (dorsal): Anterior is defined as front or "in front of." Posterior is defined as back or "in back of." For example, the nose is located on the anterior aspect of the body, and the spine is located on the posterior aspect of the body.
- **Superior** (cranial) and **inferior** (caudal): Superior is defined as "toward the head." Inferior is defined as "toward the feet." Superior may also be defined as "upper" or "above." Inferior may also be defined as "lower" or "below." For example, the lungs are superior to the diaphragm, and the intestines are inferior to the diaphragm.
- **Medial** and **lateral**: Medial is defined as "toward the midline of the body." Lateral is defined as "away from the midline of the body." For example, the great toe is on the medial side of the foot, while the little toe is on the lateral side of the foot.
- **Proximal** and **distal**: Proximal is defined as "towards the point of attachment." Distal is defined as "farthest away from the point of attachment." For example, the knee is proximal to the foot, while the hand is distal to the elbow.
- **Superficial** and **deep**: Superficial is defined as "nearer the body surface." Deep is defined as "farther away from the body surface." For example, the skin is superficial to the underlying muscles, and the bone is deep to the muscles that surround it.

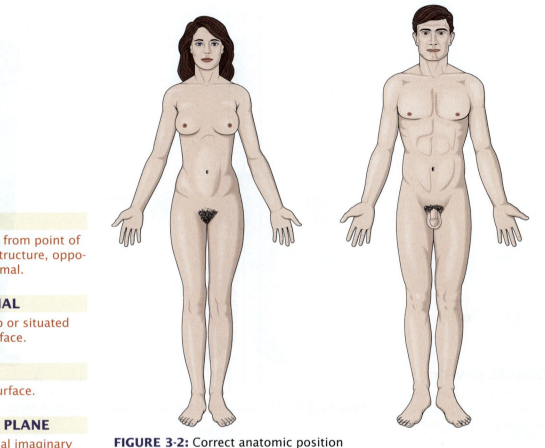

FIGURE 3-2: Correct anatomic position

DISTAL

The farthest from point of origin of a structure, opposite of proximal.

SUPERFICIAL

Pertaining to or situated near the surface.

DEEP

Below the surface.

SAGITTAL PLANE

A longitudinal imaginary line dividing the body into equal right and left parts.

MIDSAGITTAL PLANE

An imaginary line dividing the body into equal right and left halves.

FRONTAL PLANE

A plane parallel to the long axis of the body and at right angles to the median sagittal plane. The frontal plane divides the body into anterior and posterior portions.

TRANSVERSE PLANE

A plane that divides the body into a top and bottom portion.

Planes and Body Sections

In order to simplify the study of the body as a whole, it is often sectioned by imaginary lines. A section is a cut made though the body in the direction of a certain plane. To help clarify, sections and planes have been given specific names.

● Sagittal: The **sagittal plane** is a lengthwise plane running from front to back, dividing the body or any of its parts into right and left halves. If the plane starts at the crown of the head and proceeds down the chest, dividing the body into equal right and left halves, it is called a **midsagittal plane**.

● Frontal (also called the coronal plane): A **frontal plane** is a lengthwise plane running from side to side dividing the body or any of its parts into anterior and posterior portions.

● Transverse: A **transverse plane** is a horizontal or crosswise plane dividing the body or any of its parts into upper and lower regions.

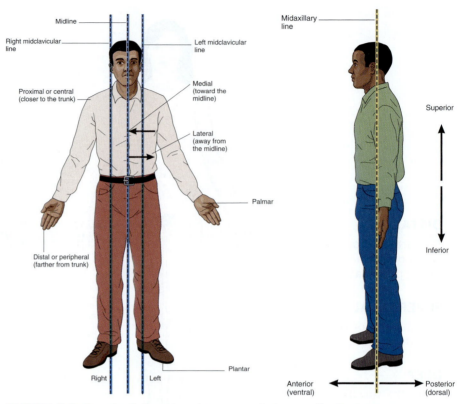

FIGURE 3-3: Standard directional terms and planes of reference

DORSAL CAVITY

The posterior cavity of the body, which houses the brain and spinal column.

CRANIAL CAVITY

The cavity that houses the brain.

SPINAL CAVITY

The cavity of the body that houses the spinal cord.

VENTRAL CAVITY

Pertaining to the belly; the opposite of dorsal. The anterior portion or the front side of the body.

MEDIASTINUM

Region of the thoracic cavity containing the heart and blood vessels, lying between the sternum (front) and vertebral column and between the lungs.

Body Cavities

Contrary to popular belief, the body is not a solid structure. The body is made up of several open spaces or cavities in which the body's organs are neatly organized (Figure 3-4). There are two major body cavities, which are further subdivided into smaller cavities.

● **Dorsal cavity**: The dorsal cavity contains the brain and spinal cord. The dorsal cavity is further subdivided into the **cranial cavity**, which houses the brain, and the **spinal cavity**, which contains the spinal cord.

● **Ventral cavity**: The ventral cavity contains the thoracic cavity (chest cavity) and the abdominopelvic cavity. The thoracic cavity is further subdivided into the right and left pleural cavities. The right lung is located in the right pleural cavity, and the left lung is located in the left pleural cavity. The central area of the thoracic cavity is known as the **mediastinum**, which is located between the lungs, from the back of the breastbone or sternum to the vertebrae of the back. The mediastinum houses the esophagus, bronchi, lungs, trachea, thymus gland, and heart. The heart is contained within a smaller cavity called the pericardial cavity.

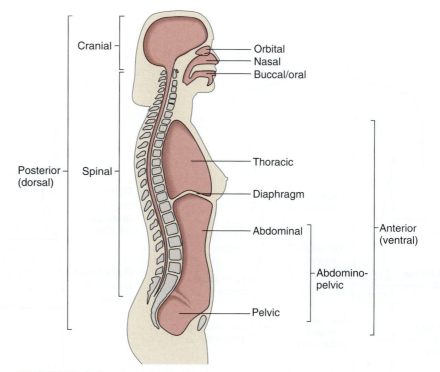

FIGURE 3-4: Cavities of the body

The abdominopelvic cavity is further subdivided into the abdominal cavity and the pelvic cavity. The abdominal cavity contains the stomach, liver, gallbladder, pancreas, spleen, small intestine, appendix, and part of the large intestine. The kidneys are located behind the abdominal cavity. The pelvic cavity contains the urinary bladder, the reproductive organs, the rectum, and the remainder of the large intestine. No physical structure separates the abdominal cavity and the pelvic cavity; however, the muscle for breathing, the diaphragm, separates the thoracic cavity from the abdominopelvic cavity.

Nine Regions of the Abdominopelvic Cavity

To locate the organs within the abdominopelvic cavity more easily, this cavity has been further subdivided into nine regions (Figure 3-5). The nine regions are located in the upper, middle, and lower areas of the abdomen.

● Upper regions: Include the epigastric region, which is located just below the sternum, and the right and left hypochondriac regions, located just below the ribs.

● Middle regions: Include the umbilical region, located around the navel or umbilicus, and the right and left lumbar regions, which extend from the anterior to the posterior of the body.

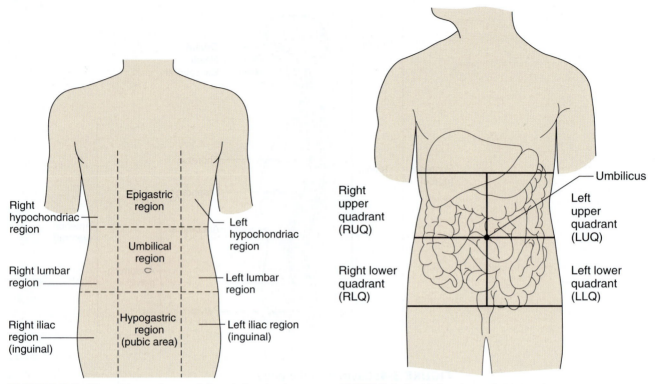

FIGURE 3-5: The nine regions of the abdominal area   **FIGURE 3-6:** Abdominopelvic quadrants

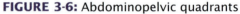

● Lower regions: Include the hypogastric region, which is also referred to as the pubic area, and the right and left iliac regions, which are also referred to as the inguinal regions.

The abdomen is also divided into quadrants (Figure 3-6): upper and lower right, and upper and lower left. The midsagittal and transverse planes passing through the umbilicus are defined as the dividing lines. RUQ—right upper quadrant, RLQ—right lower quadrant, LUQ—left upper quadrant, and LLQ—left lower quadrant are commonly used abbreviations. The phlebotomist must commit these abbreviations to memory.

● BODY FUNCTIONS

Every living organism is in a constant process of maintaining equilibrium, or balancing its internal environment, to ensure the organism's survival. This "steady state" is called **homeostasis**. Homeostasis is the state physiologists refer to as the relatively constant conditions within the internal environment of the body. Homeostasis enables all the cells of the body to obtain the nutrients and oxygen necessary to maintain life.

HOMEOSTASIS

The state of dynamic equilibrium of the internal environment of the body.

METABOLISM

Sum total of processes of digestion, absorption, and the resulting release of energy.

Metabolism is the physical and chemical reactions taking place on a cellular level, resulting in the growth, repair, energy release, and use of food by the body's cells. Metabolism consists of two processes, anabolism and catabolism. Anabolism and catabolism are opposites. Anabolism is the building up of complex materials from simpler materials such as food and oxygen. Catabolism is the breaking down and changing of complex substances, such as food molecules, into simpler ones, such as carbon dioxide and water, with a release of energy. The sum of all chemical reactions within a cell is called metabolism.

BODY ORGANIZATION
Cells

Cells are the basic unit of structure and function of all life and are responsible for all activities of the body (Figure 3-7). The human body, even though it might look like one solid structure, is actually composed of trillions of microscopic cells. Robert Hook, examining a piece of cork under a crude microscope, first discovered cells in the 1600s. The uniform unit-like pattern reminded him of a monk's room, which were called cells. A special unit of measurement called a micrometer or micron is used to determine cell size. Some cells, such as red blood cells, are as small as 7.5 microns, whereas an ovum (female sex cell) has a diameter of just less than 1,000 micrometers, about $\frac{1}{25}$ of an inch. Cells are often notably different in shape. Some cells are flat, some are brick shaped, some are threadlike, and some are irregularly shaped. Cells are sized and shaped to perform specific functions.

Even with all these differences, the basic structure of each cell is essentially the same. All cells contain **cytoplasm**. Cytoplasm is a living substance and can only be found within a cell. Each cell in the body is surrounded by a cell membrane. This membrane separates the cell contents from the diluted salt-water solution called **interstitial fluid** (tissue fluid) that bathes every cell in the body. The cell membrane functions to maintain the integrity of the cell, and even though it is a very delicate structure, only about 3/10,000,000 of an inch thick, it consists of two layers of phosphate-containing fat molecules called **phospholipids** that form the framework of the cell and keep it intact. The cell membrane acts as a gatekeeper between the fluid inside the cell and the fluid around the cell. It allows only certain substances (e.g., oxygen, nutrients) to pass through it, but bars the passage of other substances (e.g., some toxins). Each cell has a nucleus as well as smaller organelles (Box 3-1) imbedded within the cytoplasm. The

CYTOPLASM

Protoplasm of the cell body, excluding the nucleus.

INTERSTITIAL FLUID

Fluid between the tissues; surrounding a cell.

PHOSPHOLIPIDS

Fats containing carbon, hydrogen, oxygen, and phosphorous.

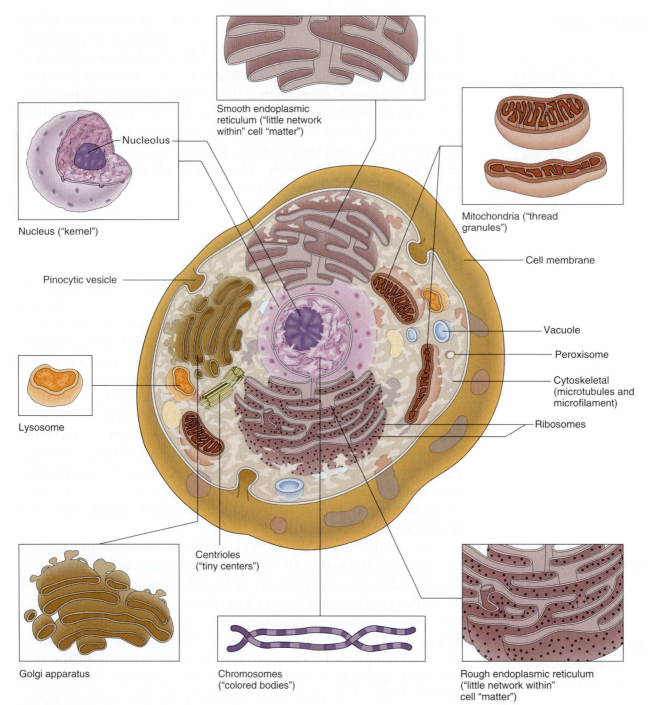

FIGURE 3-7: Human cell with organelles

nucleus is the most important organelle and functions as "the brain" of the cell to control its activities and functions to facilitate cell division. It is typically located near the center of the cell. The remaining organelles include centrioles, endoplasmic reticulum, Golgi apparatus, lysosomes, mitochondria, and ribosomes.

Box 3-1: Organelles of a Cell

- Centrioles: Two cylindrical or rod-shaped organelles, located near the nucleus, at right angles to each other. Centrioles function in cell division.

- Endoplasmic reticulum: Winding through the cytoplasm, these thin tubular structures form a network that stretches from the nucleus almost to the cell membrane. These tubular passageways carry proteins and other substances from one area of a cell to another. There are two types of endoplasmic reticulum: rough and smooth. Rough ER has ribosomes attached to its outer surface, giving it a rough appearance. Ribosomes attach to the ER as they make protein and drop it into the interior of the ER. The ER then transports the protein to processing areas. Endoplasmic reticulum often accumulates and stores large masses of protein. Areas that are too full of protein for ribosomes to attach appear smooth, hence the name smooth ER.

- Golgi apparatus: The Golgi apparatus is nicknamed the cell's chemical processing and packaging center. These organelles are most abundant in the cells of gastric, salivary, and pancreatic glands. Mucus is an example of a substance that is released from a cell. Located near the nucleus of the cell are small, flattened sacs stacked one on top of each other. These organelles synthesize carbohydrates and combine them with protein molecules, then "repackage" the new substance into small sacs called vesicles. These vesicles break away from the Golgi apparatus and slowly move toward the cell's membrane. The vesicle then breaks open and releases its contents to the outside of the cell.

- Lysosomes: Membranous, spherical bodies which appear to contain tiny particles; they contain powerful digestive enzymes. They are nicknamed "digestive bags," because not only do they help to digest proteins, but they also digest such other substances as worn-out cells and bacteria. If a lysosome ruptures, it starts to digest the cell's proteins and causes the cell to die. For this reason, lysosomes are also called "suicide bags."

- Mitochondria: Mitochondria are nicknamed the cell's "power plant." They are the site of cellular respiration and produce most of the cell's energy. Mitochondria are composed of two very tiny sacs, one inside the other. Mitochondria are very small; 15,000 of them lined up end to end are only approximately 1 inch long. Mitochondria vary in shape and number. There may be as few as one in each cell or as many as a thousand or more. Cells requiring the most energy contain the most mitochondria.

- Ribosomes: Ribosomes are very tiny particles made up of ribonucleic acid and protein. Ribosomes aid in protein synthesis and can be found throughout the cytoplasm. Because ribosomes perform the very complex function of manufacturing enzyme and protein compounds, they have been nicknamed "protein factories." As described above, they often temporarily attach to the endoplasmic reticulum.

Tissues

Tissues are made up of many similar cells working together to perform a specific function. There are four main types of tissue: epithelial, connective, muscle, and nervous. Each tissue type is different in size, shape, and function (Figure 3-8).

1. Epithelial tissue covers and protects the body and can be found in both the body's internal and external structures. Epithelial cells produce secretions, such as digestive juices, hormones, and perspiration. They also regulate the passage of materials across them. Epithelial tissue is named according to its size, shape, and structure.

2. Connective tissue is the most abundant and widely distributed tissue in the body. It is found almost everywhere in the body, including bones, cartilage, mucous membranes, muscles, nerves, skin, and all the internal organs. The functions of connective tissue vary depending on its structure and appearance. It connects tissues to each other and forms a supporting framework. For example, blood, one type of connective tissue, transports substances throughout the body. A second type of connective tissue is adipose (fat) tissue, which specializes in storing lipids. Bone and cartilage are other types of connective tissue.

CONTRACTILITY

Having the ability to contract or shorten.

3. Muscle tissue provides the body with movement; muscle cells have a higher degree of **contractility** than other types of tissue cells. There are three types of muscle tissue: skeletal muscle, smooth muscle of the internal organs and glands, and cardiac muscle. Skeletal muscle is striated and voluntary, because skeletal muscles are under conscious control of the body. Skeletal muscle attaches to bones and allows for movement and maintenance of body posture. Smooth muscle is nonstriated and its movement is involuntary. Smooth muscle tissue makes up the walls of the digestive tract, the genitourinary and respiratory tracts, blood vessels, and lymphatic vessels. Cardiac muscle is striated (having a cross-banding pattern) and involuntary, and makes up the walls of the heart.

4. Nerve tissue has the ability to react to stimulus. Nerve tissue is composed of neurons and is found in the brain, spinal cord, and in the nerves themselves.

Type of Tissue	Function	Characteristics and Location	Morphology
I. Epithelial	Cells form a continuous layer covering internal and external body surfaces, provide protection, produce secretions (digestive juices, hormones, perspiration), and regulate the passage of materials across themselves.		
	A. Covering and lining tissue These cells can be stratified (layered), ciliated, or keratinized.	1. Squamous epithelial cells These are flat, irregularly shaped cells. They line the heart, blood and lymphatic vessels, body cavities, and alveoli (air sacs) of lungs. The outer layer of the skin is composed of stratified and keratinized squamous epithelial cells. The stratified squamous epithelial cells on the outer skin layer protect the body against microbial invasion.	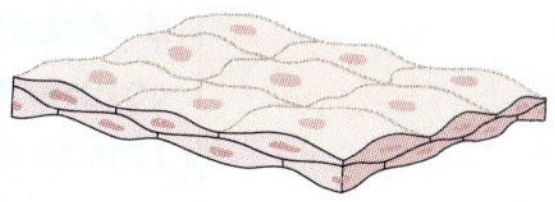
		2. Cuboidal epithelial cells These are the cube-shaped cells that line the kidney tubules, and which cover the ovaries and secretory parts of certain glands.	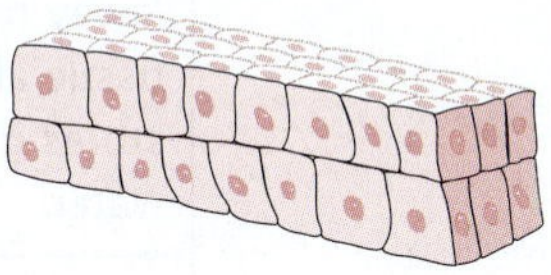
		3. Columnar epithelial cells Elongated, with the nucleus generally near the bottom and often ciliated on the outer surface. They line the ducts, digestive tract (especially the intestinal and stomach lining), parts of the respiratory tract, and glands.	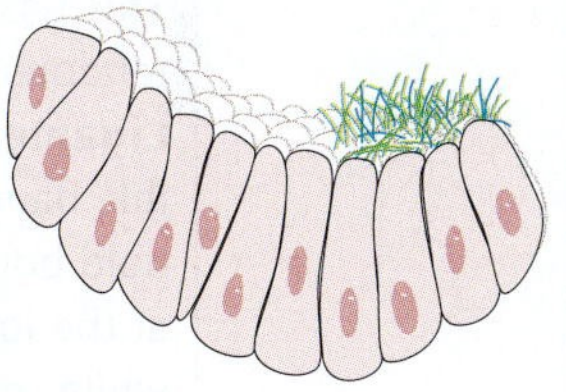
	B. Glandular or secretory tissue These cells are specialized to secrete materials such as digestive juices, hormones, milk, perspiration, and wax. They are columnar or cuboidal shaped.	Endocrine gland cells These cells form ductless glands which secrete their substances (hormones) directly into the bloodstream. For instance, the thyroid gland secretes thyroxin, while adrenal glands secrete adrenaline. Exocrine gland cells These cells secrete their substances into ducts. The mammary glands, sweat glands, and salivary glands are examples.	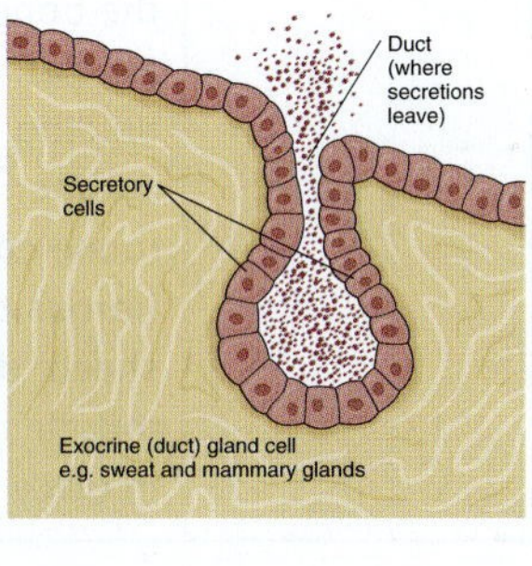

FIGURE 3-8: Tissues of the human body *(continues)*

Type of Tissue	Function	Characteristics and Location	Morphology
II. Connective	Cells whose intercellular secretions (matrix) support and connect the organs and tissues of the body.	Connective tissue is found almost everywhere within the body: bones, cartilage, mucous membranes, muscles, nerves, skin, and all internal organs.	
	A. Adipose tissue This tissue stores lipid (fat), acts as filler tissue, cushions, supports, and insulates the body.	A type of loose, connective tissue composed of sac-like adipose cells; they are specialized for the storage of fat. Adipose cells are found throughout the body: in the subcutaneous skin layer, around the kidneys, within padding around joints, and in the marrow of long bones.	
	B. Areolar (loose) connective This tissue surrounds various organs and supports both nerve cells and blood vessels which transport nutrient materials (to cells) and wastes (away from cells). Areolar tissue also (temporarily) stores glucose, salts, and water.	It is composed of a large, semifluid matrix, with many different types of cells and fibers embedded in it. These include fibroblasts (fibrocytes), plasma cells, macrophages, mast cells, and various white blood cells. The fibers are bundles of strong, flexible white fibrous protein called **collagen**, and elastic single fibers of **elastin**. It is found in the epidermis of the skin and in the subcutaneous layer with adipose cells.	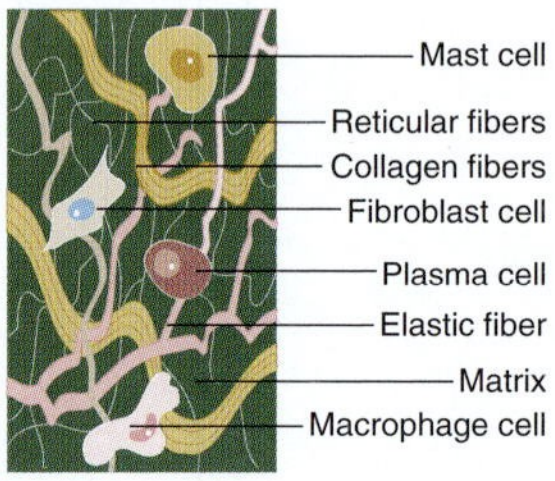
	C. Dense fibrous This tissue forms ligaments, tendons, and aponeuroses. **Ligaments** are strong, flexible bands (or cords) which hold bones firmly together at the joints. **Tendons** are white, glistening bands attaching skeletal muscles to the bones. **Aponeuroses** are flat, wide bands of tissue holding one muscle to another or to the periosteum (bone covering). **Fasciae** are fibrous connective tissue sheets that wrap around muscle bundles to hold them in place.	Dense fibrous tissue is also called white fibrous tissue, since it is made from closely packed white collagen fibers. Fibrous tissue is flexible, but not elastic. This tissue has a poor blood supply and heals slowly.	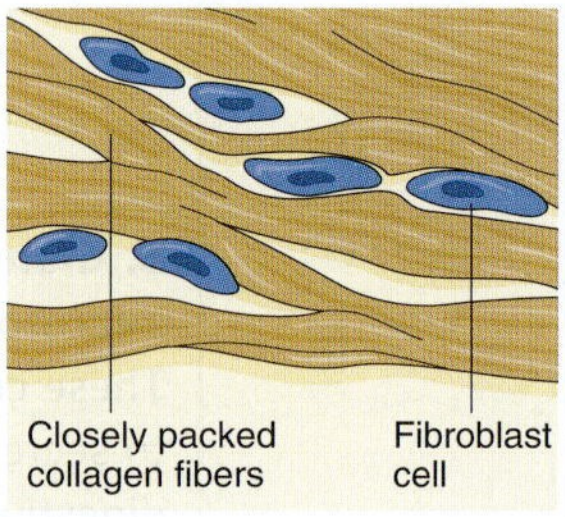

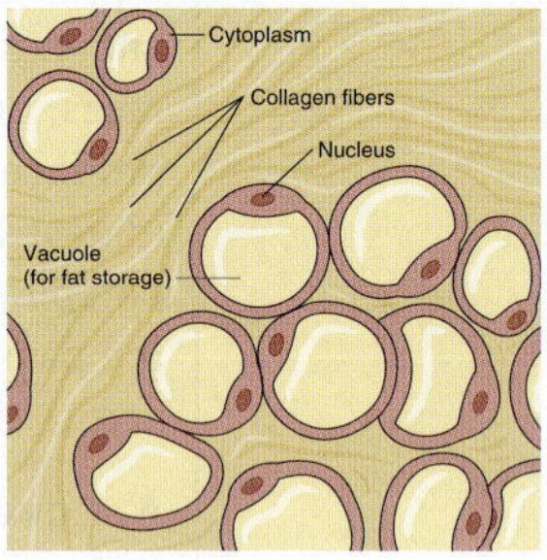

FIGURE 3-8: Tissues of the human body *(continues)*

Type of Tissue	Function	Characteristics and Location	Morphology
II. Connective *(continued)*	**D. Supportive** **1. Bone (osseus) tissue**—Comprises the skeleton of the body, which supports and protects underlying soft tissue parts and organs, and also serves as attachments for skeletal muscles.	Connective tissue whose intercellular matrix is *calcified* by the deposition of mineral salts (such as calcium carbonate and calcium phosphate). Calcification of bone imparts great strength. The entire skeleton is composed of bone tissue.	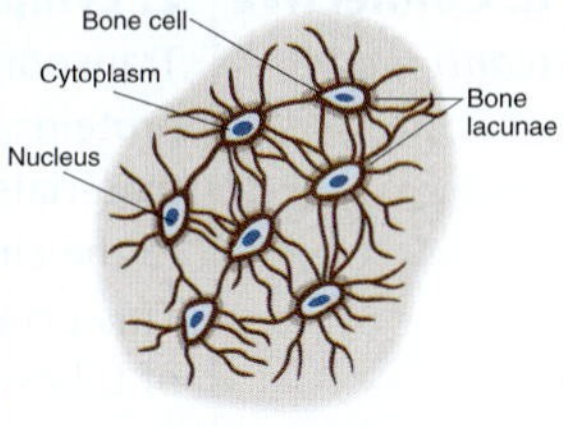
	2. Cartilage—Provides firm but flexible support for the embryonic skeleton and part of the adult skeleton. **a. Hyaline**—Forms the skeleton of the embryo.	Hyaline cartilage is found upon articular bone surfaces, and also at the nose tip, bronchi, and bronchial tubes. Ribs are joined to the sternum (breastbone) by costal cartilage. It is also found in the larynx and the rings in the trachea.	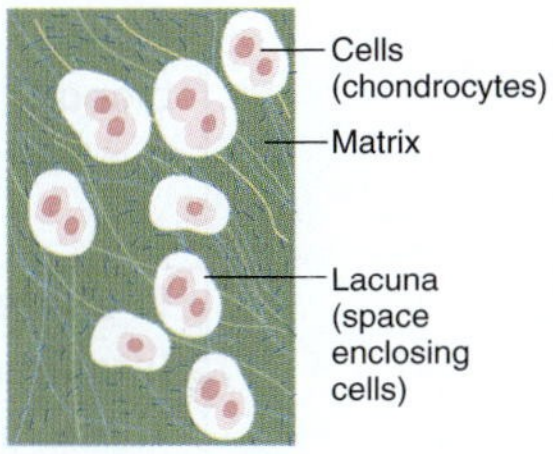
	b. Fibrocartilage—A strong, flexible, supportive substance found between bones and wherever great strength (and a degree of rigidity) is needed.	Fibrocartilage is located within inter-vertebral discs and pubic symphysis between the pubic bones.	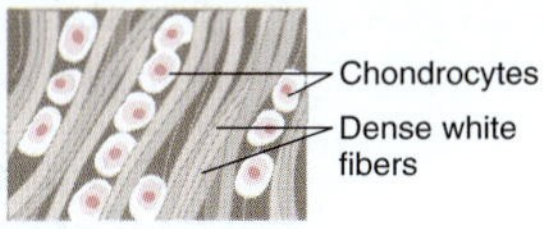
	c. Elastic cartilage—The intercellular matrix is embedded with a net-work of elastic fibers and is firm but flexible.	Elastic cartilage is located inside the auditory ear tube, external ear, epiglottis, and larynx.	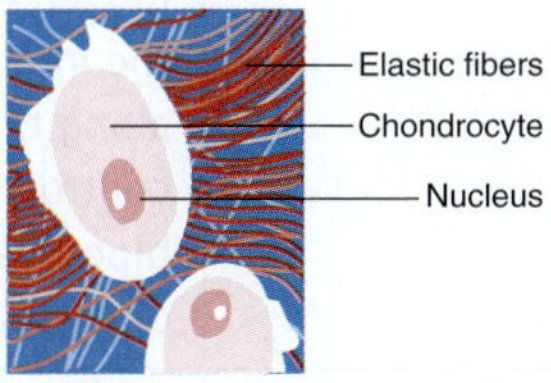
	E. Vascular (liquid blood tissue) **1. Blood**—Transports nutrient and oxygen molecules to cells, and metabolic wastes away from cells (can be considered as a liquid tissue). Contains cells that function in the body's defense and in blood clotting.	Blood is composed of two major parts: a liquid called plasma, and a solid cellular portion known as blood cells (or corpuscles). The plasma suspends corpuscles, of which there are two major types: red blood cells (erythrocytes) and white blood cells (leukocytes). A third cellular component (really a cell fragment) is called platelets (thrombocytes). Blood circulates within the blood vessels (arteries, veins, and capillaries) and through the heart.	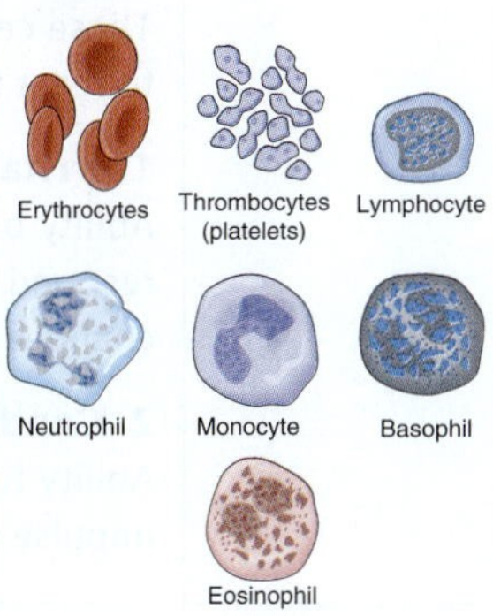

FIGURE 3-8: Tissues of the human body *(continues)*

Type of Tissue	Function	Characteristics and Location	Morphology
II. Connective (continued)	2. Lymph— Transports tissue fluid, proteins, fats, and other materials from the tissues to the circulatory system. This occurs through a series of tubes called the lymphatic vessels.	Lymph is a fluid made up of water, glucose, protein, fats, and salt. The cellular components are lymphocytes and granulocytes. They flow in tubes called lymphatic vessels, which closely parallel the veins and bathe the tissue spaces between cells.	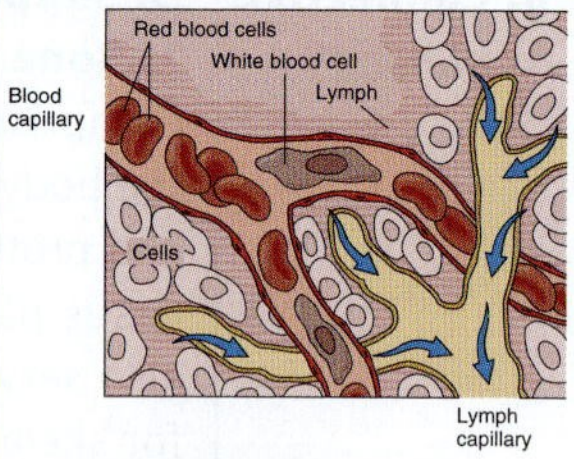
III. Muscle	A. Cardiac These cells help the heart contract in order to pump blood through and out of the heart.	Cardiac muscle is a striated (having a cross-banding pattern), involuntary (not under conscious control) muscle. It makes up the walls of the heart.	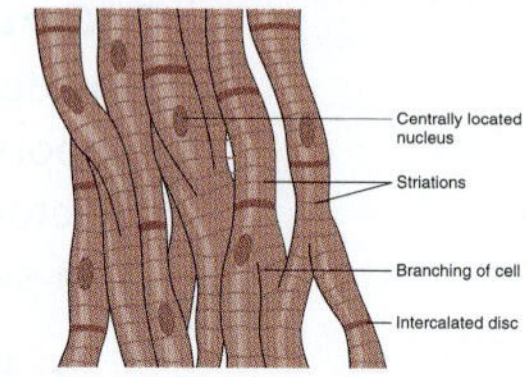
	B. Skeletal (striated voluntary) These muscles are attached to the movable parts of the skeleton. They are capable of rapid, powerful contractions and long states of partially sustained contractions, allowing for voluntary movement.	Skeletal muscle is: striated (having transverse bands that run down the length of muscle fibers); voluntary, because the muscle is under conscious control; and skeletal, since these muscles are attached to the skeleton (bones, tendons and other muscles).	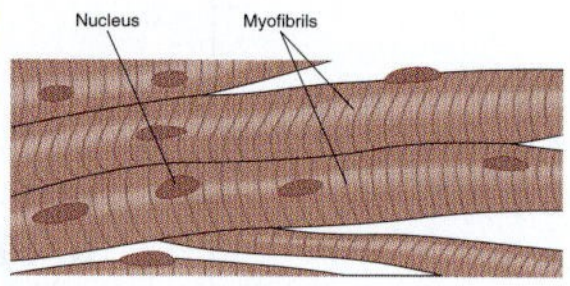
	C. Smooth (nonstriated involuntary) These provide for involuntary movement. Examples include the movement of materials along the digestive tract, controlling the diameter of blood vessels and the pupil of the eyes.	Smooth muscle is nonstriated because it lacks the striations (bands) of skeletal muscles; its movement is involuntary. It makes up the walls of the digestive, genitourinary, and respiratory tracts, blood vessels, and lymphatic vessels.	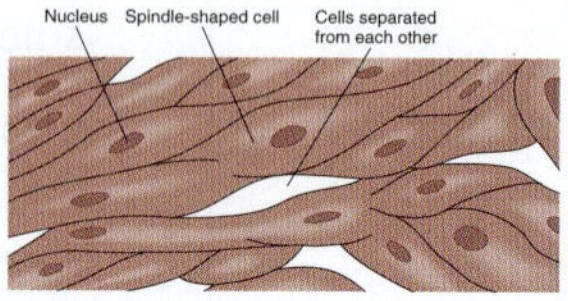
IV. Nerve	Neurons (nerve cells) These cells have the ability to react to stimuli. 1. Irritability— Ability of nerve tissue to respond to environmental changes. 2. Conductivity— Ability to carry a nerve impulse (message).	Nerve tissue is composed of neurons (nerve cells). Neurons have branches through which various parts of the body are connected and their activities coordinated. They are found in the brain, spinal cord, and nerves.	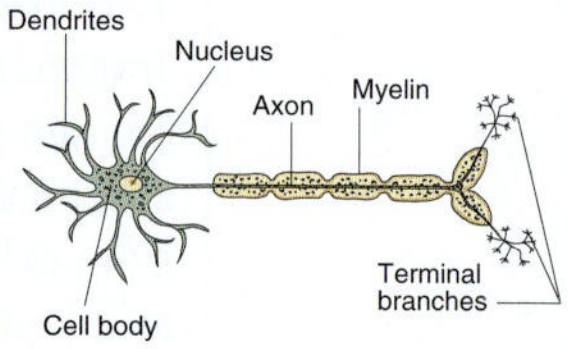

FIGURE 3-8: Tissues of the human body

Organs

Organs are composed of numerous tissues grouped together to perform a specific function. For example, the heart is an organ in the circulatory system, the lungs are organs in the respiratory system, and the stomach is an organ in the digestive system (Figure 3-9). Organs cannot function independently. They function together to create specific body systems and perform specific body functions. Organs coordinate their activities to function as a whole unit: the human body. Organs are further described as part of specific body systems.

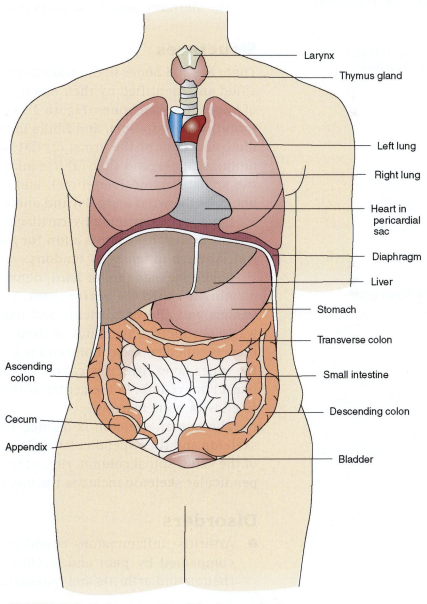

FIGURE 3-9: Various organs of the human body

SKELETAL SYSTEM

Function

The skeletal system has five specific functions:

1. Supports the body and provides the body's shape.
2. Protects internal organs (e.g., the skull protects the brain).
3. Movement and attachment of muscles.
4. Mineral storage: Minerals such as calcium and phosphorus are stored in the bones.
5. **Hemopoiesis**. The red bone marrow located in the long bones, the sternum, and the ilium is the site of blood cell formation.

HEMOPOIESIS (HEMATOPOIESIS)

The production and development of blood cells, normally in the bone marrow.

Structures

There are 206 bones in the adult body (Figure 3-10). Bones are classified and identified by their shape. There are four classifications of bones: (1) long bones (Figure 3-11), such as the bones of the extremities (femur, tibia, and fibula of the legs and the humerus, radius, and ulna of the arms; (2) flat bones, such as the skull (cranium), scapula, and ribs; (3) irregular bones, such as the bones of the spinal column (vertebrae), and (4) short bones, such as the bones of the wrist (carpals) and ankle (tarsals).

Bones are connected by cartilage at numerous joints throughout the body. These joints allow for movement initiated by muscle, which attach to bones by tendons.

Bones are made up of hard, dense tissue and are covered by a membrane called the **periosteum**. The periosteum contains blood vessels and allows nutrients and oxygen to be brought into and waste products to be removed from the bone. The outer layer of a bone is called compact bone and is a heavier, more rigid layer than the inner layer, which is called spongy bone. Spongy bone looks like a honeycomb. In the center of the bone is the medullary canal filled with bone marrow.

The human skeleton is divided into two main parts: the axial skeleton and the appendicular skeleton. The axial skeleton consists of the skull, spinal column, ribs, sternum, and hyoid bone. The appendicular skeleton includes the upper and lower extremities.

PERIOSTEUM

Fibrous tissue covering the bone.

Disorders

● Arthritis: Inflammatory condition of one or more joints, accompanied by pain and swelling. Two types of arthritis are rheumatoid arthritis and osteoarthritis.

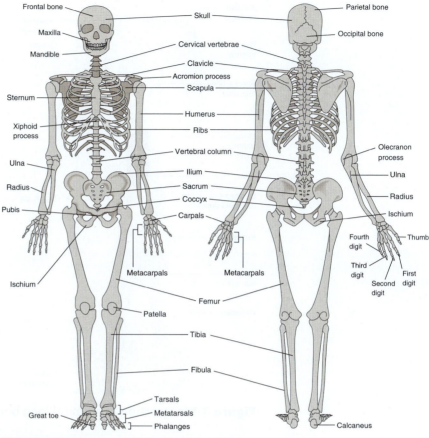

FIGURE 3-10: Bones of the human skeleton

- Bursitis: Inflammation of the fluid-filled sac, the bursa, between muscle attachments and bones.
- Gout: Increase of uric acid in the bloodstream caused by inaccurate metabolism affecting most commonly the joints of the feet. Gout is also a form of arthritis.
- Osteomyelitis: Inflammation of the bone, particularly the bone marrow, caused by bacterial infection.
- Osteochondritis: Inflammation of the bone and cartilage.
- Osteoporosis: Disorder and common condition of aging and loss of nutrients, involving loss of bone density.
- Rickets: Abnormal bone formation caused by a lack of vitamin D in the diet. This primarily affects children and causes the bones to soften and malform.
- Slipped (herniated) disc: Condition when a cartilage disc of the spine ruptures or protrudes out of place and places pressure on the spinal nerve.
- Tumors: Abnormal bone growth; may be malignant (cancer) or benign.

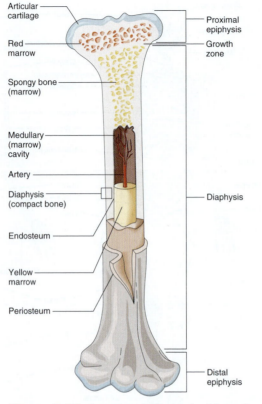

Articular cartilage

Red marrow

Spongy bone (marrow)

Medullary (marrow) cavity

Artery

Diaphysis (compact bone)

Endosteum

Yellow marrow

Periosteum

Proximal epiphysis

Growth zone

Diaphysis

Distal epiphysis

Figure 3-11: Structure of a typical long bone

Diagnostic Tests

● Alkaline phosphatase (ALP)
● Calcium
● Complete blood count (CBC)
● Erythrocyte sedimentation rate (ESR)
● Phosphorus (P)
● Synovial fluid analysis
● Uric acid
● Vitamin D

● MUSCULAR SYSTEM

Function

There are three main functions of the muscular system; it is responsible for:

1. All body movement.

2. Body form and shape (helps maintain posture).

3. Body heat, which maintains body temperature.

Structures

Muscles comprise nearly half the body's weight. All together there are 656 different muscles in the human body. They allow the body to move voluntarily from place to place and allow the involuntary movement of organs such as the heart and lungs (Figure 3-12).

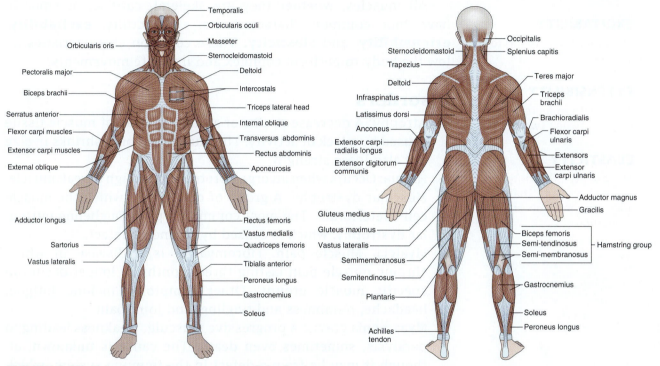

FIGURE 3-12: Principal skeletal muscles of the body

Three principal types of muscles—skeletal, cardiac, and smooth—determine all body movement. These muscles can also be described as striated, nonstriated, and spindle-shaped, because of the way the cells appear when viewed with a microscope.

Skeletal muscles are striated and are attached to bones by tendons, thereby allowing the body to move voluntarily.

Cardiac muscles are found only in the heart. They are also striated, but are involuntary. When the cardiac muscles receive a signal from the nervous system, they contract and produce a heartbeat. This occurs approximately 70 times per minute in the average adult.

Smooth muscles, or visceral muscles, are nonstriated and are spindle-shaped. They are considered smooth because of the lack of striations. Smooth muscles are involuntary, like cardiac muscles, and their actions are controlled by the autonomic nervous system. Smooth muscles can be found in the walls of the internal organs, or viscera (stomach, intestines, lungs, kidneys, and blood vessels).

Muscles maintain the body's posture, whether sitting or standing, through a series of constant partial contractions of specific muscle groups. Muscle cells producing mechanical movement of the body also contract. Adenosine triphosphate (ATP), which is manufactured in the mitochondria of the cells, produces the energy for muscle contraction. This energy is released in the form of heat.

All muscles, whether they are skeletal, cardiac, or smooth, have four common characteristics: contractility, **excitability**, **extensibility**, and **elasticity**. These common characteristics allow the body to perform complex and intricate movements.

Disorders

- Atrophy: A decrease in size or a wasting away of muscle tissue caused by a lack of activity. The muscle not only shrinks in size but also loses strength.
- Hernia: Occurs when an organ protrudes through a weak muscle.
- Muscular dystrophy: A group of diseases in which the muscle cells deteriorate. The most common type is Duchenne muscular dystrophy, which is caused by a genetic defect.
- Myalgia: Muscle pain. Fibromyalgia is a disease in which chronic muscle pain lasting three months or longer occurs in specific muscle groups. Other symptoms include fatigue, headache, numbness and tingling, and joint pain.
- Myasthenia gravis: A progressive muscular weakness leading to paralysis, sometimes even death. The cause is unknown, although it may be from a defect in the immune system, which affects myoneural function.
- Tendonitis: Inflammation of muscle tendons usually due to overexertion.
- Tetanus (lockjaw): Infectious disease characterized by continuous spasms of the voluntary muscles. Caused by the toxin *Clostridium tetani,* which enters the body through a puncture wound. Can be prevented by tetanus vaccine.
- Torticollis: Wryneck, may be caused by inflammation of the trapezius and/or sternocleidomastoid muscle.

Diagnostic Tests

- Autoimmune antibodies
- Creatine phosphokinase (CPK/CK)
- CPK/CK isoenzymes
- Lactic acid
- Lactate dehydrogenase (LDH or LD)
- Myoglobin
- Electromyography

EXCITABILITY

The ability to respond to stimuli.

EXTENSIBILITY

The ability to increase the angle between two bones.

ELASTICITY

The quality of returning to original size and shape after compression or stretching.

❶NERVOUS SYSTEM

Function

There are two main functions of the nervous system:

1. The communication and coordination of all body functions. The nervous system receives messages from both internal and external stimuli and sends these messages to the brain for interpretation. The brain responds to these messages and instructs the body to react in an appropriate manner.

   Nerve impulses and chemical substances regulate, control, integrate, and organize body functions.

2. The brain is the center for intellect and reasoning (Figure 3-13).

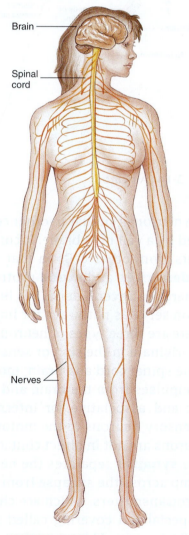

Brain

Spinal
cord

Nerves

FIGURE 3-13: The nervous system

Structures

The nervous system is composed of highly specialized cells called **neurons** (Figure 3-14). Neurons are capable of conducting messages in the form of impulses. It is estimated that the body contains over 10 billion neurons, most of which reside in the brain.

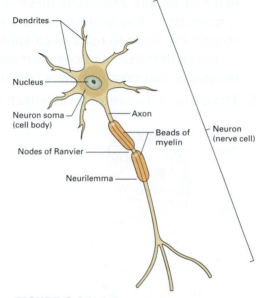

FIGURE 3-14: A neuron

The neuron is similar to other cells in that it has a cell body surrounded by a cell membrane. It contains cytoplasm and a nucleus. It differs from other cells in that it has extensions of cytoplasm called **dendrites** and **axons** protruding from the cell body. Typically there are several dendrites but only one axon. The dendrites and axon serve as pathways for impulse conduction.

There are three types of neurons: sensory, or afferent, neurons, which originate in the skin or sense organs and carry impulses toward the spinal cord and brain; motor, or efferent, neurons, which carry impulses from the brain and spinal cord to the muscles and glands; and associative, or interneurons, which carry impulses from sensory neurons to the motor neurons.

Neurons are not in direct contact with each other. A small space called a **synapse** separates the neurons. Electrical impulses literally jump across the synapse from neuron to neuron with the help of neurotransmitters, which are chemicals produced by the body.

A specialized covering called the **myelin sheath** covers the axon of a neuron. This special covering speeds up the nerve impulse as it travels along the axon. The myelin sheath is composed

DENDRITE

The nerve cell process that carries nervous impulses toward the cell body.

AXON

A process of a neuron that conducts impulses away from the cell body.

SYNAPSE

The space between adjacent neurons through which an impulse is transmitted.

MYELIN SHEATH

A phospholipid-protein membrane forming an electrical insulator that increases the velocity of impulse transmission; found surrounding nerve fibers.

SCHWANN CELL

One of the cells of the peripheral nervous system that forms the myelin sheath.

MENINGES

Membranes covering the spinal cord and brain: dura mater (external), arachnoid (middle), and pia mater (internal).

CEREBROSPINAL FLUID

(Abbr. CSF) A water cushion protecting the brain and spinal cord from physical impact.

of a fatty substance composed of **Schwann cells**, which protect the axon. This substance is called "white matter." Small indentations along the axon are called the nodes of Ranvier and are not covered by the myelin sheath. These areas are very important to the conduction of a nerve impulse. Axons of neurons of the central nervous system are nonmyelinated or not covered by the myelin sheath. They make up the nervous system's "gray matter."

The nervous system can be divided into two distinct divisions (Figure 3-15). The central nervous system (CNS) consists of the brain and spinal cord. The CNS functions as the command center and interprets all incoming impulses and dictates a response. All nerves of the body eventually terminate in the brain via the trunk of the spinal cord. A membranous covering called the **meninges** protects both the brain and spinal cord. Between the three protective layers of the meninges are fluid-filled spaces that provide the brain and spinal cord with an extra layer of cushioning. The fluid that fills these spaces is called **cerebrospinal fluid**.

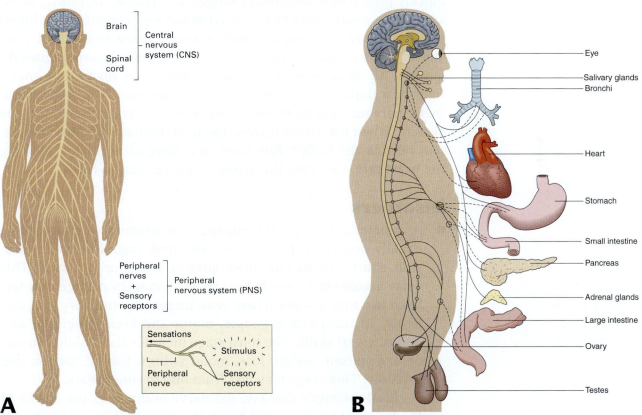

FIGURE 3-15: (A) The central and peripheral nervous systems. (B) The autonomic nervous system.

AFFERENT

Carrying impulses towards a center.

EFFERENT

Carrying away from a central organ or section, as efferent nerves.

The peripheral nervous system (PNS) consists of all the other nerves that connect to the spinal cord and brain. The peripheral nervous system can be subdivided into the sensory, or **afferent**, division and the motor, or **efferent**, division. Remember that sensory nerves carry information *to* the CNS, while motor nerves carry information *from* the CNS to organs, glands, and muscles.

The motor/efferent division can be further subdivided into the somatic/voluntary nervous system and the autonomic/involuntary nervous system. The somatic nervous system conducts impulses from the CNS to the voluntary skeletal muscles. The autonomic nervous system conducts impulses from the CNS to the involuntary smooth muscles, cardiac muscles, and glands.

The autonomic nervous system can be further subdivided into the sympathetic and parasympathetic divisions. The sympathetic nervous system produces the "fight or flight" response in emergency situations. When the body must cope with stressors such as anger, fear, hate, or anxiety, the sympathetic nervous system quickly produces widespread changes throughout the body. For example, the heart beats faster, most blood vessels constrict, blood pressure increases, sweat glands produce more sweat, and peristalsis in the digestive tract slows down, thereby slowing down digestion. All these responses make us physically ready for either a fight or a flight (i.e., running from the stressor). The parasympathetic nervous system is the opposite of the sympathetic nervous system. When the stress is over, the parasympathetic nervous system returns the body's functions to a state of normalcy, slowing the heart rate, lowering the blood pressure, and so forth.

Disorders

● Alzheimer's disease: Alzheimer's is a progressive disease that usually occurs in three stages. The first stage involves confusion, short-term memory loss, anxiety, and poor judgment. This stage usually lasts two to four years. The second stage may last from two to ten years. There is an increase in memory loss, difficulty in recognizing people, motor and logic problems, and loss of social skills. The third stage includes the inability to recognize oneself, weight loss, mood swings, loss of speech, and seizures. This stage may last from one to three years.

In Alzheimer's disease, the nerve endings in the cortex of the brain degenerate and block the signals that pass between the nerve cells.

- Bell's palsy: This condition involves the facial nerve and usually affects only one side of the face. The affected eye has difficulty closing, the mouth droops, and there is numbness on the affected side. Bell's palsy gives the patient the appearance of having had a stroke. The onset may be sudden and the cause is unknown.
- Brain tumors: A tumor may develop in any area of the brain. Symptoms vary depending on which area has been damaged and to what extent the tumor has developed. Early detection, surgery, and chemotherapy may cure most brain tumors.
- Carpal tunnel syndrome: This condition affects the medial nerve and the flexor tendons of the wrist. Carpal tunnel syndrome develops because of repetitive movement of the wrist, or when the wrist is held in an unusual position. Swelling occurs and puts pressure on the median nerve, which results in pain, muscle weakness, and numbness of the hand.
- Cerebral palsy: Cerebral palsy (CP) is caused by brain damage and causes a disturbance in voluntary muscle activity. It may occur because of an injury during the birth process or because of abnormal development of the brain. The person with CP may exhibit head rolling and grimacing, or difficulty with speech and swallowing. There is usually no impairment of the intellect; the patient frequently has normal or above normal intelligence.
- Encephalitis: Encephalitis is an inflammation of the brain and is most often caused by a virus. The symptoms include fever, lethargy, extreme weakness, and visual disturbances.
- Epilepsy: Epilepsy is a seizure disorder of the brain. It is characterized by recurrent and excessive discharge from the neurons. Seizures are believed to be the result of spontaneous uncontrolled cycles of electrical activity in the neurons of the brain. Seizures are classified as *grand mal* (severe) or *petit mal* (mild).
- Hydrocephalus: This condition is characterized by an increased volume of cerebrospinal fluid within the ventricles of the brain. This is usually caused by a blockage somewhere in the third or fourth ventricle. The condition is typically apparent at birth, with an enlargement of the infant's head. Shunts are usually surgically inserted to re-route the CSF around the blocked area.
- Meningitis: Meningitis is characterized by inflammation of the meninges covering the brain and spinal cord. Bacteria or a virus may be the cause. Symptoms include headache, fever, and stiff neck. Severe meningitis may lead to paralysis, coma, and death.

● Multiple sclerosis: Multiple sclerosis (MS) is a chronic inflammatory disease of the central nervous system in which the patient's own immune cells attack and destroy the myelin sheath of the nerve cell axons. The destruction of the myelin sheath delays or completely blocks transmission of nerve impulses to the affected areas. The cause is unknown, and there is no definitive test for MS. Symptoms include weakness of extremities, numbness, double vision, speech problems, loss of coordination, and possible paralysis.

● Neuralgia: Neuralgia is characterized by a sudden onset of a sharp, stabbing pain along a nerve. The pain is usually of short duration.

● Neuritis: Neuritis is the inflammation of a nerve or nerve trunk. Symptoms may include severe pain, loss of sensation, muscular atrophy, **paresthesia**, and hypersensitivity. The cause may be chemical, or an infectious process, or another condition such as alcoholism.

● Parkinson's disease: Parkinson's disease is characterized by tremors, a pill-rolling movement of the thumb and first finger, a shuffling gait, and muscular rigidity. A patient with Parkinson's has difficulty initiating movement.

● Poliomyelitis: Polio is a disease of the nerve pathways of the spinal cord, which results in paralysis. The Sabin and Salk vaccines have all but eliminated this disease in the United States.

● Sciatica: Sciatica is a type of neuritis which affects the sciatic nerve. It may be caused by a ruptured lumbar disc or aggravated by an arthritic condition or trauma. Symptoms include a severe pain that radiates through the buttocks and down the back of the affected leg to the foot.

● Shingles/herpes zoster: Shingles is an acute viral infection characterized by inflammation of a cutaneous nerve. Symptoms include extremely painful vesicular eruptions of the skin and mucous membrane along the route of the inflamed nerve. The causative organism is herpes zoster, which is the virus that causes chickenpox.

Diagnostic Tests

● Acetylcholine receptor antibody
● Cerebrospinal fluid (CSF) analysis (cell count, glucose, protein, culture)
● Cholinesterase
● Drug levels
● Serotonin

PARESTHESIA

An unusual sensation of tingling, crawling, or burning of the skin for no apparent reason.

INTEGUMENTARY SYSTEM

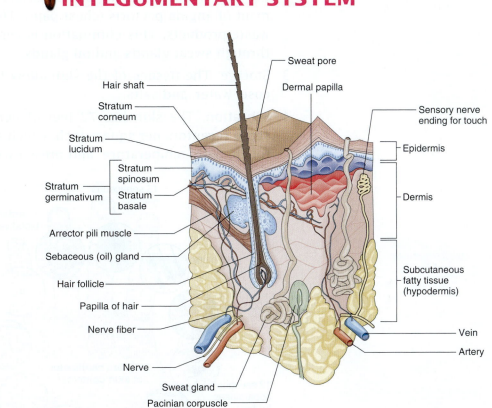

Labels:
- Hair shaft
- Stratum corneum
- Stratum lucidum
- Stratum germinativum
- Stratum spinosum
- Stratum basale
- Arrector pili muscle
- Sebaceous (oil) gland
- Hair follicle
- Papilla of hair
- Nerve fiber
- Nerve
- Sweat gland
- Pacinian corpuscle
- Sweat pore
- Dermal papilla
- Sensory nerve ending for touch
- Epidermis
- Dermis
- Subcutaneous fatty tissue (hypodermis)
- Vein
- Artery

FIGURE 3-16: A cross-section of the skin

Function

The skin is called integument, and together with its appendages, the hair and nails, comprises the integumentary system. The skin is the largest organ of the body and has four basic functions:

1. Protection: The skin protects the body from invasion by pathogens, from dehydration, and from injury by serving as a protective covering of underlying tissues. It also protects these tissues from excessive exposure to ultraviolet radiation from the sun. At the same time, it uses some of this ultraviolet light to help manufacture Vitamin D.

2. Regulation: The tissues of the skin help to regulate body temperature by controlling the amount of heat loss. Evaporation of water (perspiration) helps to cool the body when it is too hot.

   The skin also has special properties that allow for absorption of certain drugs. For example, nitroglycerin can be applied in the form of a paste on a patch to a patient's skin. This paste is then absorbed through the skin and has a systemic effect in the body, namely dilating blood vessels. It is used in the treatment of angina pectoris (chest pain). The skin also eliminates waste products. This elimination is very minimal and occurs through sweat glands and oil glands.

3. Storage: The tissues of the skin allow for storage of fat, glucose, water, and salts.

4. Sensation: The skin has 72 feet of nerves and hundreds of sense receptors per square inch, which allow for the senses of touch, pain, temperature, and pressure (Figure 3-17).

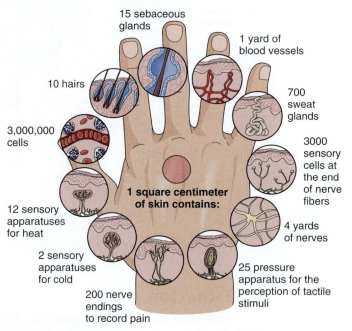

15 sebaceous glands

1 yard of blood vessels

10 hairs

700 sweat glands

3,000,000 cells

3000 sensory cells at the end of nerve fibers

1 square centimeter of skin contains:

12 sensory apparatuses for heat

4 yards of nerves

2 sensory apparatuses for cold

25 pressure apparatus for the perception of tactile stimuli

200 nerve endings to record pain

FIGURE 3-17: One square centimeter of skin

Structures

The skin consists of two basic layers attached to a third layer:

EPIDERMIS

Outermost layer of skin.

STRATUM CORNEUM

The outermost horny layer of the epidermis.

STRATUM GERMINATIVUM

The innermost layer of the epidermis.

1. The **epidermis** is the outermost and thinnest layer of the skin and is made up of stratified (layered), squamous (scalelike), keratinized (hardened), epithelial cells. The epidermis is avascular, which means it contains no blood vessels. It has two functionally significant layers: the **stratum corneum** and the **stratum germinativum**. In the stratum corneum layer, the cytoplasm of the cells keratinizes, or hardens, when a nonliving protein substance called keratin replaces it. Because of this, the skin is waterproof. The cells of this layer are flat and scalelike and flake off quite easily during normal daily activities. When these cells flake off, new cells that are produced by the stratum

germinativum layer replace them. The stratum germinativum layer is the deepest layer of the epidermis and is the only layer where mitosis (cell reproduction) occurs. The stratum germinativum layer is also where melanocytes are located. **Melanocytes** give the skin its pigmentation because they contain a substance called melanin. The more melanocytes, the darker the skin. The absence of melanin causes **albinism**.

2. The **dermis** lies underneath the epidermis and is also called the corium, or "true skin." The dermis is thicker than the epidermis and contains blood and lymph vessels, nerves, sebaceous glands, hair follicles, sudoriferous glands, connective tissue, collagen tissue bands, elastic fibers, and fat cells. It varies in thickness depending on the part of the body it covers. For example, it is thicker in the palms of the hands and soles of the feet and thinner over the eyelids. The ridges of the skin on the hands and feet are formed by papillae that originate in the dermal layer and push their way up to the stratum germinativum layer of the epidermis. These papillae form fingerprints: ridges that are distinctly different in every individual and are used as means of identification. Newborn infants are usually footprinted as a means of identification.

3. The **subcutaneous**, or hypodermal, layer lies under the dermis. However, it is not a true part of the integumentary system. The subcutaneous layer is composed of loose connective tissue and contains about one-half of the body's fat. This layer connects the integumentary system to the underlying muscles.

4. Appendages of the skin:
   ● Hair is nonliving tissue and is composed primarily of keratinized cells. Hair covers most of the body's surface except for the palms of the hands, soles of the feet, the glans penis, and the inner surfaces of the vaginal labia. The follicle from which each hair grows is situated in the epidermis. At the base of the hair follicle is a mass of tissue called the **papilla**. The papilla contains blood vessels which nourish the hair follicle cells. This is important because this is where new hair originates and where hair cells reproduce.
   ● Nails are also nonliving tissues composed of keratin. Nails cover the dorsal surfaces of the ends of the fingers and toes. Nails, like hair, grow from the roots, at the proximal end of each nail. Nail growth is continuous as long as the nail bed remains intact. Even if a nail is lost because of injury or disease, it can be replaced if the nail bed has not been damaged.

MELANOCYTE
A melanin-forming cell. Those of the skin are found in the lower epidermis.

ALBINISM
A partial or total absence of melanin pigment from eyes, hair, and skin.

DERMIS
The true skin lying immediately beneath the epidermis.

SUBCUTANEOUS
Beneath the skin.

PAPILLA
Small, nipple-shaped elevation. (*pl.* papillae)

SEBACEOUS GLAND

An oil-secreting gland of the skin.

SEBUM

A fatty secretion of the sebaceous glands of the skin.

- **Sebaceous glands** are connected to hair follicles. They secrete an oily substance called **sebum**. Sebum lubricates the skin and hair to keep them soft and supple. Sebaceous glands are often called "oil glands" because of the oiliness of sebum.

- Sudoriferous glands, also called "sweat glands," are located in the dermis. Their ducts extend through the epidermis and end in pores on the skin's surface. Sweat glands are distributed over the entire skin surface, but are present in larger numbers under the arms, on the palms of the hands, and on the soles of the feet. Sweat glands secrete a watery substance, perspiration, through the pores of the skin. Perspiration is 99% water and 1% waste products. Sweat glands can be activated by the nervous system if the body is in pain, is hot, has a fever, or is nervous. The average daily loss of water through the skin is approximately 500 milliliters. This amount can vary greatly depending on the amount of physical activity and on the temperature of the environment. With profuse perspiration, it is important to replace lost water and to prevent dehydration.

Disorders

- Acne vulgaris: A common and often chronic inflammatory disorder of the sebaceous glands and hair follicles. Excessive secretion of sebum can cause a skin pore to plug, which prevents further secretions from escaping. Leukocytes (white blood cells) fill the area and cause pus to form. This condition is most common during adolescence.

- Athlete's foot: A contagious fungal infection which affects the superficial layers of the skin. Most commonly found on the feet, it is characterized by small blisters and by cracking and scaling of the skin.

- Boils or carbuncles: A very painful bacterial infection of the hair follicles or sebaceous glands, usually caused by a staphylococcal organism.

- Burns: There are three degrees, or levels, of severity of burns. First-degree burns involve only the epidermal layer of skin and are typically caused by the sun. They are characterized by redness, swelling, and pain. Second-degree burns involve the epidermis and may also involve the dermis. Swelling, redness, pain, and blisters characterize second-degree burns. Third-degree burns completely destroy the epidermis, dermis, and subcutaneous layers. Third-degree burns are characterized by loss of skin and blackened skin. There is frequently no pain involved with third-degree burns because of the underlying damage to the nerves. Third-degree burns can be life-threatening depending on the amount of skin involved, loss of fluids, and blood loss. Third-degree burns require immediate hospitalization.

● Cancer: There are several types of skin cancer: basal cell carcinoma, squamous cell carcinoma, and malignant melanomas. Skin cancer is often attributed to excessive exposure to the sun.

● Dermatitis: Inflammation of the skin, which may be nonspecific. Dermatitis may be caused by a variety of situations or conditions, ranging from emotional stress to using a different type of laundry soap.

● Eczema: A noncontagious inflammatory skin disorder, which can be acute or chronic in nature. The skin becomes itchy, red, scaly, and dry.

● Genital herpes: A viral infection, which causes blisters in the genital area. It is usually spread through sexual contact. There are periods of remission and exacerbation.

● Herpes: A viral infection usually seen as a fever blister or cold sore. It may be spread orally or through the respiratory tract.

● Hives or urticaria: Generally a response to an allergen, such as an ingested food or drug. It is characterized by extremely itchy wheals or welts that typically have a raised white center surrounded by a pink or red area. It may appear in clusters and usually lasts one to two days.

● Impetigo: A contagious, acute inflammatory skin disease. It most commonly affects infants and small children. Staphylococcal or streptococcal organisms cause it. It is characterized by small vesicles, which rupture and develop a distinct yellow crusty appearance.

● Psoriasis: A chronic inflammatory skin disease which typically affects the skin over the elbows, knees, shins, scalp, and lower back. It is characterized by dry reddish patches covered with silvery-white scales. The cause is unknown but it is thought to be triggered by stress, trauma, or infection.

● Ringworm: A highly contagious fungal infection, characterized by itchy, raised, circular patches with crusts. It can occur on the scalp, skin, and underneath the nails.

Diagnostic Tests
● Biopsies
● KOH preparations for skin scrapings
● Microbiological cultures
● Tissue cultures

● DIGESTIVE SYSTEM

Function

There are four main functions of the digestive system:

1. To physically break down food into smaller pieces.
2. With the aid of digestive juices, to chemically change food into fats, carbohydrates, and proteins.
3. To absorb nutrients into the capillaries of the small intestines.
4. To eliminate waste products.

Structures

The following structures make up the gastrointestinal (GI) tract. The GI tract is a continuous tract, also called the alimentary canal, beginning in the mouth and ending at the anus (Figure 3-18). In an adult the GI tract is approximately 27 feet long from beginning to end.

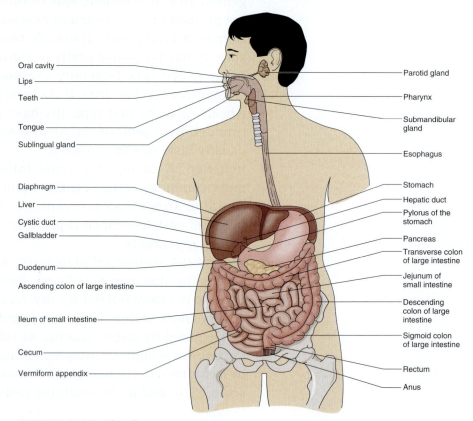

FIGURE 3-18: The digestive system

- Mouth: Food enters the GI tract at the mouth. The lips of the mouth protect the opening of the mouth and are considered to be an accessory organ of the GI tract. The mouth is lined by a mucous membrane. The roof of the mouth is composed of the hard and soft palate. The hard palate is formed from the maxillary and palatine bones, which are covered by the mucous membrane. Behind the hard palate is the soft palate, which is made from a fold of the mucous membrane. The soft palate contains blood vessels, muscle fibers, nerves, lymphatic tissue and mucous glands. It functions as a separating structure between the mouth and the nasopharynx. The **uvula** hangs from the middle of the soft palate and helps to prevent food from entering the nasopharynx. The tongue is also considered to be an accessory organ of digestion. It is attached to the floor of the mouth, and helps in both chewing and swallowing. The tongue is made of skeletal muscle and has small projections called papillae. Taste buds are formed from the papillae and respond to the bitter, sweet, salty, and sour flavors in foods. Teeth are another accessory organ of digestion. Once food has been ingested, it must be mechanically broken into smaller particles. This is the function of the teeth. The act of chewing is also called **mastication**. As food breaks into smaller and smaller pieces, the surface area of each particle increases, which allows the digestive enzymes to digest the food more efficiently.

  Three pairs of salivary glands are located in the oral cavity. The parotid salivary glands are located bilaterally in front of and below the ears. These glands carry their secretions, which are primarily salivary amylase, directly into the mouth. The submandibular glands are located below the parotid salivary glands near the angle of the lower jaw. This gland is approximately the size of a walnut and secretes two digestive enzymes, mucin and ptyalin. The last pair of salivary glands, the sublingual glands, are the smallest of the three and are located under the sides of the tongue. They mainly secrete mucus. These secretions act to further break down food particles so that additional digestion can occur.

- Pharynx: The pharynx is primarily a funnel-shaped passageway that food and air both travel through. The pharynx is more commonly referred to as the throat.

UVULA

The projection hanging from soft palate, in back of throat.

MASTICATION

Process of chewing.

● Esophagus: The esophagus is a hollow muscular tube approximately 10 inches long. It begins at the lower end of the pharynx behind the trachea, and continues downward through the mediastinum, in front of the vertebrae, through the diaphragm and into the upper end of the stomach. The walls of the esophagus have four layers: the mucosa, submucosa, and muscular and external serous layers. In the upper third of the esophagus the muscles are voluntary and in the lower two-thirds the muscles are involuntary.

● Stomach: The stomach is located just below the diaphragm in the upper left portion of the abdomen. The stomach has the same four layers as the esophagus and is divided into three sections. The uppermost section is called the fundus. The cardiac sphincter is a circular layer of muscle which controls the passage of food from the esophagus into the stomach. Each sphincter load is called a **bolus**, and when it enters the stomach, gastric enzymes further break the bolus into smaller particles. This mixture of bolus and gastric juices is called **chyme**. Chyme leaves the stomach via the pyloric sphincter, the valve located in the lower portion of the stomach, and moves into the small intestine.

● Small intestine: The small intestine has the same four layers as the esophagus and stomach. Most nutrients are absorbed into the body from the small intestine. The small intestine of an adult is approximately 20 feet long and is divided into three sections. The first section of the small intestine is the **duodenum**. It is approximately 12 inches in length and is the section of the small intestine into which the pancreatic duct and the common bile duct empty. The pancreatic duct empties digestive juices from the pancreas and the common bile duct, and bile from the liver and gallbladder. These juices further digest food.

The second section of the small intestine, the **jejunum**, is approximately 8 feet long. The third section, the **ileum**, is about 10 to 12 feet long. Absorption of nutrients takes place in the small intestine. The lining of the small intestine is not smooth but is folded into millions of microscopic projections called **villi**. Each villus contains a network of lymph and blood capillaries. The digested food passes through the villi and into the bloodstream to be carried to all areas of the body. Undigested food passes on to the large intestine to be processed as waste.

BOLUS

A rounded mass; food prepared by the mouth for swallowing.

CHYME

Food which has undergone gastric digestion.

DUODENUM

The first part of the small intestine, beginning at the pylorus.

JEJUNUM

The section of the small intestine between the duodenum and the ileum.

ILEUM

The lower part of the small intestine, extending from the jejunum to the large intestine.

VILLI

Hair-like projections, as in intestinal mucous membrane. (*sing.* Villus)

- Large intestine: The large intestine is approximately 5 feet long and 2 inches in diameter. The large intestine is often referred to as the colon. Food matter that has not been absorbed in the small intestine is passed on into the large intestine via the ileocecal valve. This valve prevents food from returning to the small intestine. The large intestine is divided into four sections: the ascending colon, the transverse colon, the descending colon, and the sigmoid colon. The sigmoid colon is the last 7 or 8 inches of the colon and is also referred to as the rectum. The sigmoid colon ends at the anus.

  Functions of the large intestine include synthesis of vitamin K and formation of feces, gas, and elimination. However, the large intestine's overriding function is to absorb water and thus help regulate the body's water balance.

  The cecum and the vermiform appendix are both blind pouches in the large intestine. The cecum is located just below the ileocecal valve. The vermiform appendix is just below the cecum and slightly to the left. Neither the cecum nor the appendix functions as part of the digestive system, but they are typically included because of their location. Because the appendix is a blind sac it fills easily with waste material. It does not empty as easily as the other sections of the intestine and is, therefore, a perfect breeding ground for bacteria. Inflammation caused by bacterial infections often leads to an appendectomy—the surgical removal of the appendix.

- Accessory organs: The liver, gallbladder, and the pancreas are considered to be part of the digestive tract because they contribute to the process of digestion.

  The liver is the largest organ of the body, other than the skin. It is located in the right upper quadrant (RUQ) of the abdomen. The liver has many functions. It manufactures bile, which aids in the digestion of fat. It produces and stores glucose in the form of glycogen. The liver detoxifies drugs and alcohol and other harmful substances. It manufactures blood proteins such as fibrinogen and prothrombin, prepares urea, a byproduct of protein metabolism, and stores vitamins A, D, and B complex.

  The gallbladder is inferior to the liver. Its function is to store and concentrate bile when the body does not need it. The pancreas is located behind the stomach and functions as both an exocrine gland and an endocrine gland. The pancreas carries digestive juices into the duodenum via the pancreatic duct.

  Food moves through both the small and large intestine by means of **peristalsis**.

PERISTALSIS

A progressive wave of contraction in tubular structures provided with longitudinal and transverse muscular fibers, as in the esophagus, stomach, and small and large intestine.

Disorders

- Appendicitis: Inflammation of the appendix typically caused by bacterial infections. If the appendix ruptures, the bacterial infection can spread to the peritoneal cavity and cause peritonitis.
- Cholecystitis: Inflammation of the gallbladder.
- Cirrhosis: A chronic, progressive inflammatory disease of the liver. Three-fourths of cirrhosis is caused by excessive alcohol consumption.
- Colitis: Also called irritable bowel syndrome (IBS). It is the inflammation of the large intestine (colon).
- Colon cancer: Typically stems from a polyplike lesion. Early detection is critical and everyone over the age of 50 is encouraged to undergo colon cancer screening. Cancerous sections of the colon may be removed. A colostomy may be performed. A colostomy is a procedure in which a small opening is made into the abdominal wall through to the colon. The cancerous portion of the colon is removed. The remainder of the colon, which is healthy tissue, is attached to an opening in the skin of the abdominal wall. The patient wears a pouch attached to the opening to collect waste material.
- Diverticulosis: A condition in which small sacs develop in the wall of the colon without inflammation or symptoms.
- Gastritis: Acute or chronic inflammation of the lining of the stomach
- Gastroesophageal reflux disease (GERD): A disorder affecting the lower sphincter muscle connecting the esophagus to the stomach. It relaxes inappropriately, allowing the contents of the stomach to flow up the esophagus, and causes irritation and a burning sensation.
- Heartburn: Acid indigestion resulting from a backflow of acid from the stomach.
- Hepatitis: Inflammation of the liver. There are several types of hepatitis: Hepatitis A, hepatitis B, hepatitis C, hepatitis D, and hepatitis E. Hepatitis A is a viral infection often referred to as infectious hepatitis and is spread through contaminated water or food. Hepatitis B and C viruses are blood-borne and spread by blood-to-blood direct contact, inoculation (needle sticks), or sexual contact. Hepatitis D is always associated with a coinfection with hepatitis B, and hepatitis E is transmitted via fecal-oral route.
- Hiatal hernia: The stomach protrudes through a rupture in the tissue of the esophagus just above the diaphragm.
- Pancreatitis: Inflammation of the pancreas, which can be caused by chronic alcohol abuse.

- Peptic ulcer: A sore or lesion that forms in the lining of the stomach or duodenum and is most frequently caused by a bacterial infection and/or stress.
- Peritonitis: The inflammation of the lining of the abdominal cavity.
- Stomach cancer: Cancer cells in the stomach rapidly grow into tumors. Malignant stomach cancer can spread to other parts of the body even if the original mass is surgically removed.

Diagnostic Tests

- Amylase
- Bilirubin "bili"
- Carcinoembryonic antigen (CEA)
- Carotene
- Cholesterol
- Complete blood count (CBC)
- Glucose
- Glucose tolerance test (GTT)
- Lipase
- Occult blood
- Ova and parasite (O&P)
- Triglycerides

● ENDOCRINE SYSTEM

Function

HORMONE

Secretion from an endocrine gland (e.g., insulin from the pancreas).

The major function of the endocrine glands is to secrete **hormones** directly into the bloodstream to be carried to the appropriate target organs and tissues (Figure 3-19). The endocrine system, like the nervous system, is a communication network. It also plays a part in homeostasis.

Structures

ENDOCRINE GLAND

A gland which secretes into the blood or tissue fluid instead of into a duct.

EXOCRINE GLAND

A gland that secretes into a duct.

The human body has two types of glands, **endocrine** (ductless glands) and **exocrine glands** (glands with ducts). The major glands of the endocrine system include pituitary, thyroid, parathyroid, thymus, adrenals, pineal, pancreas, and the gonads (ovaries in the female and testes in the male). The endocrine glands secrete hormones directly into the bloodstream. Each gland secretes one or more specific hormones that regulate a specific body function, such as: metabolism, growth, reproduction, or acid-base balance. The exocrine glands secrete substances through channels or ducts. The ducts then carry the secretions to organs or to the body surface. Exocrine secretions include sweat, saliva, mucus, and digestive juices.

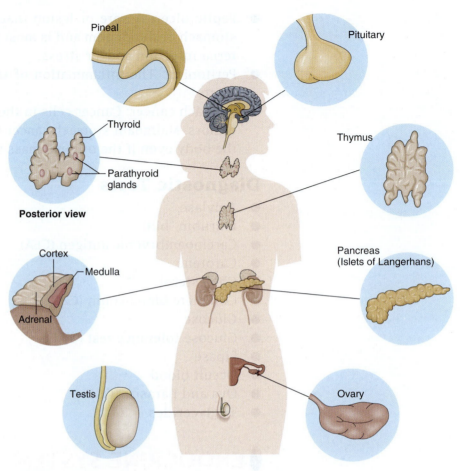

FIGURE 3-19: Locations of the endocrine glands

Disorders

● Acromegaly: Overdevelopment of the bones of the face, hands, and feet caused by oversecretion of growth hormone. Occurs during adulthood.

● Addison's disease: Caused by hypofunctioning of the adrenal cortex. Symptoms include excessive pigmentation (bronzing of the skin), decreased levels of blood glucose, hypoglycemia, low blood pressure, muscular weakness, fatigue, diarrhea, weight loss, vomiting, and decrease in sodium levels, which cause an imbalance of electrolytes.

● Cretinism: Develops in early infancy and is characterized by lack of mental and physical growth, resulting in mental retardation and malformation. Sexual development and physical growth do not progress beyond that of a seven- or eight-year-old child.

Box 3-2: Endocrine Glands

GLAND	LOCATION	HORMONE	PRINCIPAL EFFECTS
PITUITARY Anterior lobe	Undersurface of the brain in the sella turcica of the skull	Growth hormone (GH)	Normal growth of body tissues
		Thyroid stimulating hormone (TSH) (Thyrotropin)	Stimulates growth and activity of thryroid cells to produce thyroid hormone
		Adrenocorticotropic hormone (ACTH)	Stimulates the cortex of the adrenal gland
		Melanocyte-stimulating hormone (MSH)	Increases skin pigmentation
		Follicle-stimulating hormone (FSH)	Stimulates the maturity of the graafian follicle to rupture and to produce estrogen in the female. In the male it stimulates the development of the testes and the production of sperm.
		Luteinizing hormone (LH) Interstitial-cell stimulating hormone (ICSH)	Causes the development of the corpus luteum, which then secretes progesterone in the female. ICSH in the male stimulates the interstitial cells of the testes to produce testosterone
Posterior lobe		Prolactin (PR)	Develops breast tissue and stimulates secretion of milk from mammary glands
		Oxytocin	Stimulates contraction of uterus, especially during childbirth; causes ejection of milk from mammary glands
		Vasopressin or Antidiuretic hormone (ADH)	Acts on cells of kidney tubules to concentrate urine and conserve fluid in the body. Also acts to constrict blood vessels
THYROID	Lower portion of anterior neck	Thyroxine (T_4) and Triliodothyronine (T_3)	Increases metabolism; influences both physical and mental activity; promotes normal growth and development
		Thyrocalcitonin	Causes calcium to be stored in bones; reduces blood level of calcium
PARATHYROID	Posterior surface of thyroid gland	Parahormone	Regulates exchange of calcium between the bones and blood
ADRENAL Medulla	Superior surface of each kidney	Adrenaline (Epinephrine)	Increases heart rate, blood pressure, and flow of blood; decreases intestinal activity
		Aldosterone (Mineral corticoid)	Controls electrolyte balances by regulating the reabsorption of sodium and the excretion of potassium
Cortex		Glucocorticoids	Affect the metabolism of protein, fat, and glucose, thereby increasing blood sugar
		Sex hormones (Androgens)	Govern sex characteristics, especially those that are masculine
PANCREAS	Behind the stomach	Insulin	Essential to the metabolism of carbohydrates; reduces the blood sugar level
		Glucagon	Stimulates the liver to release glycogen and converts it to glucose to increase blood sugar levels
THYMUS	Under the sternum	Thymosin	Reacts upon lymphoid tissue to produce T lympho-cyte cells to develop immunity to certain diseases
PINEAL BODY	Third ventricle in the brain	Melatonin	Controls onset of puberty
OVARIES	Female pelvis	Estrogen	Promotes growth of primary and secondary sexual characteristics
		Progesterone	Develops excretory portion of mammary glands; aids in maintaining pregnancy
TESTES	Male scrotum	Testosterone	Develops primary and secondary sexual character-istics; stimulates maturation of sperm

- Cushing's syndrome: Caused by the hypersecretion of gluco-corticoid hormones from the adrenal cortex. Possible underlying causes include adrenal cortical tumors or the prolonged use of Prednisone. Symptoms include high blood pressure, muscular weakness, obesity, poor healing of skin lesions, a tendency to bruise easily, hirsutism (excessive hair growth), menstrual disorders, and hyperglycemia. The most notable characteristic is the rounded "moon face" and a "buffalo hump."

- Dwarfism: Hypofunctioning of the pituitary gland and undersecretion of growth hormone during childhood. Growth of the long bones is abnormally decreased.

- Diabetes insipidus: A condition characterized by increased thirst and increased urine production because of inadequate production of ADH (antidiuretic hormone).

- Diabetes mellitus: Caused by decreased secretion of insulin from the islet of Langerhans cells of the pancreas or by ineffective use of insulin. Without insulin the body cannot use glucose. There are two types of diabetes mellitus: insulin-dependent (IDDM), also known as type I diabetes, or noninsulin-dependent (NIDDM) or type II diabetes. Insulin-dependent diabetes is also known as juvenile diabetes, because its typical onset is in childhood or young adulthood. Type I diabetics must take insulin and monitor daily blood-glucose levels. Symptoms of type I diabetes include excessive urination, excessive thirst, excessive hunger, weight loss, blurred vision, and possible diabetic coma. Type II diabetes usually occurs later in life and typically runs in families, although the age of onset has been decreased in recent years. This is thought to be related to childhood obesity. Commonly, type II diabetics can control glucose levels by maintaining normal weight and controlling starch and sugar in the diet.

- Gigantism: Hyperfunctioning of the pituitary gland. Hypersecretion of growth hormone causing an overgrowth of the long bones during preadolescence, thus leading to abnormal stature.

- Hypothyroidism: Condition in which the thyroid gland does not secrete sufficient thyroxine. Adult hypothyroidism may be caused by insufficient dietary intake of iodine. It may cause simple goiters. This is not a common condition in North America or industrialized nations, because of the use of iodized table salt. Symptoms include dry and itchy skin, dry and brittle hair, constipation, and muscle cramps at night.

- Hyperthyroidism: Overactivity of the thyroid gland; too much thyroxine is secreted. Symptoms include weight loss even when large quantities of food are consumed, nervousness, weakened muscles, possible increase in blood pressure, and increase in blood-sugar levels. The most characteristic symptom is exophthalmos, or bulging of the eyeballs.

Diagnostic Tests

- Adrenocorticotropic hormone levels (ACTH)
- Aldosterone levels
- Antidiuretic hormone levels (ADH)
- Cortisol levels
- Erythropoietin
- Fasting blood sugar (FBS)
- Glucagon
- Glucose tolerance tests (GTTs)
- Growth hormone (GH)
- Glycosylated hemoglobin (hemoglobin A_{1c})
- Insulin
- Renin
- Serotonin
- Thyroid function (triiodothyronine—T_3, thyroxine—T_4, thyroid-stimulating hormone [TSH])

URINARY SYSTEM
Function

The urinary system has four main functions:

1. Filtering metabolic waste products from the body
2. Secreting waste products in the urine
3. Eliminating urine from the bladder
4. Helping to maintain acid-base balance

As food is metabolized and used by the body, waste products are formed. Substances that are ingested and cannot be used by the body are eliminated or excreted by means of the intestines, the skin, the respiratory system, or the urinary system. Products excreted by the urinary system include nitrogenous wastes (urea), salts, and water. One urinary system function is to regulate the levels of water, electrolytes, and nitrogenous waste products in the blood. The proper balance of these constituents is vital to life. If the urinary system is not functioning properly, the body will not be able to eliminate nitrogenous waste products, and toxicity will develop (Figure 3-20).

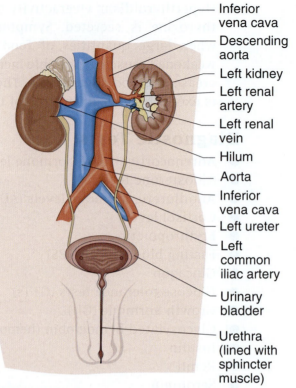

Inferior vena cava

Descending aorta

Left kidney

Left renal artery

Left renal vein

Hilum

Aorta

Inferior vena cava

Left ureter

Left common iliac artery

Urinary bladder

Urethra (lined with sphincter muscle)

FIGURE 3-20: The structures of the urinary system

GLOMERULUS

A part of the nephron; a tuft of capillaries situated within Bowman's capsule. (*pl.* glomeruli)

ELECTROLYTES

Electrically charged particles which help determine fluid and acid-base balance.

NEPHRON

A unit of structure of the kidney; contains glomerulus, Bowman's capsule, proximal distal tubule, loop of Henle, and distal tubule.

As blood passes through the kidneys, specialized units called **glomeruli** located within the nephron, filter out substances the body needs to maintain homeostasis. These filtered substances can then be reabsorbed. The remaining solutes and water are excreted as waste products.

Structures

The urinary system is composed of the following structures:

1. Two kidneys: The kidneys are bean-shaped organs situated at the dorsal aspect of the abdominal cavity, just above the waist, one on each side of the spine (vertebral column) (Figure 3-21).

   The kidneys function to maintain water and **electrolyte** balance. The kidneys also eliminate urea, the waste product of protein metabolism. The kidneys are also responsible for the production of the hormones adrenaline, aldosterone, the glucocorticoids, and the androgens.

   The functional unit of the kidneys is the **nephron**. Each kidney contains approximately one million nephrons. Most nephrons are located with the cortex of the kidney (Figure 3-22).

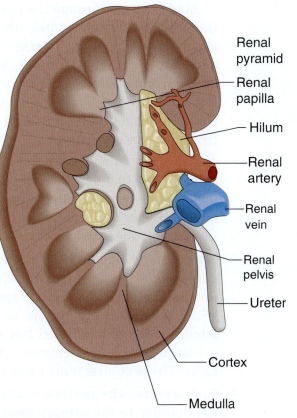

FIGURE 3-21: The structures of the kidney

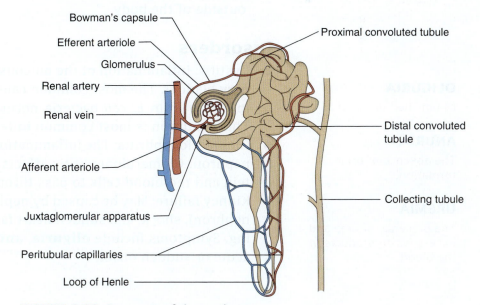

FIGURE 3-22: Structure of the nephron

Blood travels through the renal arteries and passes through the nephron's capillary bed (the glomerulus) where filtration occurs. The filtrate then passes through the Bowman's capsule and into the renal tubules where water and potassium, sodium, and calcium are reabsorbed into the bloodstream. The remaining filtrate is now called urine. The urine is transported from the renal tubules into the renal pelvis of each kidney and from there into the ureters.

2. Two ureters: One ureter passes out of each kidney and carries urine to the bladder. The ureters are approximately 10 to 12 inches in length. Because muscle fibers line the ureters they are capable of peristalsis. It is this action that pushes the urine into the bladder.

3. One urinary bladder: The urinary bladder is a hollow organ made of elastic fibers and muscle. Urine collects in the bladder until a sufficient amount triggers the elimination response. When approximately 500 ml (or about one pint) has accumulated, the bladder will feel full and the need to void becomes evident. The bladder empties by involuntary muscle contractions. These contractions force the urine into the **urethra**.

4. One urethra: The urethra is a narrow tube that extends from the bladder to the urinary meatus. In women this tube is approximately $1\frac{1}{4}$ to 2 inches in length, and in men it is approximately 5 to 6 inches long. The urinary meatus opens to the outside of the body.

Disorders

● Cystitis: Inflammation of the mucous membrane lining the urinary bladder. The most common cause of cystitis is a bacterial infection from *E. coli* bacteria normally found in the rectum. This condition is most common in females.

● Glomerulonephritis: The inflammation of the glomerulus of the nephron. Glomerulonephritis affects filtration and allows protein and red blood cells to pass through to the urine.

● Kidney failure: May be caused by nephritis (inflammation of the nephron), shock, and sudden heart failure, poisoning, or bleeding. Symptoms include **oliguria**, **anuria**, and **uremia**. May be acute or sudden onset.

URETHRA

A canal for the discharge of urine extending from the bladder to the outside.

OLIGURIA

Diminished urination.

ANURIA

The absence of urine formation.

UREMIA

The presence of urea and excess waste products in the blood.

- Kidney stones: Also called renal calculi. These are stones formed in the kidneys. Substances such as calcium phosphate, calcium urate, and uric acid may clump together to form stones. The stones grow slowly over time and may eventually block urine flowing into the ureter. The first symptom is usually extreme pain in the kidney area or lower abdomen, which progresses into the groin. Other symptoms include nausea and vomiting, frequent urge to void, chills, fever, weakness, and a burning sensation with urination. **Hematuria** may also be present.

HEMATURIA

Blood in the urine.

- Pyelonephritis: The inflammation of the kidney tissue and the renal pelvis. Generally results from an infection that has spread from the ureters. One of the symptoms is pyuria or pus in the urine.
- Urinary tract infection (UTI): Infection involving the organs or ducts of the urinary system.

Box 3-3: Dialysis

Dialysis is used when a patient's kidneys are not functioning properly or have failed completely. Dialysis cleans the blood that the kidneys are no longer capable of filtering. There are two types of dialysis: hemodialysis and peritoneal dialysis. Hemodialysis uses a machine to filter the patient's blood. The dialysis machine contains a semipermeable membrane that acts as a filter. Waste products, excess salts, and water are removed, and the device functions as a substitute kidney. Mechanical hemodialysis is usually performed 2 to 3 times a week. Each session lasts 2 to 4 hours. Patients are usually assigned to a kidney center for hemodialysis, but the procedure can be accomplished at home with the help of a family member or friend. Peritoneal dialysis uses the patient's own peritoneal lining as a filter instead of a dialysis machine. Peritoneal dialysis is a continuous process and is also called CAPD for continuous ambulatory peritoneal dialysis. The process takes about 30 minutes and most patients perform the procedure 4 times a day. Automated peritoneal dialysis can be done at night while the patient is sleeping and takes approximately 6 to 8 hours.

Diagnostic Tests

- Albumin
- Ammonia
- Blood, urea, nitrogen (BUN)
- Creatinine clearance
- Electrolytes
- Osmolality
- Urinalysis (UA)
- Urine culture and sensitivity (Urine C&S)

LYMPHATIC SYSTEM—IMMUNE SYSTEM

Function

The lymphatic system works with the circulatory system by acting as an intermediary between the blood in the capillaries and the tissues of the body. The lymphatic system has three main functions:

1. Maintaining fluid balance in the tissues by filtering blood and lymph fluid.

2. Protection of the body by filtering out harmful microorganisms. Production of lymphocytes that help to provide immunity and fight off disease.

3. Absorption of fats from the small intestine and transport to the bloodstream.

Structures

The lymphatic system is composed of the following structures (Figure 3-23):

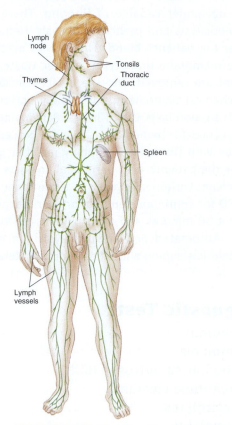

FIGURE 3-23: The lymphatic system

LYMPH

Watery fluid in the lymphatic vessels.

1. **Lymph** is a straw-colored fluid, similar to the composition of blood plasma. It is composed of water, lymphocytes, oxygen, digested nutrients, hormones, salts, carbon dioxide, and urea. It does not contain any red blood cells. Lymph is found surrounding the tissue cells of the body and is often referred to as interstitial fluid or tissue fluid. It acts as an intermediary between the blood capillaries and the tissues; and it carries nutrients, oxygen, and hormones to the cells, and waste products (carbon dioxide, urea) away from the cells back into the capillaries. Unlike the circulatory system, the lymphatic system does not have a pump like the heart; lymph is pushed through the lymphatic vessels by skeletal muscle contractions. Even the act of breathing helps to circulate lymph through the lymphatic vessels. Lymphatic vessels contain valves to prevent the backflow of lymph, like veins.

2. Lymphatic vessels are found throughout the body and closely parallel the veins of the circulatory system. Lymph capillaries are not found, however, in the nail cuticles, hair, cartilage, the central nervous system, epidermis, eyeball, inner ear, or the spleen. Lymph surrounding tissue cells enters into tiny lymph vessels, which progressively get larger and are called lymphatics. They continue to unite and become larger and larger until they flow into one of the two main lymphatics, the thoracic duct and right lymphatic duct. These ducts then empty into the large veins of the upper body.

3. Lymph nodes are tiny oval-shaped structures that range in size from that of a pinhead to that of an almond. Lymph nodes are composed of special tissue called lymphoid tissue. Some lymph nodes are found singly, while others are in groups or clusters. As lymph passes through the lymphatic vessels it eventually arrives at lymph nodes. The lymph nodes trap and destroy bacteria and foreign matter. They also produce lymphocytes. If the harmful substances that filter through lymph nodes are too numerous to be destroyed, the lymph nodes will become inflamed and may possibly be damaged. Swelling of lymph nodes (glands) is called adenitis.

4. Other components of the lymphatic system include the thymus, the spleen, and the tonsils.

   a. The thymus gland is located in the upper anterior part of the thorax, above the heart. Its main function is to produce lymphocytes. These lymphocytes are called T-cells. The thymus is an endocrine gland because it secretes the hormone thymosin, which stimulates the production of lymph cells.

b. The spleen, also composed of lymphoid tissue, is located in the upper left quadrant of the abdominal cavity, just below the diaphragm. The spleen produces lymphocytes and monocytes, and as blood passes through the spleen it is filtered. The spleen is capable of storing large numbers of red blood cells, and if the body is in need of extra blood, the spleen will contract and dump its reserves. The spleen also forms embryonic erythrocytes.

c. There are three sets of tonsils in the human body. The palatine tonsils are located on both sides of the soft palate of the mouth. The pair located in the upper part of the throat are most commonly referred to as the adenoids, and the third pair are the lingual tonsils, located at the back of the tongue.

Disorders

● Acquired immunodeficiency syndrome (AIDS): AIDS is a disease that suppresses the immune system. The causative agent is HTLV-III (human T-lymphotrophic virus type III), more commonly called HIV. A patient with AIDS cannot fight cancers or other opportunistic infections, which include: cancers such as Kaposi's sarcoma and lymphomas of the brain; parasitic infections such as *Pneumocystis carinii* pneumonia (PCP) and toxoplasmosis; fungal infections such as candidiasis and histoplasmosis; and viral infections such as cytomegalovirus disease (CMV), herpes simplex, hepatitis B, and hepatitis C.

Symptoms include prolonged fatigue; persistent fevers or night sweats; unexplained cough; thick, whitish hairlike coating in the throat or on the tongue; unexplained bleeding and easy bruising; discolored or purplish lesions of the mucous membranes or skin that do not go away and gradually increase in size; chronic diarrhea; shortness of breath; unexplained lymphadenopathy lasting over 3 months; and unexplained weight loss. There is currently no cure for this disease, although it may be medically managed up to 10 years or more.

● Autoimmune disorders: These occur when the body's immune system goes awry. The body forms antibodies to its own tissues and attacks these tissues. Examples of autoimmune disorders are rheumatic fever and lupus.

● Hodgkin's disease: A form of cancer of the lymph nodes. The most common early symptom of Hodgkin's disease is a painless swelling of the lymph nodes. This disease is most commonly seen in males.

- Human immunodeficiency virus: The causative agent of AIDS. There are three stages of HIV infections: (1) the development of full-blown AIDS, (2) development of AIDS-related Complex (ARC), and (3) asymptomatic infection.
- Hypersensitivity or allergic response: The body's defense system responds to benign substances as if they are pathogens. The substances that cause a hypersensitivity or allergic response are called allergens. Individuals can be sensitive or allergic to a variety of allergens such as ragweed pollen, ingested foods and medications, bee and wasp stings, or laundry detergents. An extremely severe and sometimes fatal reaction is called anaphylaxis or anaphylactic shock. Symptoms of anaphylaxis include extreme difficulty breathing; headache; facial, tracheal, and esophageal swelling; decreased blood pressure; stomach cramps; and vomiting. Anaphylaxis requires immediate medical attention and administration of an antidote such as adrenaline or antihistamines. If severe cases are not promptly treated, death can occur in a matter of minutes.
- Infectious mononucleosis: This disease is spread by oral contact and is often called the "kissing disease." It is caused by Epstein-Barr virus (EBV) and typically occurs in children and young adults. Symptoms include enlarged lymph nodes, fever, and physical and mental fatigue.
- Lymphadenitis: An inflammation of the lymph nodes that may occur whenever the body is fighting an infection. The term swollen gland is used frequently for this condition.
- Lymphadenopathy: Any disease of the lymph nodes, often associated with enlargement of the lymph nodes; can occur in mononucleosis.
- Lymphangitis: Inflammation of the lymph vessels.
- Lymphoma: The term used for any lymphoid tumor, either benign or malignant.
- Lymphosarcoma: Malignant lymphoid tumor.
- Splenomegaly: Enlargement of the spleen.

Diagnostic Tests
- Biopsy
- Complete blood count (CBC)
- Mononucleosis test (Monospot)
- Culture and sensitivity (C&S)
- Bone marrow biopsy

GAMETE

A mature male or female reproductive cell; the spermatozoon or ovum.

SPERMATOZOA

A mature male sex cell.

OVA

Female reproductive cell.

REPRODUCTIVE SYSTEM

All living organisms must reproduce either asexually or sexually. The human reproductive system is sexual and produces **gametes**, which in the male are called **spermatozoa**, or sperm, and in the female are called **ova**, or eggs. Reproduction occurs when a sperm from the male fertilizes the ovum of the female and the fetus is carried to term.

Function

The reproductive system has two basic functions:

1. Provides the organs necessary for reproduction.
2. Manufactures the hormones necessary for development of the reproductive organs and of secondary sex characteristics.

Structures

The structures of the reproductive system vary from male to female and are addressed separately.

Female

- Ovaries: The ovaries are the primary sex organs of the female. They are located on both sides of the uterus, in the lower abdominal cavity (Figure 3-24). Each ovary is approximately the size and shape of an almond, about 3 cm long and from 1.5 to 3 cm wide. The ovaries perform two functions. They produce the female germ cells, or ova, and the female sex hormones estrogen and progesterone.

- Fallopian tubes: The fallopian tubes are approximately 10 centimeters in length, and are not directly attached to the ovaries. However, the top of the fallopian tube that curves over the top edge of each ovary is surrounded by a number of fringelike folds called **fimbriae**. By peristaltic action, the fimbriae sweep the ova released from the ovary into the fallopian tube, where fertilization takes place. The ovum then passes down into the uterus.

FIMBRIA

The longest fringe-like extremity of a fallopian tube extending from the uterine tube to almost the ovary.

- Uterus: The uterus is a hollow, thick-walled, pear-shaped, and highly muscular organ. The uterus lies behind the urinary bladder and in front of the rectum. The nonpregnant uterus measures approximately 7.5 cm in length, 5 cm wide, and about 2.75 cm thick (3" long, 2" wide, 1" thick). The uterus is divided into three parts: the fundus (the bulging, rounded upper part), the body, and the cervix.

- Cervix: The cervix is the cylindrical, lower, narrow portion of the uterus that extends into the vagina.

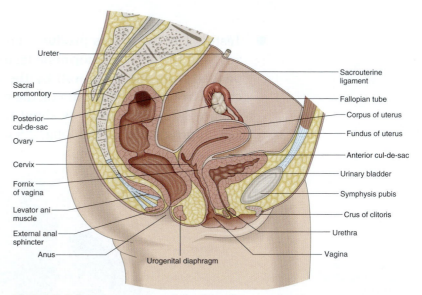

Ureter

Sacral promontory

Posterior cul-de-sac

Ovary

Cervix

Fornix of vagina

Levator ani muscle

External anal sphincter

Anus

Urogenital diaphragm

Sacrouterine ligament

Fallopian tube

Corpus of uterus

Fundus of uterus

Anterior cul-de-sac

Urinary bladder

Symphysis pubis

Crus of clitoris

Urethra

Vagina

FIGURE 3-24: Structures of the female reproductive system

- Vagina: The vagina is a short canal which extends from the cervix of the uterus to the vulva. The vagina is composed of smooth muscle with a mucous membrane lining. This muscle tissue allows the vaginal canal to accommodate the penis during sexual intercourse; it also permits a baby to pass through during birth.

- Vulva: The vulva contain the external organs of the female reproductive system. It consists of the mons pubis, clitoris, labia minora, and labia majora. At the entrance to the vagina are Bartholin's glands, which contain mucus. The area between the vaginal opening and the rectum is called the perineum. In childbirth an episiotomy incision may be made to the perineum to help facilitate childbirth.

- Breasts/mammary glands: Female breasts are accessory organs to the female reproductive system. They are composed mainly of fatty tissue but contain clusters of secreting cells surrounding tiny ducts. Each tiny duct opens in the nipple. Prolactin from the anterior lobe of the pituitary gland stimulates the mammary glands to secrete milk following childbirth.

Male

● Testes: The two testes produce the male gametes or spermatozoa, and the male sex hormone testosterone. The testes are suspended from the body wall by the spermatic cord and are enclosed in a pouch lying outside the male body called the scrotum
(Figure 3-25). Each testis is about the size and shape of a small
egg, approximately 4 cm long, 2.5 cm wide, and 2 cm thick.

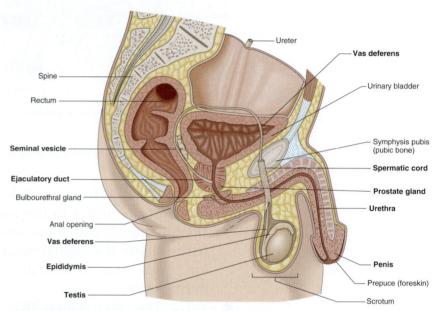

Ureter

Vas deferens

Spine

Urinary bladder

Rectum

Seminal vesicle

Symphysis pubis
(pubic bone)

Spermatic cord

Ejaculatory duct

Prostate gland

Bulbourethral gland

Urethra

Anal opening

Vas deferens

Epididymis

Penis

Prepuce (foreskin)

Testis

Scrotum

FIGURE 3-25: Structures of the male reproductive system

● Epididymis: The testes are attached to an overlying structure
called the epididymis. The epididymis consists of a convoluted
tube 13 to 20 feet long. It functions as the first part of the se-
cretory duct of each testis.

● Vas deferens: There are two vas deferens, a right and a left.
They are continuous with the epididymis. They serve as a storage site for sperm cells and as the excretory duct of the testis.

● Seminal vesicles: The seminal vesicles are two highly convoluted membranous tubes that produce secretions which help to
nourish and protect the sperm. A duct leads from the seminal
vesicles to the ductus deferens to form the ejaculatory ducts on
either side. At the moment of ejaculation, seminal fluid is
added to the sperm cells as they leave the ejaculatory ducts.

● Ejaculatory ducts: The ejaculatory ducts are very short and narrow. They descend into the prostate gland and join to the urethra, into which they discharge semen.

- Prostate gland: The prostate gland is located in front of the rectum just under the urinary bladder surrounding the opening of the urethra. The prostate gland is about the size and shape of a chestnut and is covered by a dense fibrous capsule. The prostate gland secretes a thin, milky alkaline fluid that enhances sperm motility. It also gives semen its characteristic strong, musky odor. Because the fluid in the ductus deferens is very acidic and the female vaginal secretions are acidic, the alkaline secretions of the prostate help to neutralize the fluids, which enhances the viability and motility of the sperm cells.
- Penis: The external male genitalia consist of the scrotum and the penis. The penis contains erectile tissue that during sexual arousal becomes enlarged and rigid to allow for insertion into the female vagina, to deliver sperm for fertilization of the ovum. Loose-fitting skin, called the foreskin or prepuce, covers the end of the penis. This skin can be surgically removed in a simple operation called a circumcision. Circumcision is commonly performed on newborn male infants although not deemed medically necessary by the American Association of Physicians.
- Urethra: The male urethra serves two functions: to empty the bladder of urine, and to expel semen during sexual intercourse. The urethra runs the length of the penis, and opens at the urinary meatus.
- Bulbourethral glands (also known as Cowper's glands): Lie on either side of the urethra below the prostate. Their function is to add an alkaline secretion to the semen. This secretion helps the sperm to live longer when presented with the acidity of the female reproductive tract.

Disorders

- Cervical cancer: Cervical cancer is often seen in women between the ages of 30 and 50 and can most often be detected by a Pap (Papanicolaou) smear. A sample of cells from the cervix is obtained by scraping the cervix and cervical canal, and is examined under a microscope.
- Infertility: A condition in which conception does not occur. Infertility may be caused by damage to fallopian tubes, a low sperm count, hormonal imbalances, and several other disorders.
- Impotence: The inability to have or sustain an erection during intercourse.
- Ovarian cancer: Cancer of the ovaries. It usually occurs between the ages of 40 and 65. Early diagnosis is difficult and treatment is aggressive surgery to remove all reproductive organs. It is the leading cause of cancer death in women.

- Ovarian cyst: A growth on the ovary that is typically non-malignant.
- Prostate cancer: The most common type of cancer in males over the age of 50. Symptoms include frequency of urination, dysuria, urgency, nocturia, and occasionally hematuria. Males over the age of 40 should have annual rectal examinations, which can detect enlargement of the prostate. A prostate-specific antigen blood screening test (PSA), which detects an abnormal substance released by cancer cells, should also be done annually.
- Sexually transmitted diseases: STDs are transmitted through sexual contact and the exchange of body fluids. The most common STDs are chlamydia, genital herpes, genital warts, syphilis, and gonorrhea.
- Uterine cancer: Endometrial cancer is the most common type of uterine cancer and typically occurs after menopause.

Diagnostic Tests

- Acid phosphatase
- Estrogen
- Follicle stimulating hormone (FSH)
- Human chorionic gonadotropin (HCG)
- Luteinizing hormone (LH)
- Microbiological cultures
- PAP smear
- Prostate-specific antigen (PSA)
- Rapid plasmin reagin (RPR)
- Testosterone
- Tissue analysis

❚RESPIRATORY SYSTEM

Function

Every cell requires oxygen to function. The human body can sustain life for only a few minutes without a constant supply of oxygen. The respiratory system provides this oxygen supply to the body, and has two main functions:

1. Provides the structures for the exchange of oxygen and carbon dioxide in the process of respiration. Respiration is divided into external, internal, and cellular respiration.

2. Provides the structures allowing the body to produce sound. The vocal chords of the larynx produce sound when air is passed over them (Figure 3-26).

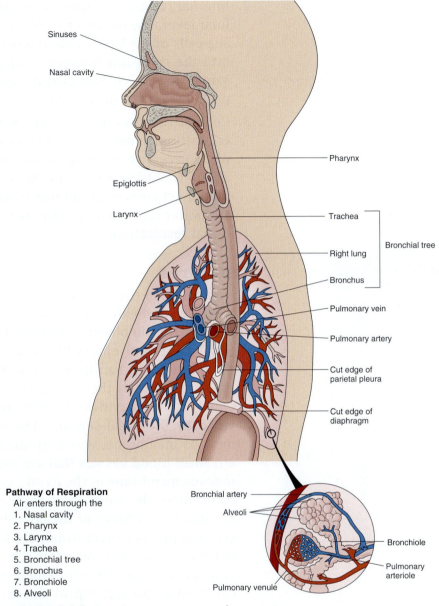

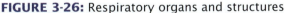

Pathway of Respiration
Air enters through the
1. Nasal cavity
2. Pharynx
3. Larynx
4. Trachea
5. Bronchial tree
6. Bronchus
7. Bronchiole
8. Alveoli

FIGURE 3-26: Respiratory organs and structures

Respiration

1. External respiration: The exchange of oxygen and carbon dioxide taking place between the lungs of the body and the outside environment. Each respiration consists of one inspiration (inhalation) and one expiration (exhalation). During inspiration, air carrying a high concentration of oxygen enters the body and is warmed, moistened, and filtered as it passes into the lungs. During exhalation, air leaves the body carrying a higher concentration of carbon dioxide.

2. Internal respiration: Internal respiration takes place at the cellular level. The oxygen-rich blood transports oxygen to the tissue cells of the body. Through osmosis, oxygen is transported into the cells and released, and at the same time, using the same process, carbon dioxide and waste materials are transported from the tissue cells back to the blood.

3. Cellular respiration: Involves the use of oxygen to release energy stored in nutrient molecules such as glucose. Cellular respiration occurs inside the cells and provides the body with the ability to release energy in the form of heat. This process, oxidation, creates waste products in the form of carbon dioxide and water vapor, which are removed through the process of internal respiration.

Structures

The structures of the nasal cavity form a continuous tract in which air is inhaled and exhaled. The tract starts with the nose and then continues with the pharynx, larynx, trachea, bronchi, and lungs.

● Nasal cavity: Air enters the body through the nasal cavity. Although humans can inhale and exhale through their mouths, the nasal cavity is the main route of respiration. The nose is divided into two cavities, the right and left nostrils, which are divided by the nasal septum. The nasal cavities are lined with mucous membrane, which produces mucus that moistens the air. Small blood vessels that are located near the surface of the mucous membrane in the nasal cavity help to also warm the air as it enters the nasal passage. Small hairs called cilia are located at the entrance of the nostrils. Cilia trap larger dirt particles and prevent them from entering. Nerve endings located in the mucous membranes near the end of the nasal cavity provide us with the sense of smell (olfactory nerves). The nasal cavity, or sinuses, also provides the voice with resonance. If the sinuses are blocked or inflamed, the voice is distorted.

● Pharynx: The nasal cavities lead into the pharynx, more commonly known as the throat. The pharynx is a funnel-shaped passageway approximately 5 inches long that is used for both food and air. When food is swallowed, a flap of cartilage called the **epiglottis** closes over the opening to the larynx so that food goes to the esophagus and not into the trachea.

● Larynx: The larynx is also called the voice box. The vocal chords are small rings of cartilage. The largest ring is called the Adam's apple. As air is pushed over the vocal chords, sound is produced. The movement of the lips and teeth produce words. The larynx

EPIGLOTTIS

Elastic cartilage which prevents food from entering the trachea.

is lined with mucous membrane, which is continuous throughout the nasal cavities and pharynx down to the tracheal lining. The end of the vocal chords is the dividing feature between the upper respiratory tract and the lower respiratory tract.

- Trachea: The trachea, also called the windpipe, is a tube approximately 4.5 inches in length. It extends from the larynx, lying in front of the esophagus and continuing down until it branches into the bronchi. The trachea is composed of alternating bands of membrane and 15 to 20 bands of c-shaped cartilage. These rings are nearly indestructible, so that the airway always remains open. However, the trachea can become blocked with large pieces of food, inflamed lymph nodes, or tumors. The walls of the trachea are lined with mucous membrane and cilia. Their function is to trap dust particles and then sweep them upward to the pharynx. Coughing and sneezing are methods the body uses to rid itself of these particles. The lower end of the trachea splits into the right and left bronchi.

- Bronchi and Bronchioles: The bronchi are similar in structure to the trachea because they are composed of mucous membrane, cartilage, and cilia. The right and left divisions of the bronchus form a y-shaped structure that further carries air toward the lungs. The bronchi become smaller and smaller as they get closer to the lungs. These smaller divisions of the bronchi are called bronchioles. The bronchioles have thinner walls and lose the cartilage plates. They are composed of smooth muscle and elastic tissue but are still lined with cilia. Bronchioles end in small sac-like clusters called alveolar sacs (**alveoli**) that terminate in the lungs.

ALVEOLI

Air cells of the lungs.

- Alveoli: Each alveolar sac contains thousands of alveoli. Alveoli are composed of a single layer of epithelial tissue, surrounded by a thin membrane. Normally the pressure exerted on these thin walls would cause them to collapse, but because of a coating of fluid called **surfactant**, the walls of the alveoli are able to withstand the constant pressure placed on them. If there is an insufficient amount of surfactant, as occurs in some premature babies, the walls of the alveoli will collapse. The adult human body contains approximately 500 million alveoli, which is about three times more than is necessary to maintain life. Gas exchange between the lungs and the blood occurs in the alveoli. A network of capillaries surrounds each alveolus. In the process of respiration, oxygen is transferred from the alveoli to the blood cells, and carbon dioxide and waste products are transferred from the blood cells to the alveoli.

SURFACTANT

A surface-active agent that lowers surface tension.

● Lungs: The human body has two lungs—a right lung with three lobes and a left lung with two lobes (the two lobes of the left lung allow space for the heart). The lungs are separated from each other by the mediastinum and are covered by a thin pleural membrane. The pleural membrane is composed of two layers. The layer directly lining the lungs is called the visceral pleura. The second layer, called the parietal layer, lines the thoracic cavity. There is a tiny space between the two layers filled with pleural fluid. This fluid prevents the two linings from rubbing against each other.

The lungs are large cone-shaped organs that are soft and spongy and extend from just beneath the collarbone to the diaphragm. The lungs are not muscular organs and depend on the muscles of the diaphragm and the surrounding muscles of the rib cage to enlarge and contract the chest during respiration. Adult lungs hold approximately 3 to 4 liters of air, depending on the activity of the person.

● Gas exchange and transport: The red blood cells transport oxygen and carbon dioxide throughout the body by using the protein molecule called hemoglobin. Hemoglobin binds oxygen and carbon dioxide directly to the red blood cell, which increases the red blood cell's capacity to carry oxygen by approximately 70%. When oxygen is bound to the hemoglobin, it is called oxyhemoglobin; when it is bound to carbon dioxide, it is called carbaminohemoglobin. Because of the thin walls of the blood capillaries and alveoli, the gases can be diffused from an area of higher concentration to the area of lower concentration. For example, when the blood cells pass through the tiny capillaries surrounding the alveoli, they are very low in their concentrations of oxygen and high in their concentrations of carbon dioxide. Because the alveoli contain high concentrations of oxygen and low concentrations of carbon dioxide, the oxygen molecules diffuse into the blood in the capillaries where the concentrations are low, and the carbon dioxide molecules diffuse out of the blood capillaries into the alveoli. Thus, exchange of gases has taken place.

Disorders

● Apnea: A temporary cessation of breathing.
● Asthma: A disease where the airway becomes obstructed by an inflammatory response triggered by a stimulus, which may be exercise, an allergen, or a psychological stressor. Symptoms include difficulty breathing accompanied by wheezing and spasms, and tightness in the chest.

- Bronchitis: An inflammation of the mucous membrane of the trachea and bronchial tubes, which produces excessive mucus. Bronchitis may be acute or chronic and often follows an infection of the upper respiratory tract.
- Cancer of the lungs: Lung cancer begins in a small cell called an oat cell, and spreads rapidly to other cells and organs. Individuals who smoke have a higher incidence of acquiring this type of lung cancer. There are two other types of lung cancer, which do not spread as rapidly. They are squamous cell and adeno-carcinoma. Symptoms include a cough and weight loss.
- Cystic fibrosis: A genetic endocrine disorder causing an excessive production of mucus.
- Diphtheria: A highly infectious disease caused by the *Corynebacterium diphtheria.* Children are routinely immunized against diphtheria. Adults may also be at risk for contracting diphtheria; therefore, they should receive booster doses. This is commonly done via a tetanus-diphtheria vaccination.
- Dyspnea: Difficult, labored, or painful breathing.
- Emphysema: A type of chronic obstructive pulmonary disease (COPD). In patients with emphysema, the alveoli of the lungs become overdilated. They lose their elasticity and cannot rebound. The alveoli may eventually rupture. Air becomes trapped and it becomes increasingly difficult to exhale.
- Eupnea: Normal or easy breathing with quiet inspirations and expirations.
- Hyperpnea: Increase in the depth and rate of breathing accompanied by abnormal exaggeration of respiratory movements.
- Hyperventilation: A condition that can be caused by disease or stress. It is marked by rapid breathing, which causes the body to lose carbon dioxide quickly. Symptoms include dizziness and possible fainting, to carpal/pedal spasms of the hands and feet.
- Hypoxia: A deficiency of oxygen.
- Infant respiratory distress syndrome (IRDS): A severe impairment of respiratory function in a newborn due to a deficiency of surfactant in the baby's lungs
- Influenza (flu): A viral infection characterized by an inflammation of the mucous membranes of the respiratory system. Influenza is usually accompanied by a fever, a mucus discharge, muscular pain, and extreme exhaustion.
- Laryngitis: An inflammation of the larynx, or voice box. Often secondary to other respiratory infections. Symptoms include hoarseness or loss of voice and dysphagia (difficulty in swallowing).

- Pertussis (whooping cough): Characterized by severe coughing attacks that end with a whooping noise. Children are routinely immunized against pertussis and this has greatly decreased its occurrence in the United States. Currently it is most commonly spread by unvaccinated and undiagnosed adults.
- Pleurisy: Inflammation of the pleural membrane surrounding the lungs.
- Pneumonia: An infection of the lung. Pneumonia can be caused by bacterial or viral infections. The alveoli become filled with a thick fluid (exudate) containing red blood cells and pus. Symptoms include chest pain, fever, chills, and dyspnea.
- Pulmonary edema: Accumulation of fluid in the lungs.
- Tuberculosis (TB): An infectious disease of the lungs, caused by tubercle bacillus, *Mycobacterium tuberculosis.* Symptoms include a cough, low-grade fever in the afternoon, weight loss, and night sweats.
- Rhinitis: Inflammation of the nasal mucous membranes.
- Tachypnea: An abnormally rapid and shallow rate of breathing.
- Tonsillitis: Inflammation of the tonsils. May cause obstruction of the respiratory tract and diminish the ability to breathe normally.
- Upper respiratory infection (URI): An infection of the nose, throat, larynx, or upper trachea. May be caused by one of many cold viruses.

Diagnostic Tests

- Alkaline phosphatase (ALP)
- Arterial blood gases (ABGs)
- Bronchial washings
- Capillary blood gases (CBGs)
- Complete blood count (CBC)
- Drug levels
- Electrolytes ("lytes")
- Microbiology cultures
- Pleuracentesis
- Skin tests: PPD (tuberculosis or TB test)
- Sputum cultures

⬤CARDIOVASCULAR SYSTEM

All the systems of the body are connected by the cardiovascular system, because it transports oxygen and nutrients via blood to every living cell in the body. As the cardiovascular system is the primary body system the phlebotomist directly works with, there are three elements of the cardiovascular system that the phlebotomist must thoroughly understand: the heart, the blood, and the vessels.

The Heart

Function

The heart functions as the body's pump, circulating blood to all parts of the body. It is a double pump, pumping approximately 2 ounces of blood with each heartbeat, 5 quarts per minute, 75 gallons per hour. The heart contracts about 72 times per minute, or about 100,000 times each day.

Structures

The heart is a hollow, muscular organ, just slightly larger than a closed fist, approximately 3.5" wide, and 5" long, weighing less than one pound. It is located just slightly to the left of the midline of the thoracic cavity. The heart has four chambers. The two upper chambers are called **atria**, and are the receiving chambers of the heart. The two lower chambers are the **ventricles** and are the heart's pumping chambers (Figure 3-27).

The heart is separated into right and left halves by a wall of cartilage called the septum. The septum completely separates the blood on the right side of the heart from the blood on the left.

- The atria: The two upper chambers of the heart are referred to as the right and left atrium (*pl.* atria) or right and left auricles. The atria are the receiving chambers. The right atrium receives **deoxygenated** blood from the body. The left atrium receives oxygenated blood from the lungs.
- The ventricles: The two lower chambers of the heart are referred to as the right and left ventricles. The ventricles are the pumping chambers of the heart. The right ventricle pumps deoxygenated blood to the lungs and the left ventricle pumps oxygenated blood to the body.

ATRIUM

An upper chamber of the heart. (*pl.* atria)

VENTRICLE

A small cavity or chamber as in the heart or the brain.

DEOXYGENATED

The state of having oxygen removed from a compound or tissue.

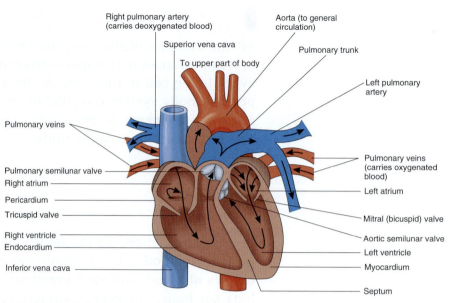

Right pulmonary artery
(carries deoxygenated blood)

Aorta (to general
circulation)

Superior vena cava

Pulmonary trunk

To upper part of body

Left pulmonary
artery

Pulmonary veins

Pulmonary veins
(carries oxygenated
blood)

Pulmonary semilunar valve

Right atrium

Left atrium

Pericardium

Tricuspid valve

Mitral (bicuspid) valve

Right ventricle

Aortic semilunar valve

Endocardium

Left ventricle

Inferior vena cava

Myocardium

Septum

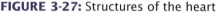

FIGURE 3-27: Structures of the heart

TRICUSPID VALVE

A three-part valve located between the right atrium and right ventricle.

BICUSPID VALVE

Also called the mitral valve. Atrioventricular valve of the left side of the heart.

PULMONARY SEMILUNAR VALVE

The half-moon shaped valve between the right ventricle and the pulmonary artery.

AORTIC SEMILUNAR VALVE

The valve between the left ventricle and the ascending aorta, made up of three half-moon–shaped cups.

● Valves: The heart has four valves, which permit the blood to flow in only one direction. The valves open and close with the contraction of the heart. The atrioventricular valves are located between the atria and the ventricles. The **tricuspid valve** is located between the right atrium and the right ventricle. Its name is derived from the fact that it has three (tri) cusps or flaps. It allows blood to flow from the right atrium to the right ventricle, but not back. The **bicuspid valve**, also called the mitral valve, is located between the left atrium and the left ventricle. It is named for its two cusps. The bicuspid valve allows blood to flow from the left atrium to the left ventricle and, like the tricuspid valve, prevents backflow. When the atrioventricular valves close they are responsible for the *"lubb"* sound heard when listening to the heart through the chest wall.

The semilunar valves are located at the point where blood leaves the heart. They also prevent the blood from flowing backwards. The **pulmonary semilunar valve** is located in the right ventricle, at the opening to the pulmonary artery that leads to the lungs. The **aortic semilunar valve** is located in the left ventricle at the opening of the aorta, leading from the heart out to the body. The semilunar valves make the *"dupp"* sound when they close. Abnormal heart sounds caused by malfunction of the valves are called murmurs.

Layers of the Heart

The heart has three layers of tissue. The outermost layer of protective fibrous tissue is called the **pericardium**. The pericardium consists of two layers of tissue. Between the two layers is a thin space filled with pericardial fluid. Pericardial fluid prevents the two layers from rubbing together and creating friction, much like the pleural fluid of the lungs. The layer closest to the heart is called the visceral pericardium and the tough outer layer is called the parietal pericardium. The second layer of heart tissue is called the **myocardium**. The myocardium is the main cardiac muscle tissue of the heart. The third layer and inner lining of smooth tissue is called the **endocardium**. The endocardium lines the heart valves and the blood vessels.

The Electrical Conduction System

The electrical conduction system of the heart is covered in Chapter 7—Electrocardiography.

Disorders

● Angina pectoris: Angina pectoris is characterized by severe chest pain caused by a lack of oxygen to the heart tissues. Angina pectoris is not a disease in and of itself, but an underlying symptom of problems with coronary circulation. The chest pain typically radiates through the chest and to the left shoulder, and down the left arm. Angina can be induced by stress and exertion, often with sudden onset, and is relieved with rest or nitroglycerin.

● Arrhythmia: Also called dysrhythmia. A term used to describe any change or deviation from a normal heart rate or rhythm.

● Bacterial endocarditis: Inflammation of the endocardial lining of the heart and heart valves. May lead to the development of blood clots, which can often be fatal.

● Bradycardia: Term used for a slow heart rate of less than 60 beats per minute.

● Congestive heart failure (CHF): Abnormal condition that reflects impaired cardiac pumping, causing pulmonary congestion and systemic venous congestion and peripheral edema.

● Heart failure: Occurs when the ventricles of the heart are unable to contract effectively and blood pools in the chambers of the heart. Symptoms vary depending on which ventricle is affected. If the right ventricle is affected, the organs fill with venous blood, and edema will occur. If the left ventricle is affected, dyspnea occurs.

PERICARDIUM

The closed membranous sac surrounding the heart.

MYOCARDIUM

Muscle of the heart.

ENDOCARDIUM

Membrane lining the interior of the heart.

ARTERIOSCLEROSIS

The hardening of arteries, resulting in thickening of walls and loss of elasticity.

ATHEROSCLEROSIS

The hardening of arteries caused by deposits of fat-like material in the lining of the arteries.

● Murmurs: Indicate defects in the valves of the heart. When the heart valves do not close properly a gurgling or hissing sound occurs. Murmurs are classified by the valve involved. If the murmur occurs with contraction it is called a systolic murmur. If the murmur occurs during relaxation it is called a diastolic murmur. Murmurs can be corrected surgically.

● Myocardial infarction: More commonly known as a "heart attack" or "MI." Myocardial infarctions occur when there is a lack of blood supply to the myocardium. A blockage of the coronary artery resulting from a blood clot or a narrowing of the artery caused by **arteriosclerosis** or **atherosclerosis** can cause an MI. The heart muscle can become damaged from the lack of oxygen. Symptoms include a crushing, severe chest pain radiating to the left shoulder, arm, neck, and jaw. Patients may also complain of nausea, increased perspiration (diaphoresis), difficulty breathing, and fatigue. The pain is not relieved with rest or nitroglycerin.

● Pericarditis: Inflammation of the outer lining of the heart. Symptoms include chest pain, dyspnea, rapid pulse, fever, and a cough.

● Tachycardia: Term used for a rapid heart rate of more than 100 beats per minute.

Diagnostic Tests

● ABGs
● AST (SGOT)
● Cholesterol
● CK (CPK)
● ECG (EKG)
● Potassium (K)
● Triglycerides

The Blood Vessels and Circulation

The heart pumps blood to all the tissues of the body through numerous methods of circulation: cardiopulmonary, systemic, coronary, portal, or fetal circulation.

Cardiopulmonary Circulation

Cardiopulmonary circulation is the process whereby blood circulates through the heart, taking deoxygenated blood from the heart through the lungs where carbon dioxide is exchanged for oxygen, and oxygenated blood is then pumped out to the body (Figure 3-28). Deoxygenated blood from the body is pumped into the right atrium of the heart; it then passes through the tricuspid valve into the right ventricle. When the right ventricle contracts, it pumps blood through the pulmonary semilunar valve into the pulmonary trunk. The pulmonary trunk branches into right and left pulmonary arteries, which transport blood to the right and left lungs. Inside the lungs, the pulmonary arteries branch into smaller arteries called **arterioles**. The arterioles connect to the smaller vessels of the capillary beds, which lie in close proximity to the alveoli of the lungs. It is at this level that the exchange of gases takes place. Carbon dioxide leaves the blood cells and is picked up by the alveoli. Oxygen attached to the hemoglobin in the alveolar red blood cells is carried first by the small venules attached to the capillary network, and then to larger veins, and finally to the pulmonary veins into the left atrium. From the left atrium, the blood is pumped through the bicuspid (mitral) valve and into the left ventricle. The left ventricle pumps the blood out to the systemic circulation via the aortic semilunar valve, through the aortic arch, and then through aorta. At this point the circulation leaves the heart and lungs and becomes systemic.

ARTERIOLE

A small branch of an artery.

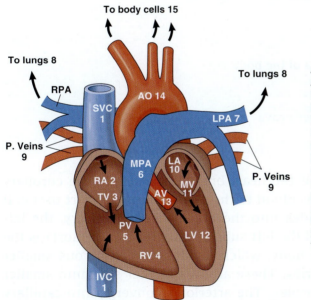

FIGURE 3-28: The flow of blood

AO — Aorta
AV — Aortic valve
IVC — Interior vena cava
LA — Left atrium
LPA — Left pulmonery artery
LV — Left ventricle
MPA — Main pulmonary artery
MV — Mitral valve
PV — Pulmonary valve
P. VEINS — Pulmonary veins
RA — Right atrium
RPA — Right pulmonary artery
RV — Right ventricle
SVC — Superior vena cava
TV — Tricuspid valve

1. Blood reaches heart through superior vena cava (SVA) and inferior vena cava (IVC)
2. To right atruim
3. To tricuspid valve
4. To right ventricle
5. To pulmonary valve (semi-lunar)
6. To main pulmonary artery
7. To left pulmonary artery and right pulmonary artery
8. To lungs—blood receives O_2
9. From lungs to pulmonary veins
10. To left atrium
11. To mitral (bicuspid) valve
12. To left ventricle
13. To aortic valve (semi-lunar valve)
14. To aorta (largest artery in the body)
15. Blood with oxygen then goes to all cells of the body

Systemic Circulation

Systemic circulation (Box 3-4) serves several purposes. It circulates oxygen, water, nutrients, and secretions to the body's tissues and back to the heart. It carries carbon dioxide and other waste products away from the body's tissues. It helps to balance body temperature, and aids in protecting the body from harmful bacteria (Figure 3-29).

Box 3-4: The Flow of Blood—Quick Reference to Trace a Drop of Blood Through the Heart

- Right atrium
- Tricuspid valve
- Right ventricle
- Pulmonary semilunar valve
- Pulmonary arteries
- Pulmonary arterioles
- Pulmonary capillaries—alveoli of the lungs
- Gas exchange
- Pulmonary venules
- Pulmonary veins
- Left atrium
- Bicuspid (mitral) valve
- Left ventricle
- Aortic semilunar valve
- Aorta
- Arteries
- Arterioles
- Capillaries—tissues of the body
- Venules
- Veins
- Superior/inferior vena cava
- Right atrium

The aortic arch of the heart branches first into the coronary artery, which supplies blood to the myocardium or heart tissue. It then further subdivides into the brachiocephalic artery, the left common carotid, and the left subclavian arteries. The aorta is the largest artery of the body, which divides into numerous smaller branches called arteries. These arteries further split into smaller branches called arterioles. The arterioles converge into capillary beds where the gas exchange takes place on a cellular level, depositing oxygen and nutrients and picking up carbon dioxide and waste products. Traveling through the capillary network, the now oxygen-depleted blood makes its way through the smallest of veins, called venules, through progressively larger veins, and then ultimately through the superior or inferior vena cava back to the right atrium of the heart.

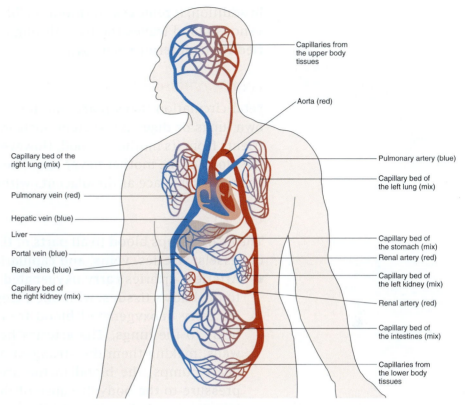

FIGURE 3-29: The systemic, pulmonary, renal, and portal blood circuits

Coronary Circulation

Coronary circulation takes oxygenated blood directly to the cells of the heart muscle. The coronary arteries branch off the aorta and encircle the heart muscle, becoming smaller and smaller vessels reaching every heart cell. The blood returns to the right atrium, by way of the coronary veins, directly through a pocket in the wall of the right atrium, called the coronary sinus.

Portal Circulation

Portal circulation is a division of systemic venous circulation. Veins from the pancreas, stomach, small intestine, colon, and spleen empty their blood into the portal vein, which travels to the liver. It is very important that venous blood makes this detour through the liver before it returns to the heart because the liver removes excess glucose from digested food, converting it to glycogen for later use. This detour helps keep the body's glucose concentration balanced. The liver also removes toxins and drugs, removes hormones the body no longer needs, and produces urea.

In addition, it removes worn-out red blood cells. The deoxygenated venous blood leaves the liver through the hepatic vein and is carried to the inferior vena cava.

Fetal Circulation

Fetal circulation takes place in a fetus. The fetus does not use its own lungs or digestive system. Instead, it obtains oxygen and nutrients from its mother's blood. However, the blood of the fetus and the blood of the mother never mix. The gas, nutrient, and waste exchange takes place at the placenta within the mother's uterus.

Blood Vessels

The heart pumps blood to all parts of the body through three types of vessels: arteries, veins, and capillaries.

● Arteries: Arteries carry oxygenated blood away from the heart to the body's tissues, with one exception: the pulmonary arteries carry deoxygenated blood from the right ventricle of the heart to the lungs. The arteries have thick, elastic, muscular walls, making them the strongest of the blood vessels. As the heart pumps, the blood in the arteries is transported under pressure to the body. Because of this pressure, a pulse can be felt at arterial sites close to the surface of the skin. This pressure also distinguishes the arteries from veins. Because the blood of the arteries is oxygenated, normal arterial blood appears a bright cherry-red in color. The smaller branches are called arterioles. The largest artery in the body is the aorta.

● Veins: Veins carry deoxygenated blood toward the heart. The one exception is the pulmonary vein, which carries oxygenated blood from the lungs back to the heart. Veins have thinner walls than arteries and do not have the pressure of the ventricular contractions to move blood along. Movement of blood in the veins occurs mainly because of the movement of the skeletal muscles. The veins contain valves much like the valves in the heart. Even though the blood is moving against the flow of gravity, these valves help to prevent backflow and keep the blood moving in the direction of the heart. Because the blood in the veins is low in oxygen it is a darker, somewhat bluish-red color. Because the vessel walls are thin, veins collapse more easily than arteries do. The smallest veins of the body are called venules and the largest veins are the superior and inferior vena cava. The longest vein in the body is the great saphenous vein, located in the leg.

● Capillaries: Capillaries are microscopic vessels, one cell thick. They connect with arterioles and venules (Figure 3-30), so blood in the capillaries is a mixture of both venous and arterial blood. The walls of the capillaries are so thin that it is possible for tissue cells and blood cells to exchange oxygen and other nutrients, and carbon dioxide and other waste products.

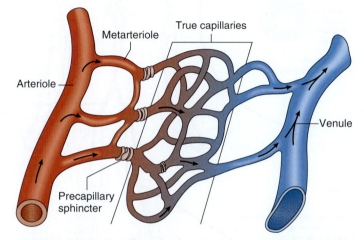

FIGURE 3-30: Capillary bed connecting an arteriole with a venule

The Structure of Blood Vessels

Arteries and veins are composed of three layers (Figure 3-31). Vessel thickness depends on the size and location of the vessel. The internal opening of a blood vessel is called the **lumen**.

● **Tunica adventitia**: This is the outermost layer, often referred to as the *tunica externa.* It is composed of fibrous connective tissue and, in the arteries, bundles of muscle fibers, which produce the elasticity of the arteries. The tunica adventitia is thicker in arteries than in veins.

● **Tunica media**: This is the middle layer and is made up of smooth muscle tissue arranged in a circular pattern with some elastic fibers. Again, this layer is also thicker in the arteries than in the veins.

● **Tunica intima**: Also referred to as *tunica interna.* It is the inner lining of a blood vessel. It is composed of three smaller layers: a single layer of endothelial cells, a layer of connective tissue, and an elastic internal membrane, which gives the artery a smooth lining allowing blood to flow freely.

The walls of the capillaries are extremely thin and are composed of a single layer of endothelial cells enclosed in a basement membrane.

LUMEN

Passageway or opening to a tubular structure such as a blood vessel, phlebotomy, or hypodermic needle.

TUNICA ADVENTITIA

The outermost fibroelastic layer of a blood vessel.

TUNICA MEDIA

The middle layer in the wall of a blood vessel composed of circular or spiraling smooth muscle and some elastic fibers.

TUNICA INTIMA

The lining of a blood vessel composed of an epithelial layer and the basement membrane, a connective tissue layer, and usually an internal elastic lamina.

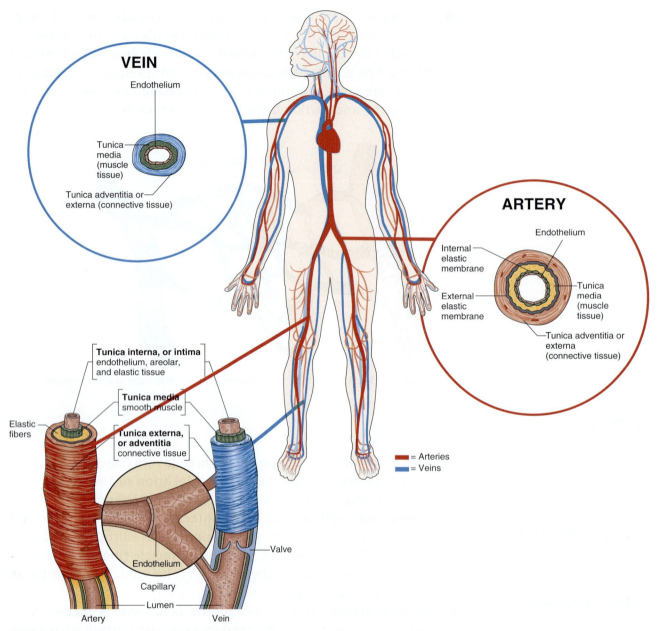

FIGURE 3-31: Structure of arteries and veins

Blood Vessels Related to Venous and Atrial Puncture

Venous Puncture: The veins most frequently used for venipuncture are located in the area referred to as the **antecubital fossa**. The antecubital (or AC) fossa is located on the anterior surface of the arm at the bend of the elbow. Several major veins lie close to the surface of the skin in this area, making them easier to visualize, palpate, and penetrate. These veins are collectively referred to as the antecubital veins (Figure 3-32).

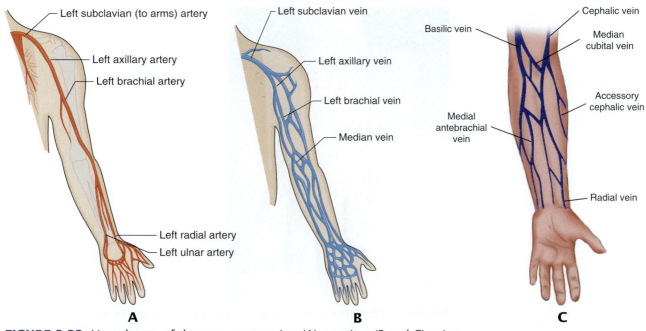

FIGURE 3-32: Vasculature of the upper extremity: (A) arteries; (B and C) veins

● Antecubital veins (listed in order of preference for venipuncture):

Median cubital vein: This vein is usually large and well anchored. This makes it the first choice for venipuncture because it typically is a less painful site which is less likely to
bruise, and is the easiest to visualize.

Cephalic vein: The second choice for venipuncture. This
vein is usually well anchored. However, it is often harder to
palpate in obese patients.

Basilic vein: This vein is usually often easy to palpate but it
is not well anchored, which causes it to roll and bruise more
easily than the median cubital vein or the cephalic vein.
Puncturing this vein is often more painful to the patient. It
is also located quite close to the median nerve and the
brachial artery, both of which can accidentally be punctured
during the draw.

● Other veins of the hands and arms: When antecubital veins are
unsuitable or unavailable, other veins of the arms and hands
may be used (Figure 3-33).

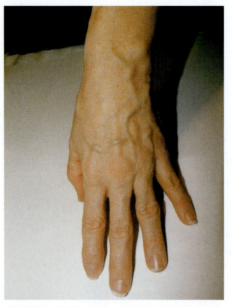

FIGURE 3-33: Veins of the hand (Courtesy of Mark Zeringue)

● Veins of the leg, ankle, and foot: Veins of the leg, ankle, or foot (Figure 3-34) are only used when no other veins are available, and then only with permission from the patient's physician. When the femoral veins are used for venipuncture, only a physician or specifically trained medical professional is authorized to perform the procedure.

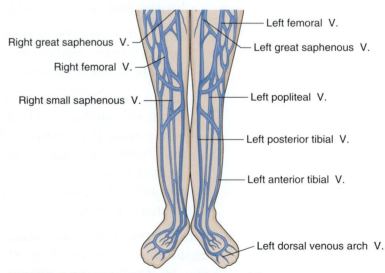

Right great saphenous V.
Right femoral V.
Right small saphenous V.

Left femoral V.
Left great saphenous V.
Left popliteal V.
Left posterior tibial V.
Left anterior tibial V.
Left dorsal venous arch V.

FIGURE 3-34: Veins of the leg, ankle, and foot

Arterial

Only specifically trained medical professionals are authorized to perform arterial punctures. They are more painful to the patient and carry a higher risk of injury than venipuncture. Puncture of arteries is typically performed for collection of arterial blood gases (ABGs). The arteries used in the arm are the radial and brachial arteries. The femoral artery of the leg may be used in an emergency or when no other arterial sites are available. Arterial puncture procedures are discussed in Chapter 12.

Disorders

- Aneurysm: An aneurysm occurs when a weakened artery bulges or balloons out. Symptoms include pain and pressure. Aneurysms most often occur in the aorta.
- Arteriosclerosis: A disease that accompanies the process of aging. Arterial walls thicken and harden, thus losing elasticity.
- Atherosclerosis: A form of arteriosclerosis which occurs when deposits of lipids (fatty substances) form along the walls of the arteries. In both arteriosclerosis and atherosclerosis the lumen of the artery is narrowed. Diet and exercise play an important role in prevention of both atherosclerosis and arteriosclerosis.
- Cerebrovascular accident (CVA/stroke): A sudden interruption of blood supply to the brain. This results in a loss of oxygen to brain cells, impairment of the brain functions, and/or death.
- Embolism: Obstruction of a blood vessel by a traveling blood clot (embolus). A pulmonary embolism is a blood clot in the lungs.
- Hemorrhoids: Varicose veins in the walls of the lower rectum and tissues around the anus.
- Phlebitis: The inflammation of the lining of a vein, accompanied by clotting of blood in the vein. Symptoms include edema of the affected area, pain, and redness along the length of the vein.
- Thrombophlebitis: The inflammation of a vein, in addition to thrombus (blood clot) formation.
- Thrombus: A stationary blood clot in a blood vessel.
- Transient ischemic attacks (TIAs): Temporary interruptions of blood flow to the brain that occur when the carotid artery is narrowed or occluded by fat deposits. Patients experience symptoms similar to those of a stroke.
- Varicose veins: Occur when blood flow back to the heart is impeded. Blood can back up in the veins if the muscles do not massage them. The condition often develops because of hereditary weakness in vein structure, poor posture, pregnancy, prolonged standing, and physical exertion. The condition most commonly occurs in the veins of the legs.

Diagnostic Tests

- Disseminated intravascular coagulation (DIC) screen
- Lipoproteins
- Prothrombin time (PT)
- Partial thromboplastin time (PTT/APTT)
- Triglycerides

The Blood

The average adult human body contains approximately 8 to 10 pints or 4 to 5 quarts of blood.

Function

Blood is the viscous transporting fluid that provides the body with oxygen, nutrients, hormones, and removal of waste products. It also aids in the maintenance of body temperature and is important in regulating acid-base balance and in fighting infection.

Structure

The blood is composed of plasma and cellular elements. Plasma, which makes up about 55% of the total blood volume, is the straw-colored liquid portion of blood minus the cellular elements. It is approximately 92% water. The remaining 8% contains the following seven substances called **solutes**: proteins, gases, nutrients, electrolytes, hormones, vitamins, enzymes, and metabolic waste products.

SOLUTE

A dissolved substance in a solution.

Plasma Solutes

- Plasma proteins: Three proteins are found in blood plasma. The first, fibrinogen, is necessary for blood clotting. The second protein, albumin, is a product of the liver and helps to maintain the blood's osmotic pressure and volume. The third protein, globulin, is formed in the liver and also in the lymphatic system. These proteins help in the synthesis of antibodies, which fight infection. Globulin proteins called prothrombins help blood to coagulate.
- Gases such as oxygen, carbon dioxide, and nitrogen are carried in blood plasma.
- Nutrients such as carbohydrates, glucose, fatty acids, cholesterol, and amino acids are absorbed from the digestive tract and are circulated in the plasma to provide energy to the body.

- Electrolytes such as sodium (Na^+), potassium (K^+), calcium (Ca^{2+}), and magnesium (Mg^{2+}) are found in the plasma. Sodium helps to maintain fluid balance; calcium and potassium are necessary for the proper functioning of the heart. Potassium is also essential for proper muscle activity and the conduction of nerve impulses. Calcium is used for the growth of bone and teeth, nerve conduction, and muscle contraction. Calcium is also essential in the blood-clotting process.
- Hormones, vitamins, and enzymes are found in small amounts in blood plasma and help to control its chemical reactions.
- The plasma carries metabolic waste products to the excretory organs.

Box 3-5: Serum—Plasma—Whole Blood

Some laboratory tests can only be performed on blood that has not been allowed to clot or separate. In other words, the test must be performed on whole blood that is in the same form as blood that circulates in the body. In order to maintain whole blood in the collection tube, an anticoagulant is added to the specimen. The anticoagulant is mixed with the whole blood for a minimum of 2 minutes. Testing must occur within 1 hour of collection.

Other tests must be performed on plasma. Most coagulation tests and some chemistry test results that are needed STAT use a plasma specimen. The blood is prevented from clotting by adding an anticoagulant to it. When a blood specimen containing an anticoagulant is centrifuged, it separates into three distinct layers. The top layer is a clear, straw-like fluid called plasma. The middle layer, called the buffy coat, contains white blood cells and thrombocytes, and the bottom layer is red blood cells. The plasma layer can be separated from the cells and used for testing. This layer of plasma looks exactly like a layer of serum. The difference is that serum lacks fibrinogen, which is necessary for clotting.

Serum is blood that has been removed from the body and allowed to coagulate or clot for 30 to 60 minutes before being centrifuged. Fibrinogen from the plasma traps RBCs and forms a fibrin network. Chemistry and immunological tests are performed on serum, although many laboratory tests can now be performed on either serum or plasma.

ERYTHROCYTE

A mature red blood cell (RBC).

LEUKOCYTE

A white blood cell or corpuscle (WBC).

THROMBOCYTE

Platelet.

Cellular Elements

Also called *formed elements,* these consist of **erythrocytes**, **leukocytes**, and **thrombocytes** (Figure 3-35), and are described as follows:

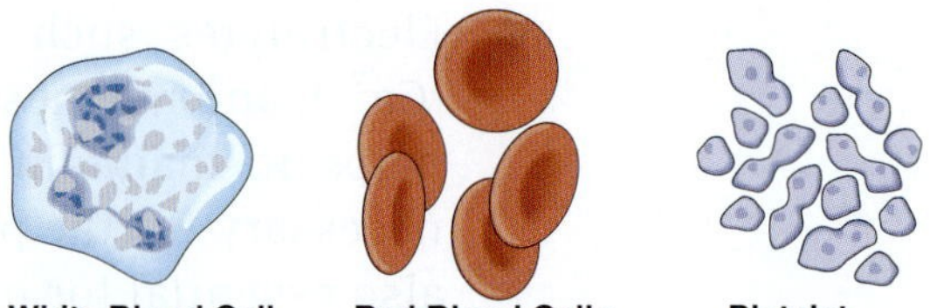

	White Blood Cell (Leukocyte)	Red Blood Cells (Erythrocyte)	Platelet (Thrombocyte)
Function	Body defense (extravascular)	Transport of oxygen and carbon dioxide (intravascular)	Stoppage of bleeding
Formation	Bone marrow, lymphatic tissue	Bone marrow	Bone marrow
Size/shape	9–16 micrometers; different size, shape, color, nucleus (core)	6–7 micrometers; bioconcave disc. Normally no nucleus in circulatory blood	1–4 micrometers; fragments of megakaryocytes
Life cycle	Varies, 24 hours–years	100–120 days	9–12 days
Numbers	5–10,000/ cubic millimeter	4.5–5.5 million/ cubic millimeter	250–450,000/ cubic millimeter
Removal	Bone marrow, liver, spleen	Bone marrow, spleen	Spleen

FIGURE 3-35: Cellular elements of blood

● Erythrocytes are biconcave (indented on both sides), disc-shaped cells, better known as red blood cells (RBCs). RBCs are 7 to 8 microns in diameter and are anuclear (no nucleus). The average adult has 4.5 to 5 million RBCs per cubic millimeter of blood. Their main function is to carry oxygen from the lungs to the cells. They also carry carbon dioxide from the cells back to the lungs. Their capacity to carry oxygen and carbon dioxide is greatly increased because each RBC carries protein molecules called globins and iron compounds called heme, combined together as **hemoglobin** (Hgb). The hemoglobin gives erythrocytes their typical red color. Every red blood cell contains several million hemoglobin molecules. Red blood cells are produced in the bone marrow. At first they contain a nucleus, but once they are mature enough to leave the bone marrow and enter the bloodstream, they have lost their nuclei. If an immature red blood cell enters the bloodstream it may contain remnants of the nucleus. Such cells are called reticulocytes. Mature red blood cells have a life span of approximately 120 days, after which they begin to disintegrate and are removed from the bloodstream by the spleen or liver. **Hemolysis** occurs when red blood cells rupture. Sometimes a reaction to a blood transfusion can cause hemolysis; at other times it is caused by disease.

HEMOGLOBIN

Oxygen-carrying pigment of the blood.

HEMOLYSIS

The bursting of red blood cells.

Leukocytes, or white blood cells (WBCs), are larger than RBCs and vary in size (Figure 3-36). Each leukocyte contains a nucleus. The average adult has approximately 5,000 to 10,000 WBCs per cubic millimeter of blood. White blood cells are formed in the bone marrow and lymphatic tissue, where RBCs stay within the blood vessels. WBCs can travel into surrounding tissues, which greatly affects the WBCs' life span. WBCs may only stay in the blood stream for 6 to 8 hours, but can live in the tissues for weeks, months, even years. The main function of white blood cells is to destroy pathogens. At times this is accomplished by **phagocytosis**. The pathogen is surrounded and engulfed by the white blood cell, and then literally eaten by the cell. At other times, white blood cells produce antibodies that destroy pathogens either directly or indirectly by releasing substances that attack the pathogen.

WBCs are classified by size, shape, and shape of the nucleus, and by whether they contain granules. They can be stained with Wright's stain and differentiated when viewed with a microscope. Cells that contain granules in the cytoplasm are called **granulocytes**, and cells without granules are called **agranulocytes**.

PHAGOCYTOSIS

The ingestion of foreign substances or other particles, such as worn-out cells, by certain white blood cells.

GRANULOCYTE

A white blood cell having granules in its cytoplasm.

AGRANULOCYTE

A nongranular white blood cell.

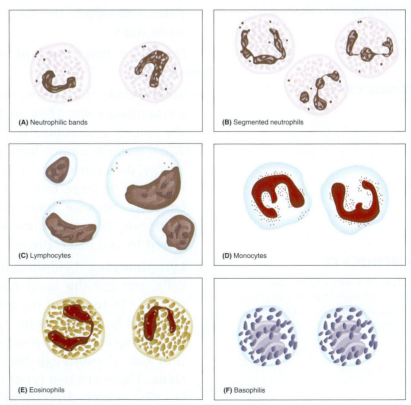

(A) Neutrophilic bands

(B) Segmented neutrophils

(C) Lymphocytes

(D) Monocytes

(E) Eosinophils

(F) Basophilis

FIGURE 3-36: Various divisions of leukocytes

NEUTROPHIL

Many-lobed nucleus, white blood cell that phagocytizes bacteria, sometimes called "polys or segs."

EOSINOPHIL

White blood cells whose granules stain a bright orange-red with eosin or other acid dyes. They increase in an allergic response.

BASOPHIL

One type of granulocytic white blood cell. Basophils make up less than 1% of all leukocytes but are essential to nonspecific immune response to inflammation. They have an attraction for basic dyes.

MONOCYTE

Large mononuclear leukocyte with deeply indented nucleus, and slate-gray cytoplasm.

LYMPHOCYTE

A type of white blood cell; makes up less than 1% of the circulating blood cells.

There are three different granulocytes:

1. **Neutrophils**: Approximately 65% of all WBCs are neutrophils. These cells have fine granules in the cytoplasm that stain lavender with Wright's stain. Neutrophils are polymorphonuclear leukocytes, which mean the nucleus has several lobes or segments. They may be referred to as PMNs, Polys, or Segs. Neutrophils are phagocytic and their numbers increase in patients with bacterial infections. Their life span can be approximately 6 hours to a few days long.

2. **Eosinophils**: The beadlike granules of the eosinophils stain a bright orange-red. The nucleus has two lobes. Eosinophils comprise approximately 3% of the total white blood cells and are often referred to as "Eos" (pronounced ee-ohs). Eos levels increase in allergic reactions and in parasitic infestations. They ingest and detoxify foreign proteins. The life span of Eos is from 8 to 12 days long.

3. **Basophils**: Basophils ("Basos") comprise only 1% of the total white blood cell count. The granules of the basophils are large and often obscure the nucleus. They stain a dark blue-purple to black. The nucleus of a basophil is frequently shaped like an "S." Basos release histamine and heparin, and help in the inflammatory process. They live only a few days.

There are two types of agranulocytes: monocytes and lymphocytes.

1. **Monocytes**: Monocytes, or "Monos," are the largest of the white blood cells. They are formed in the bone marrow and the spleen, and comprise 1% to 7% of the total WBC count. When stained, monos have a light, blue-gray cytoplasm and a large, dark nucleus. The cytoplasm of a monocyte contains vacuoles, or large holes, in which debris can occasionally be seen, because monocytes are phagocytic and ingest pathogens. When a monocyte leaves the bloodstream it is referred to as a macrophage. Its life span is several months.

2. **Lymphocytes**: Lymphocytes are the smallest white blood cells, but are the most numerous of the WBCs. Approximately 15% to 30% of the total WBC count are lymphocytes. A typical lymphocyte, or "lymph," has a large, round, dark purple nucleus that occupies the bulk of the cell. Only a thin rim of robin-egg blue cytoplasm surrounds the nucleus. There are two types of lymphocytes: T-lymphocytes (T-cells), which directly attack infected cells, and B-lymphocytes (B-cells), which produce antibodies. Lymphocytes

reside mainly in lymphatic tissue, and play a major role in immunity. The life span of a lymphocyte varies from a few hours to several years.

● Thrombocytes: Thrombocytes are better known as platelets, and are the smallest of the formed elements. Platelets are originally part of very large cells called megakaryocytes, which are formed in the red bone marrow. The average adult has approximately 250,000 to 450,000 platelets per cubic millimeter of blood. Platelets are first on the scene at the site of an injury and are essential to the coagulation of the blood. Their life span is approximately 10 days. Old platelets disintegrate in the bone marrow.

Coagulation/Hemostasis

When a blood vessel is injured, the process whereby blood coagulates and bleeding stops is called **hemostasis**. Coagulation takes place in four stages. The first two stages are called primary hemostasis and the second two stages are called secondary hemostasis. In stage one **vasoconstriction** occurs. The flow of blood to the injured area decreases as the vessel constricts. In stage two, a platelet plug forms. Whenever there is an injury to a vessel or tissue, platelets and the injured tissue release **thromboplastin**. Thromboplastin causes the platelets to clump and stick to one another. This process is called platelet aggregation, which forms the platelet plug. A bleeding time test assesses the speed of platelet plug formation.

Thromboplastin is released because an injury to the vessel makes the vessel's lining rough. As platelets in the blood flow over the roughened area, they disintegrate and release thromboplastin. In order for a platelet plug to form, calcium and prothrombin, as well as thromboplastin, must be present. Prothrombin is a plasma protein that is synthesized in the liver. Thromboplastin and calcium act together as an enzyme and cause a reaction that converts the prothrombin into thrombin. Thrombin is not normally present in the blood and only occurs when there is bleeding.

If the injury to the vessel is minimal, such as a needle puncture, the platelet plug formation is sufficient to stop the flow of blood. If the injury is larger, the process continues to secondary hemostasis.

In the first stage of secondary hemostasis, the thrombin that was formed at the end of stage two, in primary hemostasis, acts as an enzyme, changing fibrinogen into fibrin. The gel-like fibrin threads layer themselves over the cut, creating a fine meshlike network (fibrin clot). This network traps red blood cells, platelets, and plasma, and forms a blood clot. At first, serum oozes out of the injury, and as it dries, a crust (scab) forms over the fibrin threads,

HEMOSTASIS

An arrest of bleeding or of circulation.

VASOCONSTRICTION

A decrease in the caliber of blood vessels.

THROMBOPLASTIN

The substance secreted by platelets when tissue is injured; necessary for blood clotting.

completing the clotting process. In the second stage of secondary hemostasis, fibrinolysis occurs. During the clotting process, substances are released that convert plasminogen to plasmin. Plasmin is an enzyme that breaks the fibrin into small fragments, which are then removed by reticuloendothelial or phagocytic cells.

The liver plays an important role in the process of coagulation. It is responsible for manufacturing most of the coagulation factors, including fibrinogen, prothrombin, and heparin. It also helps the absorption of Vitamin K by producing bile salts. If the liver is diseased, coagulation factors are affected and prolonged bleeding may result.

Blood Type

ANTIGEN

A protein or oligosaccharide marker on the surface of cells that identifies the cell as *self* or *nonself*; identifies the type of cell (e.g., skin, kidney).

There are four major blood types: A, B, AB, and O (Box 3-6). Blood types are inherited, and are determined by the presence or absence of one of two blood proteins, called agglutinogens or **antigens**, located on the surface of red blood cells. People who have type A blood have the A antigen on the surface of their red blood cells. People with type B have the B antigen. People with AB blood have both the A and the B antigen on the surface of their red blood cells. Those with type O blood have neither antigen.

Box 3-6: Blood Types

Blood Type	Percent of U.S. Population	Antigen on Red Blood Cells	Antibody in Plasma	Can Receive	Can Donate To
A	41%	A	B	A or O only	A or AB only
B	12%	B	A	B or O only	B or AB only
AB	3%	A & B	None	A, B, AB, O (universal recipient)	AB only
O	44%	None	A & B	O only	A, B, AB, O (universal donor)

There is also a protein present in the plasma of a person's blood referred to as agglutinin, or antibody. A person with type A blood has B antibodies. Type B blood has A antibodies, type AB has no antibodies, and type O contains both A and B antibodies.

The antigens in the blood react with antibodies of the same type. These reactions cause red blood cells to clump together in a process called agglutination. For example, if a person with type B blood were transfused with type A blood, the A antibodies of the recipient would clump with A antigens of the donor. In an emergency, a person with type A blood could receive type A and type O blood, because type O blood carries no A or B antigens. Therefore, there would be no reaction because of the lack of antigens. If there were, the blood vessels would clog, impeding circulation and possibly causing death.

Because type O blood lacks antigens, it can be donated to all four blood types. Therefore, type O blood is the **universal donor**. By the same token, type AB blood lacks antibodies in its plasma, so it cannot agglutinate the red blood cells of any donor. Therefore, type AB blood is the **universal recipient**; it can receive all four blood types. This would only be done in emergency situations, as the same blood type should be given to avoid serious complications.

This is why it is vitally important to know a patient's blood type before surgeries or blood transfusions. A test called Type and Crossmatch is performed prior to a blood transfusion or surgery. This test identifies the blood type of both the recipient and the donor so that they are properly matched, to avoid a mismatch emergency.

Rh Factor

The outer membrane of human red blood cells may also contain a D antigen, better known as the Rh factor, in addition to AB antigens. The Rh factor/D antigen was first discovered in Rhesus monkeys, hence the term Rh. People who possess the Rh factor are said to be Rh positive (Rh+), and those who do not are Rh negative (Rh–). It is critical that the same Rh type be given from donor to recipient. If Rh+ blood is transfused to an Rh– patient, he may develop antibodies to it. The antibodies take approximately 2 weeks to develop. There is usually no problem with the first transfusion, but if subsequent transfusions occur, the accumulated Rh antibodies in the patient's blood could react with the Rh antigen of the donor's blood. Clumping and its potentially lethal consequences could occur.

The same problem may arise when an Rh– mother is pregnant with an Rh+ fetus. The mother's blood can develop anti-Rh antibodies to fetal Rh antigens. This typically does not affect the first-born child. However, subsequent pregnancies may be affected because the mother's accumulated anti-Rh antibodies will clump with the fetus's red blood cells. If the condition is left untreated, the baby could be born with a condition called erythroblastosis fetalis (hemolytic disease of the newborn). This condition is preventable because a special injection of immune globulin, RHO-Gam can be

UNIVERSAL DONOR

An individual with Type O blood, which has no A or B antigens and can be donated to all blood types.

UNIVERSAL RECIPIENT

An individual belonging to the AB blood group who can accept blood from all blood types.

given to an Rh– mother within 72 hours after delivery of a viable or nonviable fetus or a miscarriage. The RHO-Gam antibodies will destroy any Rh+ fetal cells which may have entered the mother's bloodstream. Therefore, the mother's immune system will not be stimulated to produce antibodies.

Disorders

● Anemia: A deficiency in the number or percentage of red blood cells and the amount of hemoglobin in the blood. There are a variety of different anemias, including iron-deficiency anemia, pernicious anemia, aplastic anemia, sickle cell anemia, and Cooley's anemia. Each type of anemia has its own cause and symptoms, but all types of anemia result from an abnormal reduction in the number of RBCs in the circulating blood.

● Hemophilia: A hereditary disease in which the blood clots slowly or abnormally, which causes prolonged bleeding with even a minor cut or scrape. Hemophilia occurs mainly in males and is transmitted genetically by females to their sons.

● Leukemia: A cancerous or malignant condition in which there is a great increase in the number of white blood cells. These WBCs are often abnormal in size and shape. Immature WBCs replace RBCs, interfering with the transportation of oxygen to the cells. They can also hinder the synthesis of new red blood cells from the bone marrow. The acute form develops quickly and runs its course rapidly. It occurs most often in children and young adults.

● Leukocytosis: An abnormal increase in WBCs in the circulating blood.

● Leukopenia: An abnormal decrease in WBCs.

● Polycythemia: A condition in which too many red blood cells are formed. This condition may be temporary and can occur at high altitudes as the body tries to compensate for low oxygen levels in the air. It may also occur as a serious disease. An increase in the number of RBCs can thicken the blood and form clots. The treatment for this condition is "bloodletting," or phlebotomy.

● Septicemia: The presence of pathogenic organisms or toxins in the blood.

● Thrombocytosis: An increase in the number of platelets, which can cause the blood to clot excessively.

● Thrombocytopenia: A blood disease in which the number of platelets is decreased. In this condition blood does not clot properly.

Diagnostic Tests

- ABO and Rh type
- Bone marrow
- Complete blood count (CBC)
- Crossmatch
- Differential
- Eosinophil (Eos) count
- Erythrocyte sedimentation rate (ESR)
- Ferritin
- Hematocrit (Hct)
- Hemoglobin (Hgb)
- Hemogram
- Indices (MCH, MCV, MCHC)
- Iron (Fe)
- Reticulocyte (retic) count
- Total iron binding capacity (TIBC)

● SUMMARY

The human body is a complicated and unique structure. A basic understanding and working knowledge of the cell and the ten body systems are crucial for every medical professional. The phlebotomist performs a variety of collection procedures and tests on patients who may have conditions and/or illnesses of any or all body systems. Understanding how these systems operate independently and together as a whole gives the phlebotomist a deeper appreciation and knowledge base from which to draw when working with patients. Especially important to the phlebotomist is a thorough understanding of the cardiovascular system, its functions, structures, disorders, and diagnostic tests.

● STUDY AND REVIEW EXERCISES
Defining Key Terms

Write the definition for each of the following key terms.

1) afferent _____

2) agranulocytes _____

3) albinism _____

4) alveoli _____

5) anatomy _____

6) antecubital fossa _____

7) anterior _____

8) antigen _____

9) anuria _____

10) aortic semilunar valve _____

11) arteriole _____

12) arteriosclerosis _____

13) atherosclerosis _____

14) atrium _____

15) axon _____

16) basophil _____

17) bicuspid valve _____

18) bilateral symmetry _____

19) bolus _____

20) cerebrospinal fluid _____

21) chyme _____

22) contractility _____

23) cranial cavity _____

24) cytoplasm _____

25) deep _____

26) dendrite _____

27) deoxygenated _____

28) dermis _____

29) distal _____

30) dorsal cavity _____

31) duodenum _____

32) efferent _____

33) elasticity _____

34) electrolytes _____

35) endocardium _____

36) endocrine gland_____

37) eosinophil _____

38) epidermis_____

39) epiglottis _____

40) erythrocytes _____

41) excitability_____

42) exocrine gland _____

43) extensibility _____

44) fimbria_____

45) frontal plane _____

46) gamete_____

47) glomerulus_____

48) granulocytes _____

49) hematuria_____

50) hemoglobin _____

51) hemolysis_____

52) hemopoiesis _____

53) hemostasis_____

54) homeostasis _____

55) hormones _____

56) ileum _____

57) inferior _____

58) interstitial fluid _____

59) jejunum_____

60) lateral_____

61) leukocytes _____

62) lumen_____

63) lymph _____

64) lymphocyte _____

65) mastication _____

66) medial _____

67) mediastinum _____

68) melanocytes _____

69) meninges _____

70) metabolism _____

71) midsagittal plane _____

72) monocyte _____

73) myelin sheath _____

74) myocardium _____

75) nephron _____

76) neuron _____

77) neutrophil _____

78) oliguria _____

79) ova _____

80) papilla _____

81) paresthesia _____

82) pericardium _____

83) periosteum _____

84) peristalsis _____

85) phagocytosis _____

86) phospholipids _____

87) physiology _____

88) posterior _____

89) prone _____

90) proximal _____

91) pulmonary semilunar valve _____

92) sagittal plane _____

93) Schwann cell _____

94) sebaceous gland _____

95) sebum _____

96) solute _____

97) spermatozoa _____

98) spinal cavity _____

99) stratum corneum _____

100) stratum germinativum_____

101) subcutaneous _____

102) superficial_____

103) superior_____

104) supine_____

105) surfactant _____

106) synapse _____

107) thrombocyte _____

108) thromboplastin_____

109) transverse plane_____

110) tricuspid valve _____

111) tunica adventitia _____

112) tunica intima_____

113) tunica media _____

114) universal donor _____

115) universal recipient _____

116) uremia _____

117) urethra_____

118) uvula_____

119) vasoconstriction_____

120) ventral cavity _____

121) ventricles _____

122) villi _____

Reviewing Key Points

1) Describe the correct anatomic position.

2) Identify the body's planes, cavities, and regions using the correct directional terms by labeling the diagrams.

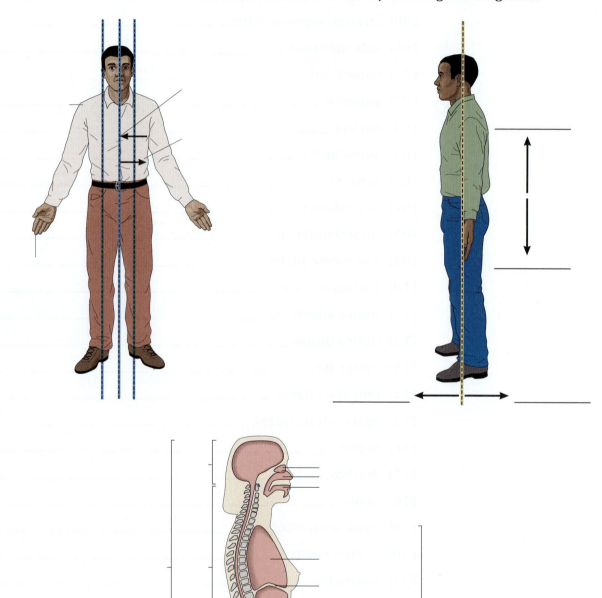

3) Describe the process of homeostasis.

4) List four types of circulation and briefly describe each process.

5) Trace a drop of blood from the right atrium of the heart through the body and back to the right atrium.

Sentence Completion

1) The study of the structure of an organism and the relationship of that organism to other parts of the body is the study of _____.

2) _____ is the study of physical and chemical reactions taking place on a cellular level, resulting in the growth, repair, energy release, and use of food by the body's cells.

3) The _____ is the basic unit of structure and function of all life and is responsible for all activities of the body.

4) The _____ is located just below the diaphragm in the upper left portion of the abdomen and is divided into three sections: the fundus, body, and pyloric sphincter.

5) _____ has the ability to bind oxygen directly to a red blood cell, increasing its oxygen carrying capacity by 70%.

6) The average healthy adult has approximately 5,000 to 10,000 _____ per cubic millimeter of blood.

7) The myelin sheath is composed of a fatty substance containing _____, which protects the axon.

8) The human adult body contains _____ bones.

9) A metabolic disorder and common condition of aging involving loss of nutrients and diminishing bone density is _____.

10) A decrease in size or a wasting away of muscle tissue caused by a lack of activity is a condition called _____.

11) The communication and coordination of all body functions is performed by the _____ system.

12) The specific, highly specialized cells of the nervous system are called _____.

13) The muscle for breathing is called the _____.

14) The first section of the small intestine is the _____.

15) The medical term for muscle pain is _____.

16) The outermost layer of skin is called the _____.

17) The sweat glands are also called _____.

18) The major function of the endocrine glands is to secrete _____.

19) A condition called _____ develops in early infancy and is characterized by the lack of mental and physical growth, resulting in mental retardation and malformation.

20) The _____ are two bean-shaped organs situated at the dorsal aspect of the abdominal cavity.

21) The need to void can be felt when the bladder contains approximately _____ mL of urine.

22) _____ is a straw-colored fluid found surrounding the tissue cells of the body.

23) The _____ is located in the upper anterior part of the thorax. Its main function is to produce lymphocytes.

24) The male gametes are spermatozoa; the female gametes are called _____.

25) In a male the _____ is located in front of the rectum just under the urinary bladder surrounding the opening of the urethra.

26) Bronchioles end in small, saclike clusters called _____.

Multiple Choice

1) The great toe is on the _____ side of the foot.
   A. lateral
   B. ventral
   C. dorsal
   D. medial

2) _____ is a living substance and can only be found within a cell.
   A. Protoplasm
   B. Ectoplasm
   C. Interstitial fluid
   D. Cytoplasm

3) The body system that supports the body and protects its internal organs is the _____ system.
   A. muscular
   B. nervous
   C. skeletal
   D. integumentary

4) Bones are made up of hard, dense tissue and are covered by a membrane called the _____.
   A. pericardium
   B. periosteum
   C. spongiosum
   D. myelin sheath

5) _____ comprise(s) nearly half of the body's weight.
   A. Water
   B. Bones
   C. Muscles
   D. Skin

6) Cardiac muscle is _____ and _____.
   A. striated—involuntary
   B. non-striated—voluntary
   C. non-striated—involuntary
   D. striated—voluntary

7) The _____ is/are a protective membranous covering that protects both the brain and the spinal cord.
   A. cerebrospinal membrane
   B. cranial membrane
   C. meninges
   D. white matter

8) The _____ nervous system conducts impulses from the CNS to the consciously controlled skeletal muscles.
   A. autonomic
   B. somatic
   C. sympathetic
   D. parasympathetic

9) A seizure disorder.
   A. Carpal tunnel syndrome
   B. Bell's palsy
   C. Cerebral palsy
   D. Epilepsy

10) A contagious fungal infection affecting the superficial layers of the skin.
    A. Acne vulgaris
    B. Athlete's foot
    C. Carbuncles
    D. Dermatitis

11) Inflammation of the gallbladder.
    A. Colitis
    B. Cirrhosis
    C. Appendicitis
    D. Cholecystitis

12) The function of the _____ system is to filter waste products and then secrete the waste products.
    A. endocrine
    B. urinary
    C. digestive
    D. reproductive

13) _____ is a form of cancer of the lymph nodes.
    A. Hodgkin's disease
    B. Human immunodeficiency virus
    C. Lupus
    D. Lymphadenopathy

14) A very painful bacterial infection of the hair follicles or sebaceous glands usually caused by a staphylococcal organism is called _____.
    A. acne vulgaris
    B. dermatitis
    C. carbuncle
    D. eczema

15) The liver, gallbladder, and the pancreas are considered accessory organs of the _____ system.
    A. endocrine
    B. digestive
    C. lymphatic
    D. cardiovascular

16) A condition caused by hypofunctioning of the adrenal cortex. Symptoms include bronzing of the skin, decreased levels of blood glucose, fatigue, weight loss, and decreased sodium levels.
    A. Cushing's syndrome
    B. Cretinism
    C. Acromegaly
    D. Addison's disease

17) A condition caused by decreased secretion of insulin from the islets of Langerhans cells of the pancreas.
    A. Diabetes mellitus
    B. Diabetes insipidus
    C. Cushing's syndrome
    D. Addison's disease

18) Inflammation of the kidney tissue and the renal pelvis is called _____.
    A. kidney stones
    B. pyelonephritis
    C. hematuria
    D. urinary tract infection

19) The _____ system works hand in hand with the circulatory system by acting as an intermediary between the blood in the capillaries and the tissues of the body.
    A. respiratory
    B. digestive
    C. lymphatic
    D. endocrine

20) The organ(s) of the female reproductive system which is hollow, thick-walled, pear shaped and highly muscular is/are the _____.
    A. ovaries
    B. uterus
    C. fallopian tube
    D. cervix

21) The leading cause of cancer death in women is:
    A. breast cancer
    B. cervical cancer
    C. uterine cancer
    D. ovarian cancer

22) The type of respiration that occurs inside a cell is called:
   A. cellular respiration
   B. internal respiration
   C. external respiration
   D. environmental respiration

23) The adult lungs hold approximately _____ liters of air, depending on the activity of the individual.
   A. 1 to 2
   B. 3 to 4
   C. 5 to 6
   D. 4 to 5

24) A patient experiencing _____ will have severe chest pain, which may radiate down the left arm, caused by a lack of oxygen to the heart tissues.
   A. congestive heart failure
   B. bacterial endocarditis
   C. angina pectoris
   D. bradycardia

25) The main function of white blood cells is to destroy pathogens. This is accomplished by _____.
   A. pinocytosis
   B. phagocytosis
   C. biotic genesis
   D. cellular respiration

Label the Diagrams

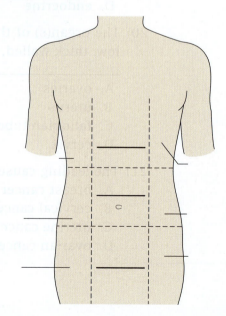

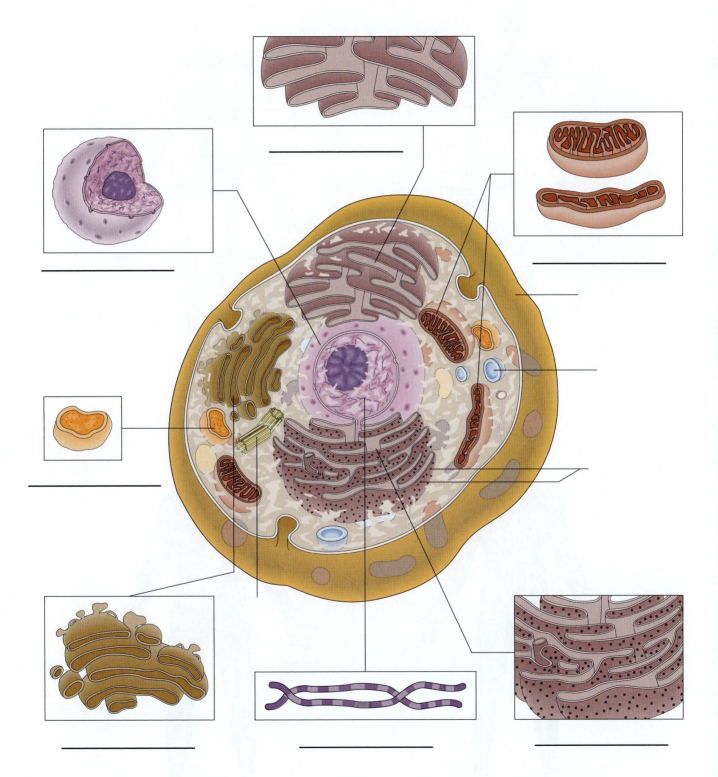

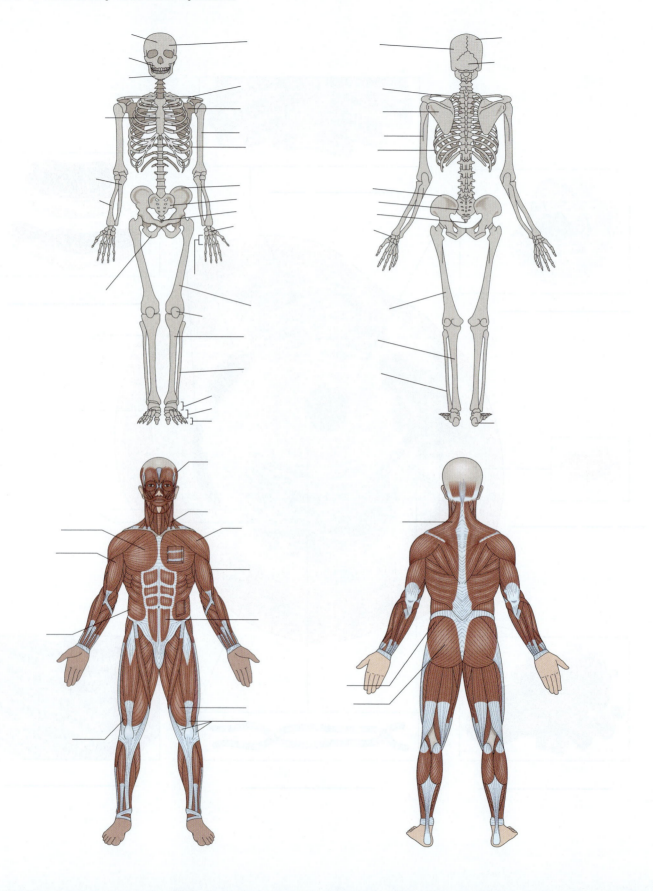

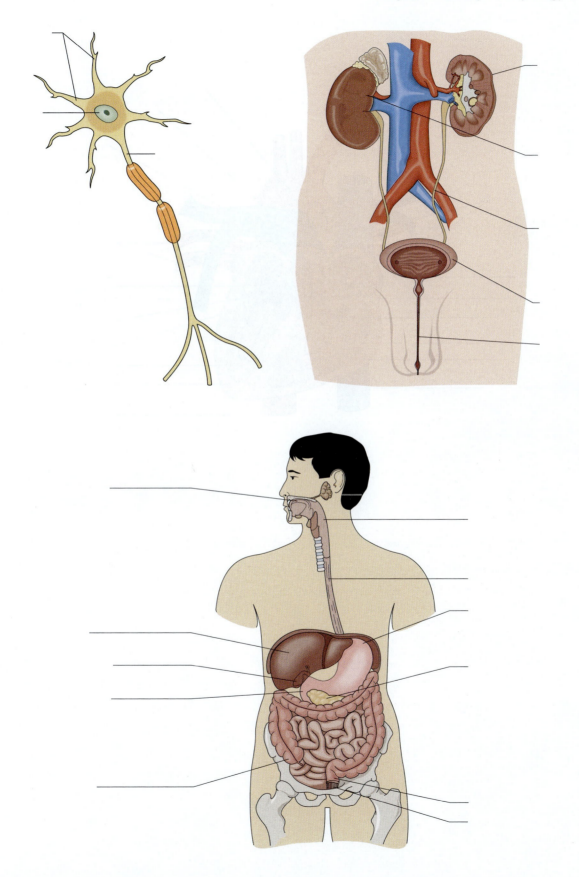

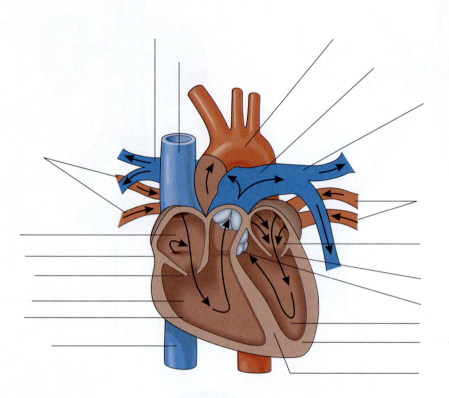

Infection Control—
Safety Procedures

OBJECTIVES

Upon completion of this chapter the student should be able to:

- Correctly spell and define the key terms.
- Describe the infection cycle.
- Describe the chain of infection and identify its key components.
- List and describe the seven types of infection isolation techniques.
- Understand the difference between Universal Precautions, Barrier Substance Isolation, and Standard Precautions.
- Identify personal protective equipment and demonstrate the ability to don, wear, and remove each article of protective gear.
- Demonstrate the correct procedure for handwashing.
- Describe the correct procedure for working with patients in isolation.
- Differentiate between medical and surgical asepsis, listing components of both practices.
- Demonstrate the correct procedure for opening a sterile package.
- Identify laboratory hazards and describe the safety procedures that apply to each hazard.
- List general laboratory safety rules.
- Describe and list the components of a Personal Exposure Control Plan.
- Describe the correct procedure for cleaning up a contaminated spill.

INFECTION

The presence and growth of a microorganism that produces tissue damage.

MICROORGANISM

A minute living body not perceptible to the naked eye, such as a bacterium or protozoan.

MICROBE

A unicellular or small multicellular microscopic organism not visible to the naked eye.

NONPATHOGENIC

A microbe which is nondisease producing.

PATHOGENIC

Capable of causing disease.

PATHOGEN

An organism or substance capable of causing a disease, condition, or infection.

CHAIN OF INFECTION

A series of related events that lead to an infection.

CAUSATIVE ORGANISM

The organism responsible for causing an infection.

THE INFECTION CYCLE

The risk of contracting and/or spreading **infection** is an occupational hazard in health care. The phlebotomist must fully understand the risks of infection and be prepared to prevent and control the spread of infection and disease. The phlebotomist, knowing how the infection cycle works and what precautions to take to stop the spread of infection and disease, decreases this risk when obtaining samples from patients, particularly those with known communicable diseases and infections.

Every day in the places we live, work, and play, we encounter many thousands of **microorganisms**. These microorganisms are referred to as **microbes**. Microbes are classified as bacteria, virus, fungi, or protozoa. The majority of these microbes are **nonpathogenic**; in fact we need them to stay healthy. However, some microbes are **pathogenic** and capable of causing disease and/or infection. In order for a pathogen to cause an infection or disease the conditions must be favorable. Environmental conditions are very specific for a **pathogen** to survive.

The environment must meet the following criteria: 1) nutrients, 2) water, 3) oxygen (or the lack thereof), 4) proper pH, 5) proper temperature, and 6) darkness. Once the criteria have been established, the **chain of infection** can begin and a **causative organism** (pathogen) takes up residence in the **reservoir host**. The reservoir host may or may not display symptoms of infection or disease. If symptoms are not present the reservoir host is defined as a **carrier**. The next link in the chain is a **means of exit**. This is the route by which the pathogen leaves the reservoir host to be trans-

RESERVOIR HOST

Any person, animal, arthropod, plant, soil, or substance in which an infectious agent normally lives, reproduces, and depends on for survival, that allows transmission to a susceptible host. In essence, a reservoir host is the breeding ground for transmission of pathogens to others.

CARRIER

A person who harbors a specific pathogenic organism, has no discernible symptoms or signs of the disease, condition, or infection, and is potentially capable of spreading the organism to others.

MEANS OF EXIT

The route microorganisms can take to leave a host (i.e., eyes, mouth, nose, open wound, blood).

SUSCEPTIBLE HOST

A person who has little resistance to an infectious disease.

MEANS OF TRANSMISSION

The method by which microorganisms can be transmitted from one host to another. The five main routes of transmission are: contact, droplet, airborne, common vehicle, and vector-borne.

mitted to a **susceptible host**. Examples of a means of exit include the mouth, the respiratory tract, the digestive tract, wounds, and blood. Pathogens require a **means of transmission**, which is the method by which it can be transmitted from one host to another. There are five main routes of transmission (Box 4-1): contact, droplet, airborne, common vehicle, and vector-borne.

Box 4-1: Routes of Transmission

1. **Contact Transmission:** Contact transmission is the most important and most frequent mode of transmission and is divided into two subcategories.

   a) **Direct Contact:** Involves the direct physical transference of pathogens from a reservoir host to a susceptible host. Direct physical contact must be made, such as kissing, skin-to-skin contact (e.g., shaking hands or hugging), or contact that involves exchange of body fluids (i.e., sexual intercourse). Not all pathogens can be transmitted by all means of direct contact. For example, staphylococcus bacteria may be transmitted by a handshake, but the AIDS virus can only be transmitted by direct contact of body fluids containing blood.

   b) **Indirect Contact:** Involves exposing a susceptible host to a pathogen by means of an inanimate object. Examples of this include pens, pencils, or telephones that have been contaminated, contaminated needles, items that have blood or body fluids on it, such as blood tubes, syringes, bloody dressings, and gloves that are not changed between patients.

2. **Droplet Transmission:** Droplet transmission, in theory, is a form of contact transmission. However, the method of transmission is unique and is considered a separate route of transmission. Droplets are generated from the source person primarily during coughing, sneezing, and talking. Transmission occurs when droplets containing microorganisms generated from the infected person are propelled a short distance through the air and deposited on the host's conjunctivae, nasal mucosa, or mouth. Because droplets do not remain suspended in the air, special handling and ventilation are not required to prevent droplet transmission. Do not confuse droplet transmission with airborne transmission.

3. **Airborne Transmission:** Airborne transmission occurs by dissemination of either airborne droplet nuclei (small particle residue of evaporated droplets containing microorganisms that remain suspended in the air for long periods of time) or dust particles containing the infectious agent. Microorganisms carried in this

(continues)

Box 4-1: Routes of Transmission *(continued)*

manner can be dispersed widely by air currents and may become inhaled by a susceptible host within the same room or over a longer distance from the source patient, depending on environmental factors. Therefore, special handling and ventilation are required to prevent airborne transmission. Microorganisms transmitted by airborne transmission include *Mycobacterium tuberculosis* and the rubeola and varicella viruses.

4. **Common Vehicle Transmission:** Common vehicle transmission applies to microorganisms transmitted by contaminated items such as food, water, medications, devices, and equipment.

5. **Vector-Borne Transmission:** Vector-borne transmission occurs when vectors such as mosquitoes, flies, rats, and other vermin transmit microorganisms; this route of transmission is of less significance in hospitals in the United States than in other regions of the world.

The next link in the chain of infection is a means of entry into a susceptible host. The route of entry is the same route taken as the route of exit from the reservoir host's mouth, respiratory tract, digestive tract, wounds, and blood. The last link in the chain is the susceptible host. A susceptible host is a person capable of being infected by the pathogen. The susceptible host must meet all the criteria for pathogen growth listed above, as well as one, or a combination of, the following: malnourishment, suppressed immune system, or general ill health. The infection cycle can now begin again with the susceptible host becoming the reservoir host.

● BREAKING THE CHAIN OF INFECTION

To break the chain of infection the pathogen must be stopped at one of the links of the chain, either by eliminating the means of transmission or reducing the susceptibility of the host (Figure 4-1). To reduce the susceptibility of a potential host, proper nutrition, sleep, stress reduction, and immunizations are required. In addition, there are a variety of methods to eliminate transmission of pathogens, including handwashing, wearing **personal protective equipment** (gloves, gowns, and masks), disposing of contaminated waste properly, insect and rodent control, and decontamination of equipment, instruments, and surfaces such as countertops, examination tables, and blood drawing stations. Isolation procedures also prevent the transmission of pathogens.

PERSONAL PROTECTIVE EQUIPMENT

Disposable gloves, lab coats or aprons, and/or protective face gear, such as masks and goggles with side shields, required by OSHA to be worn when handling body fluids.

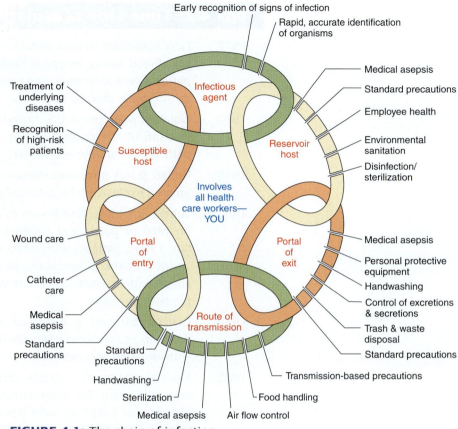

FIGURE 4-1: The chain of infection

● ISOLATION PROCEDURES

The Centers for Disease Control (CDC), Occupational Safety and Health Administration (OSHA), Joint Committee for Accrediting Healthcare Organizations (JCAHO), and The Hospital Infection Control Practices Advisory Committee (HICPAC) all assist hospitals, clinics, and laboratories to maintain up-to-date isolation practices and to establish guidelines and enforce regulations governing infection control.

Isolation procedures have been documented throughout history. The first published recommendations for isolation precautions in the United States appeared in a hospital handbook in 1877. The document recommended placing patients with infectious diseases in separate facilities. These facilities became known as infectious disease hospitals. Small progressions were made over the next hundred years (Box 4-2).

Box 4-2: Time Line of Isolation Techniques

1877   First published recommendations for isolation precautions in the United States. Hospital handbook recommended placing patients with infectious diseases in separate facilities, known as infectious disease hospitals.

1910   Isolation practices in U.S. hospitals were altered by the introduction of the cubicle system of isolation, which placed patients in multiple-bed wards.

1950s   United States infectious disease hospitals, except those designated exclusively for tuberculosis, began to close.

1960s   Tuberculosis hospitals began to close, partly because general hospital or outpatient treatment became preferred. In the late 1960s, patients with infectious diseases were housed in wards in general hospitals, whether in specially designed, single-patient isolation rooms or in regular single or multiple-patient rooms.

1970   CDC published a detailed manual entitled *Isolation Techniques for Use in Hospitals* to assist general hospitals with isolation precautions.

1975   Revised edition of *Isolation Techniques for Use in Hospitals* was published. The manual could now be applied in small community hospitals with limited resources, as well as in large, metropolitan, university-associated medical centers.

1980   Hospitals began experiencing new endemic and epidemic nosocomial infection problems, caused by multidrug-resistant microorganisms and newly recognized pathogens, requiring different isolation precautions.

1983   The CDC *Guideline for Isolation Precautions in Hospitals* was published to take the place of the 1975 isolation manual. Many important changes were made, such as the increased emphasis on decision making on the part of users, and the modification of the specific categories of isolation.

1985   Isolation practices in the United States were dramatically altered by the introduction of a new strategy for isolation precautions, which became known as Universal Precautions.

1986   New system of isolation, called Body Substance Isolation (BSI), was proposed after three years of study.

1988   Updated recommendations for management of patients with suspected hemorrhagic fever were published.

1990   Recommendations for Tuberculosis (AFB) Isolation were updated.

1991	Final rule on occupational exposure to blood-borne pathogens was published.
	HICPAC was established to provide advice and guidance regarding the practice of hospital infection control and strategies for surveillance, prevention, and control of nosocomial infections in U.S. hospitals.
	Standard Precaution guidelines were developed, combining the major features of Universal Precautions and Body Substance Isolation into a single set of precautions to be used for the care of *all* patients.
1994	Criteria for respirators used as AFB protection was finalized.

In 1970, the CDC published a detailed manual entitled "Isolation Techniques for Use in Hospitals." The manual introduced the category system of isolation precautions. This system was divided into seven categories: 1) Strict Isolation, 2) Discharge Precautions, 3) Protective Isolation, 4) Enteric Precautions, 5) Wound and Skin Precautions, 6) Respiratory Isolation, and 7) Blood Precautions. Box 4-3 describes each category.

Box 4-3: Category Specific Isolation

Isolation Category	Description and Barrier Precautions Required
Strict Isolation	Complete isolation is required for all patients with highly contagious diseases, which may be spread through direct contact and/or by air. Examples are: Ebola, rabies, diphtheria, chickenpox, anthrax, measles, and streptococcal and staphylococcal pneumonia. Strict isolation requires wearing gloves, mask, and gowns by anyone entering the patient's room. All items taken into the room must be left in the room and/or disposed of properly in biohazardous waste containers.
Contact Isolation	Contact isolation was designed for highly transmittable diseases spread primarily by direct contact, not warranting strict isolation. Examples of these conditions are antibiotic-resistant pathogens, and respiratory disorders, such as bronchitis, croup, epiglottitis, and pneumonia. Contact isolation protocols require the wearing of gloves, masks, and gowns if soiling is likely.
Respiratory Isolation	Respiratory isolation is required for patients with infections that can be spread from short distances through the air by means of droplet transmission. Examples of these conditions are whooping cough (pertussis), meningococcal meningitis, *Haemophilus influenzae*, mumps, and measles. Masks must be worn by anyone coming in close contact with these patients. All supplies should be disposed of inside the patient's room.

(continues)

Box 4-3: Category Specific Isolation *(continued)*

Isolation Category	Description and Barrier Precautions Required
AFB Isolation	AFB (acid-fast bacilli) isolation is required for patients with infectious tuberculosis. It is referred to as AFB isolation in part to protect the patient's right to confidentiality. OSHA implemented a new policy in 1993, requiring the use of a high-efficiency particulate air (HEPA) respirator as a minimum level of respiratory protection for all health care workers who care for AFB patients. Gowns and gloves are also required as part of the barrier precautions. All supplies must be disposed of inside the patient's room.
Drainage/Secretion Isolation	Drainage/secretion isolation is required for patient with skin infections, open wounds, or burns and sometimes following surgery. Patients are restricted to their rooms and anyone entering the room is required to wear gowns and gloves. Masks, gowns, and gloves should all be worn if soiling will occur.
Enteric Isolation	Enteric isolation procedures are used with patients with intestinal infections that may be transmitted by ingestion. Examples include *Salmonella, Shigella, Escherichia coli, Staphylococcus, Campylobacter,* and for any other organisms causing diarrhea or dysentery. Masks, gowns, and gloves are required of anyone entering the room. The patient's bathroom facilities should not be used by anyone other than the patient. All contaminated materials must be disposed of in the patient's room.

The precautions recommended for each category were determined primarily because of their routes of transmission. By the mid-1970s, 93% of U.S. hospitals had adopted the isolation system recommended in the manual. In 1975 a revised edition of the manual appeared.

In 1983, the CDC *Guideline for Isolation Precautions in Hospitals* was published, replacing the 1975 edition. It contained many important changes, including the increased emphasis on decision making on the part of the user.

In the category-specific section of the guideline, existing categories were modified, new categories were added, and many infections were reassigned to different categories. The old category of Blood Precautions, primarily directed toward patients with chronic carriage of hepatitis B virus (HBV), was renamed Blood and Body Fluid Precautions and was expanded to include patients with AIDS and body fluids other than blood. The old category of Protective Isolation was deleted because of studies demonstrating its lack of efficiency in general clinical practice in preventing the immunocompromised patient from acquiring infections. The 1983 guideline contained the following categories of isolation: Strict Isolation, Contact Isolation, Respiratory Isolation, Tuberculosis (acid-fast bacillus [AFB]) Isolation, Enteric Precautions, Drainage/Secretions Precautions, and Blood and Body Fluid Precautions.

NOSOCOMIAL

Infection acquired in a hospital.

HUMAN IMMUNODEFICIENCY VIRUS (HIV)

A retrovirus that causes acquired immunodeficiency syndrome (AIDS).

HEPATITIS B (HBV)

A blood-borne pathogen that causes a severe acute infection and may progress to chronic infection and permanent liver damage. It is caused by the hepatitis B virus, an enveloped, double-stranded DNA virus.

BLOOD-BORNE PATHOGEN

The term describing any infectious microorganism present in blood and/or other body fluids and tissues. It is most commonly applied to the hepatitis B virus and the human immunodeficiency virus.

Recommendations for Tuberculosis (AFB) Isolation were updated in 1990 because of heightened concern about **nosocomial** transmission of multidrug-resistant tuberculosis and an increased incidence in immunocompromised patients.

● UNIVERSAL PRECAUTIONS VERSUS BODY SUBSTANCE ISOLATION VERSUS STANDARD PRECAUTIONS

In 1985, largely because of the HIV epidemic, isolation practices in the United States were altered dramatically by the introduction of a new strategy for isolation precautions, which became known as Universal Precautions (UP). Universal Precautions, as defined by the CDC, are a set of precautions designed to prevent transmission of **human immunodeficiency virus (HIV)**, **hepatitis B virus (HBV)**, and other **blood-borne pathogens** when providing first aid or health care. Under Universal Precautions, blood and certain body fluids of *all* patients are considered potentially infectious for HIV, HBV, and other blood-borne pathogens, regardless if a diagnosis for an infectious disease has been made.

In 1987 and again in 1988 the report was updated. The 1988 report emphasized two important points: 1) blood was the single most important source of HIV, HBV, and other blood-borne pathogens in the occupational setting, and 2) infection control efforts for preventing transmission of blood-borne pathogens in health care settings must focus on preventing exposures to blood, as well as during delivery of HBV immunization. The report stated that UP applied to blood, to body fluids that had been implicated in the transmission of blood-borne infections (semen and vaginal secretions), to body fluids from which the risk of transmission was unknown (amniotic, cerebrospinal, pericardial, peritoneal, pleural, and synovial fluids), and to any other body fluid visibly contaminated with blood. The report further stated that UP did not apply to feces, nasal secretions, sputum, sweat, tears, urine, or vomit unless they contained visible blood.

In 1987, after a three-year study by infection control personnel at the Harborview Medical Center in Seattle, Washington, and the University of California at San Diego, California, a new system of isolation, called Body Substance Isolation (BSI), was proposed as an alternative to diagnosis-driven isolation systems. BSI focused on the isolation, primarily through the use of gloves, of all moist and potentially infectious body substances (blood, feces, urine, sputum, saliva, wound drainage, and other body fluids) from *all* patients, regardless of their presumed infection status. Personnel were instructed to don clean gloves just before contact with mucous membranes and nonintact skin, and to wear gloves for anticipated contact with moist body substances. In addition, a "Stop Sign" alert was used to instruct persons wishing to enter the room of patients with infections to first check with the floor nurse for appropriate precautions before entering. Personnel were to be immune from or immunized against select infectious diseases transmitted by airborne or droplet routes (measles, mumps, rubella, and varicella), or they were not allowed to enter the rooms of patients with these diseases.

Some of the advantages cited for BSI stated that it was simple, easy to learn, and easy to administer. It avoided the assumption that individuals without known or suspected diagnoses of transmissible infectious diseases were free of risk to patients and personnel, and that only certain body fluids were associated with transmission of infections. The disadvantages of BSI included the added cost of increased barrier equipment, particularly gloves, the difficulty in maintaining routine application of the protocol for all patients, and the uncertainty about the precautions to be taken when entering a room with a "Stop Sign" alert.

The BSI system was not without controversy. BSI appeared to replace some, but not all, of the isolation precautions necessary to prevent transmission of infection. BSI did not contain adequate provisions to prevent 1) droplet transmission of serious infections, 2) direct or indirect contact transmission from dry skin or environmental sources, and 3) true airborne transmission of infections.

BSI and UP shared many similar features designed to prevent the transmission of blood-borne pathogens in hospitals. However, there was an important difference in the recommendation for glove use and handwashing. UP guidelines stated that gloves were recommended for anticipated contact with blood and specified body fluids, and hands were to be washed immediately after gloves were removed. BSI guidelines stated that gloves were recommended for anticipated contact with any moist body substance, but handwashing after glove removal was not required unless the hands were visibly soiled. Using gloves as a protective substitute for handwashing may have provided a false sense of security. Using gloves resulted in less handwashing, and increased the risk of nosocomial transmission of pathogens. This was caused in part by the fact that hands can become contaminated even in the process of removing gloves.

In the early 1990s, confusion about which body fluids or substances required precautions under UP and BSI became a cause for concern. Many hospitals espousing UP really were using BSI and vice versa. In view of these concerns, no simple adjustment to the existing approaches of UP or BSI appeared likely. A new synthesis of the various systems was needed to provide a more comprehensive guideline.

Based on these concerns, the following "Standard Precautions" guidelines were subsequently developed. Standard Precautions combine the major features of Universal Precautions and Body Substance Isolation into a single set of precautions to be used for the care of *all* patients regardless of their presumed infection. Standard Precautions apply to 1) blood; 2) all body fluids, secretions and excretions, (except sweat), regardless of whether or not they contain visible blood; 3) non-intact skin; and 4) mucous membranes. Standard Precautions are designed to reduce the risk of transmission of microorganisms from both recognized and unrecognized sources of infection (Figure 4-2).

In 1991, the Hospital Infection Control Practices Advisory Committee (HICPAC) was established. This agency provides advice and guidance regarding the practice of infection control and strategies for surveillance, prevention, and control of nosocomial infections in hospitals in the United States. HICPAC also advises the Center for Disease Control (CDC) on the periodic updating of guidelines and other policy statements regarding prevention of nosocomial infections. For example, HICPAC's latest revision of *Guidelines for Isolation Precautions in Hospitals* contains two parts: Part I, "Evolution of Isolation Practices," and Part II, "Recommendations for Isolation Precautions in Hospitals." This new guideline supercedes previous CDC recommendations for isolation precautions in hospitals.

The revised guideline contains two tiers of precautions. In the first and most important tier are those precautions designed for the care of all patients in hospitals regardless of their diagnosis or presumed infection status. This first tier is "Standard Precautions." The second tier, "Transmission-Based Precautions," is designed for patients documented or suspected to be infected or colonized with highly transmissible or epidemiologically important pathogens. This second tier is critically important, as additional precautions beyond Standard Precautions are needed to interrupt the transmission of disease in hospitals. Within the second tier of "Transmission-Based Precautions," there are three types of precautions: Airborne Precautions, Droplet Precautions, and Contact Precautions. These precautions may be combined for diseases that have multiple routes of transmission. When used either singularly or in combination, they are to be used in addition to Standard Precautions.

STANDARD PRECAUTIONS

FOR INFECTION CONTROL

Wash Hands (Plain soap)
Wash after touching **blood, body fluids, secretions, excretions**, and **contaminated items**.
Wash immediately **after gloves are removed** and **between patient contacts**.
Avoid transfer of microorganisms to other patients or environments.

Wear Gloves
Wear when touching **blood, body fluids, secretions, excretions**, and **contaminated items**.
Put on **clean** gloves just **before touching mucous membranes** and **nonintact skin**.
Change gloves between tasks and procedures on the same patient after contact with material that may contain high concentrations of microorganisms. Remove gloves promptly after use, before touching noncontaminated items and environmental surfaces, and before going to another patient, and wash hands immediately to avoid transfer of microorganisms to other patients or environments.

Wear Mask and Eye Protection or Face Shield
Protect mucous membranes of the eyes, nose and mouth during procedures and patient–care activities that are likely to generate **splashes** or **sprays** of **blood, body fluids, secretions**, or **excretions**.

Wear Gown
Protect skin and prevent soiling of clothing during procedures that are likely to generate **splashes** or **sprays** of **blood, body fluids, secretions**, or **excretions**. Remove a soiled gown as promptly as possible and wash hands to avoid transfer of microorganisms to other patients or environments.

Patient-Care Equipment
Handle used patient–care equipment soiled with **blood, body fluids, secretions**, or **excretions** in a manner that prevents skin and mucous membrane exposures, contamination of clothing, and transfer of microorganisms to other patients and environments. Ensure that reusable equipment is not used for the care of another patient until it has been appropriately cleaned and reprocessed and single use items are properly discarded.

Environmental Control
Follow hospital procedures for routine care, cleaning, and disinfection of environmental surfaces, beds, bedrails, bedside equipment and other frequently touched surfaces.

Linen
Handle, transport, and process used linen soiled with **blood, body fluids, secretions**, or **excretions** in a manner that prevents exposures and contamination of clothing, and avoids transfer of microorganisms to other patients and environments.

Occupational Health and Bloodborne Pathogens
Prevent injuries when using needles, scalpels, and other sharp instruments or devices; when handling sharp instruments after procedures; when cleaning used instruments; and when disposing of used needles.

Never recap used needles using both hands or any other technique that involves directing the point of a needle toward any part of the body; rather, use either a one-handed "scoop" technique or a mechanical device designed for holding the needle sheath.

Do not remove used needles from disposable syringes by hand, and do not bend, break, or otherwise manipulate used needles by hand. Place used disposable syringes and needles, scalpel blades, and other sharp items in puncture–resistant sharps containers located as close as practical to the area in which the items were used, and place reusable syringes and needles in a puncture–resistant container for transport to the reprocessing area.

Use **resuscitation devices** as an alternative to mouth–to–mouth resuscitation.

Patient Placement
Use a **private room** for a patient who contaminates the environment or who does not (or cannot be expected to) assist in maintaining appropriate hygiene or environmental control. Consult Infection Control if a private room is not available.

The information on this sign is abbreviated from the HICPAC Recommendations for Isolation Precautions in Hospitals.

Form No. **SPR**   BREVIS CORP., 3310 S 2700 E, SLC, UT 84109   © 1996 Brevis Corp.

FIGURE 4-2: Standard Precautions (Courtesy of Brevis Corp.)

PERSONAL PROTECTIVE EQUIPMENT (PPE)

To prevent skin and mucous membrane exposure during contact with patient blood or body fluids, Standard Precautions require all health care workers to routinely use appropriate barrier precautions called Personal Protective Equipment (PPE). Personal Protective Equipment includes gloves, masks, gowns, aprons, protective eye wear, and face shields.

Gloves

Gloves are worn for three important reasons. First, they provide a protective barrier and prevent gross contamination of the hands when touching blood, body fluids, secretions, excretions, mucous membranes, and nonintact skin. OSHA mandates that gloves be worn in specified circumstances to reduce the risk of exposures to blood-borne pathogens. Second, gloves are worn to reduce the likelihood of microorganisms on the hands of personnel being transmitted to patients during invasive or other patient-care procedures that involve touching a patient's mucous membranes and nonintact skin. Third, gloves are worn to reduce the likelihood that hands of personnel contaminated with microorganisms from patients or **fomites** are not transmitting microorganisms to another patient. Gloves must be changed between patient contacts, and hands should be washed immediately or as soon as patient safety permits, after gloves are removed.

Wearing gloves does not replace the need for handwashing, because gloves may be torn during use or may have small, unapparent defects. Hands may also become contaminated during glove removal. Failure to change gloves between patient contacts is an infection control hazard.

Although gloves reduce the risk of contamination from blood and/or other body fluids, they do not prevent needle sticks, or punctures from other sharp instruments, or replace the need for scrupulous handwashing.

The phlebotomy technician must wear gloves every time contact is made with a potentially infectious material, such as blood, body fluids, nonintact skin, or mucous membranes. Gloves must be worn for collection of all specimens. If the phlebotomist has cuts, scratches, or other breaks in his or her skin they must also be bandaged prior to wearing gloves. Torn or damaged gloves must be replaced immediately. Disposable gloves are never washed and reused. Appropriately remove and dispose of gloves in a **biohazardous** waste container.

FOMITES
Objects such as clothing, towels, and utensils that possibly harbor a disease agent and are capable of transmitting it.

BIOHAZARDOUS
Anything that is harmful or potentially harmful to humans, other species, or the environment.

PROCEDURE 4-1

Glove Removal

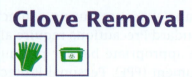

Equipment/Supplies
● Biohazardous waste container
● Gloves

Method/*Rationale*

1. Hold gloved hands over biohazardous waste container.

   To decrease the risk of contaminating other surfaces with debris from the gloves, they are discarded in the biohazardous waste container immediately upon removal.

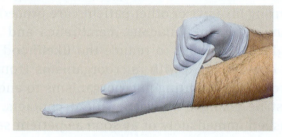

2. Grasp the contaminated outside wrist area of your gloved dominant hand with your gloved nondominant hand approximately 1 to 2 inches from the cuff.

   Prevents contamination of exposed skin.

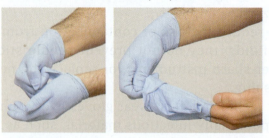

3. With a fluid motion, pull the glove down your hand so that it pulls inside out. Do not put the gloved, nondominant hand inside the glove being removed.

   Keeps contaminated side of glove away from skin.

4. Immediately discard the glove in the biohazardous waste container.

   Prevents spread of pathogens.

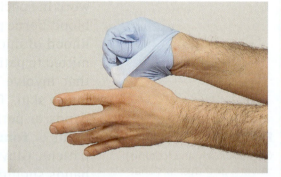

5. Insert the bare fingertips of your dominant hand inside the glove of your nondominant hand. Grasp the glove from the inside without touching the contaminated portion of the glove.

   Prevents contamination.

6. With a fluid motion, pull the glove down the hand so that it pulls inside out. Immediately discard in biohazardous waste container.

   Prevents spread of pathogens.

7. Wash hands immediately.

   Standard Precautions.

Masks, Respiratory Protection, Protective Eye Wear, Face Shields

Wearing masks, protective eye wear (goggles), and face shields in specified circumstances to reduce the risk of exposures to blood-borne pathogens is mandated by the OSHA blood-borne pathogens final rule. A surgical mask is generally worn to provide protection from the spread of infectious large-particle droplets. Large-particle droplets that are transmitted by infected patients, who are coughing or sneezing in close contact, generally travel only short distances (up to 3 feet). Make sure that the mask covers the nose and mouth completely. Masks must be changed between patients and discarded in a biohazardous waste container.

An area of major concern since the mid-1990s has been the role and selection of respiratory protection equipment and the implications of a respiratory protection program for prevention of transmission of tuberculosis in hospitals. In 1990 however, the CDC tuberculosis guidelines stated that surgical masks may not be effective in preventing the inhalation of droplet nuclei. They recommended the use of disposable particulate respirators or high-efficiency particulate air (HEPA) filter respirators certified by the CDC National Institute for Occupational Safety and Health (NIOSH). HEPA respirators must be fitted specifically to each individual wearer to be effective. Other respirators meeting the CDC requirements, such as the N95, are also acceptable.

Protective Apparel

Protective apparel such as gowns, aprons, and laboratory coats are worn to prevent contamination of clothing and to protect the skin of personnel from blood and body fluid exposures. Gowns specially treated to make them impermeable to liquids, leg coverings, boots, or shoe covers provide greater protection of the skin when splashes of large quantities of infectious material are present or anticipated. Wearing gowns and protective apparel in specified circumstances to reduce the risk of exposures to blood-borne pathogens is mandated by the OSHA blood-borne pathogens final rule (Figure 4-3).

Gowns are also worn in isolation procedures, where patients have compromised immune systems, when collecting specimens in surgical recovery rooms, or any other situations requiring extra attention to infection control. Gowns may be disposable, and discarded in a biohazardous container, or nondisposable, and laundered on the premises.

Laboratory coats are considered a part of PPE. Lab coats are worn to prevent contamination of the phlebotomist's clothing dur-

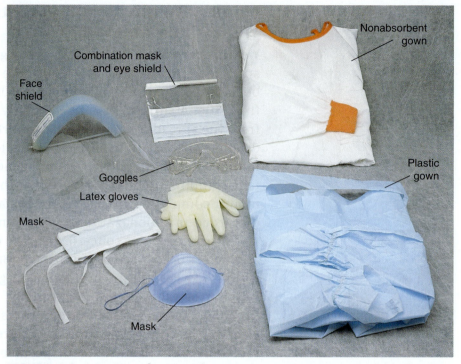

FIGURE 4-3: A variety of personal protective equipment is available for the phlebotomy technician to use in infection control.

ing laboratory procedures. Lab coats are never worn when the phlebotomist is on break or lunch, or outside of the clinical setting. Laboratories must provide the phlebotomist with a laboratory coat, which remains at the laboratory and is laundered on the premises or is disposable.

When putting on complete personal protective equipment, the gown is put on first, followed by the mask. Gloves are pulled on last to ensure they are pulled over the sleeves of the gown. Personal protective equipment is removed in the opposite direction: gloves first, then the mask, and the gown last. Be very careful when removing PPE to ensure all items are removed in an aseptic manner to prevent contamination. Wash hands immediately after removing all PPE.

HANDWASHING

Handwashing is the first line of defense in the fight against the spread of infection. Handwashing is performed before and after *every* patient contact, between different procedures on the same patient, whenever hands are visibly contaminated, before and after using the lavatory, before leaving the laboratory, before and after breaks and lunch, and before and after wearing and removing gloves. Handwashing involves the use of running warm water and antibacterial or antimicrobial soap.

MEDICAL/SURGICAL ASEPSIS

Asepsis, by definition, is a condition free from germs, infection, and/or any form of life. Aseptic technique is any method used medically or surgically to prevent contamination. The phlebotomist must fully understand and be able to implement the principles and procedures used to maintain asepsis.

There are two types of asepsis: medical and surgical. A phlebotomist uses principles of both.

● Medical asepsis is the process of destroying microorganisms after they leave the body to prevent the transmission of microorganisms from one person to another. It is employed when coming in contact with a body part that is not normally sterile, such as performing a throat culture. To maintain medical asepsis, hands and wrists are washed for a minimum of 2 minutes with antimicrobial or antibacterial soap.
● Surgical asepsis is the process of destroying microorganisms before they enter the body. This process maintains sterility when entering a normally sterile part of the body, such as inserting a needle into a patient's vein to obtain a blood specimen. All items required to be sterile (i.e., needles, syringes, sterile gloves) are sterilized and prepackaged by the manufacturer. The phlebotomist maintains the integrity of a "sterile field" by following specific guidelines called "sterile techniques." A sterile field is a designated area free from all organisms.

STERILE TECHNIQUES

The phlebotomist is responsible for using antiseptics for patient preparation and for using sterile supplies for skin punctures and venipunctures. Alcohol pads are used to cleanse skin sites for venipuncture. Although alcohol pads destroy most of the bacteria, they do not destroy all microorganisms. When a sterile site is required, such as for blood cultures, a further decontamination technique is employed. This procedure will be discussed in detail in Chapter 12.

INVASIVE PROCEDURE

A procedure that requires penetrating intact skin or mucous membranes.

All items used for **invasive procedures** must be sterile. This is accomplished by several methods. An important point to remember when maintaining surgical asepsis is, "When in doubt—throw it out." In other words, if you are not sure that an item is sterile, throw it away and use another item you know is sterile.

PROCEDURE 4-2

Handwashing

Equipment/Supplies
- Running water
- Antibacterial or antimicrobial soap
- Disposable towels (paper)

Method/*Rationale*

1. Remove jewelry (rings and watches).

   Jewelry traps contaminates and prevents thorough handwashing.

2. Turn on faucets and adjust water temperature.

   Water should be warm, not hot. Warmer water helps to kill pathogens. However, the water should not be too hot, as it will cause burns.

3. Standing away from the sink, wet your hands. Keep your fingers pointing downward into the sink. Do not touch the sink.

   Touching the sink will contaminate your hands. Keeping your fingers pointed downward allows contaminates to run off the fingertips rather down your arms. Your forearms are typically less dirty than your hands. Concentrate on cleaning your hands.

4. Apply antibacterial soap. By rubbing your hands together to create friction, lather is created. Scrub every part of your hands. Start by rubbing the palm of one hand on the back of the other hand and then repeating the procedure with the other hand. Scrub between every finger. Pay particular attention to your fingertips, nails, and palms.

   Brisk rubbing helps to loosen dead skin and to remove debris and pathogens. All areas of your hands are potentially contaminated. Clean debris from under your nails with an orange stick or similar device.

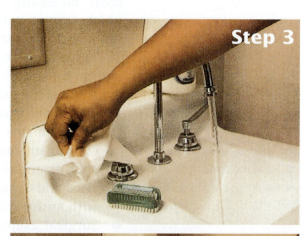

Step 3

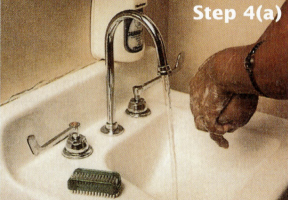

Step 4(a)

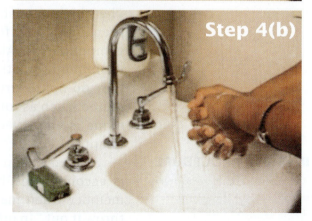

Step 4(b)

5. Scrub vigorously for a minimum of two minutes.

   Two minutes should be adequate time to completely scrub all areas of your hands.

6. Rinse all soap from hands.

   Keep fingers pointed downward without touching the sink or faucet. Rinse from wrist to fingertips.

7. Dry hands with paper towels.

   Using disposable towels helps prevent the spread of disease because the towels are discarded and not reused. Pat dry to prevent chaffing of hands.

8. Turn off faucets.

   Using additional clean paper towels to turn off the faucets prevents further contamination. Make sure that the towel used to turn off the faucet is dry. Contaminates can travel through a wet paper towel to recontaminate the phlebotomist's hands.

9. Discard all waste and take care not to contaminate your hands.

   Orange sticks, scrub brushes, and paper towels are not generally discarded in a biohazardous waste container unless blood or body fluid has contaminated them.

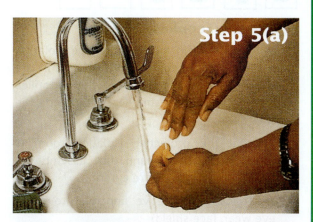

Step 5(a)

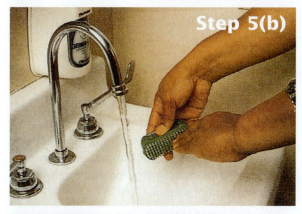

Step 5(b)

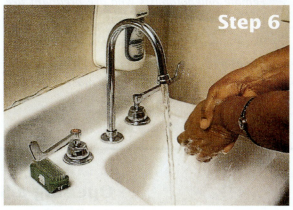

Step 6

PROCEDURE 4-3

Isolation Techniques

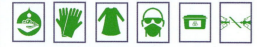

Equipment/Supplies

All equipment taken into a protective isolation room must remain there. Isolation rooms are equipped with either an anteroom where supplies are kept or a cart with supplies just outside the patient's door.

Ensure that the protective isolation room is equipped with a needle and tube assembly, a tourniquet, and a pen before entering.

- PPE (gloves—protective apparel, protective eye wear, face shield)

- HEPA respirator (for AFB isolation)

- Specimen collection supplies

- Biohazardous waste containers

- Isolation bag(s)

Method/*Rationale*

1. Prior to entering the isolation room, check with the nurse's station for patient diagnosis and/or the isolation sign posted on the door to the patient's room.

   Female phlebotomists who are pregnant are not to enter isolation rooms.

2. Place a mask over your nose and mouth.

   For AFB isolation, a fitted high-efficiency particulate air (HEPA) respirator must be worn.

3. Wash hands.

   Reduces the spread of infection.

4. Put on a sterile gown, touching only the inside of the gown. Make sure the gown covers your entire uniform and is tied securely. The sleeves of the gown must cover your wrists.

   To protect isolated patients from outside pathogens the gown is put on using sterile techniques. Gowns need not be sterile for other isolation precautions. They are worn to protect the phlebotomist from pathogens of the patient.

5. Put on disposable sterile gloves. Pull gloves up over the sleeves of the gown.

   When entering a protective isolation room using surgical asepsis.

6. Invert the isolation bag halfway inside-out placing it outside the door on the cart. Take only the equipment you will need into the room. Leave the laboratory requisition slip on the cart or counter outside the room.

   Only the equipment needed for the requested procedure should be taken into the room. Waste material is disposed of inside the isolation room. Nothing is brought out of the room when you leave.

7. Identify the patient by checking the patient's identification bracelet. Label the tubes with the information from the identification bracelet.

   A pen should already be in the room. If you brought a pen in with you it must remain in the room.

Opening a Sterile Package

Needles, lancets, syringes, butterfly infusion sets, and sterile gloves are types of sterile packages the phlebotomist might be required to open.

8. Collect the appropriate specimens.

9. Dispose of needles in the "sharps" container inside the patient's room. Dispose of all other waste products in the biohazardous waste container inside the patient's room.

   Prevents the spread of infection to other patients and persons outside the isolation room.

10. Before placing the tubes in the isolation bag for transport to the laboratory, remove any blood that might be on the outside of the tubes by wiping with an alcohol wipe. While still standing in the isolation room, place the tubes inside the isolation bag, touching only the insides of the bag. Make sure that you touch nothing else outside of the isolation room with your gloved hands.

    Prevents the spread of infection to the outside of the isolation room.

11. Wash your *gloved* hands in the patient's room. Dry your hands and turn off the faucet with a dry paper towel.

    Reduces the risk of contaminates on your hands prior to removing your gloves.

12. Remove your gown by breaking the ties. As you remove the gown, touch only the inside of the gown. As you remove the gown, fold the contaminated side (outside) to the inside and discard it in a biohazardous waste container.

Touching only the inside of the gown and folding the contaminated side to the inside reduces the risk of contamination.

13. Remove your gloves as described previously in this chapter. Discard gloves in a biohazardous waste container.

14. Wash your hands and use a clean, dry paper towel to turn off the faucet.

    Using a clean, dry paper towel to turn off the faucet reduces the risk of recontaminating your hands. If the paper towel is wet, "strike through" occurs.

15. Leave the isolation room: Use a clean, dry paper towel to turn the door handle and open the door. Hold the door open with one foot and discard the paper towel in the wastebasket beside the door inside the isolation room.

    Leaves all material used inside the isolation room.

16. Place the tubes inside the isolation bag into a second biohazardous material bag, touching only the outside of the bag. Check the tubes against the requisition slip to confirm the tubes were drawn from the correct patient.

    Ensures that tests are performed on the correct patient.

17. Wash hands, again, at the nurse's station prior to the next patient or returning to the laboratory.

    Standard Precautions.

STRIKE THROUGH

Contamination caused by pathogens being transported through a wet barrier from a nonsterile area to a sterile area.

● Needles/lancets: Needles/lancets are prepackaged. Needles are contained in either a peel-apart plastic and paper package or a hard plastic tube. When opening the peel-apart packages, grasp each flap of the package with the thumb and first finger of each hand. With the package pointed away from you, gently but firmly pull the flaps apart. If packaged in a plastic tube, twist the paper seal until the needle is released from the case. Once the covering of a needle or a lancet is removed, the needle or lancet must not touch anything until it punctures the skin. If it accidentally touches anything prior to contact with the skin, it must be discarded in an appropriate "sharps" container. A new sterile needle must be used. If an unsuccessful skin puncture or venipuncture occurs, a new needle is used for subsequent attempts. Do not touch the exposed hub end of the needle; touching this end will contaminate the needle. If this occurs, the contaminated needle must be discarded and a new sterile needle must be used. Attach needles to evacuated tube holders or syringes immediately after opening to prevent possible accidental contamination.

● Syringes, butterfly infusion sets, and sterile gloves: All these items are prepackaged in peel-apart packages. Follow the instructions described above to open. Prior to opening a syringe for use, the entire syringe is sterile both inside and out. Once the syringe is picked up for use, the outside of the syringe becomes contaminated. The inside remains sterile, as well as the area of needle attachment, called the hub. Touching the hub or inside of a syringe contaminates it, and the syringe must be discarded and a new syringe opened for use.

LABORATORY SAFETY

A working environment that is safe for employees and patients alike is not only the goal of every health care facility, but employers are mandated by OSHA to provide a safe working environment for their employees. This does not mean that the laboratory is free from hazards, but guidelines are implemented to minimize the risks of these hazards. Precautions are taken to prevent accidents. It is important that the phlebotomist familiarize herself with the specific guidelines of the facility in which she works and adhere to the policies established. The following is a list of general laboratory safety rules:

● *Never* eat, drink, chew gum, or smoke in the laboratory.
● *Never* put anything in your mouth such as pens, pencils, or fingers, while working in the laboratory.
● *Never* store food or beverages in the laboratory refrigerator used to store reagents or specimens.
● *Never* apply cosmetics, handle contact lenses, or rub eyes in the laboratory.
● *Never* wear excessive jewelry, such as long chains, large or dangling earrings, or loose bracelets.

PROCEDURE 4-4

Opening a Sterile Package

Equipment/Supplies

● Sterile package

Method/*Rationale*

1. Wash hands.

   Reduces the risk of contamination.

2. Locate the peel-apart end of the pack.

   Peel-apart end is clearly labeled on most packages.

3. Grasp each side of the package by a flap using your thumb and first finger.

   Touch as little of the packaging as possible to prevent contamination.

4. Direct the package opening away from your body.

   Reduces the risk of contamination by an article of your clothing.

5. Gently, slowly, but firmly pull the package apart.

   Do not let the contents of the package fall out onto a contaminated surface.

6. Remove the item from the package, maintaining the integrity of the item.

   If the item must remain sterile, place onto a sterile field. Only touch further if you have put on sterile gloves.

   If the item is to be used in part as nonsterile, such as a syringe, then use appropriately by touching only the areas that may safely be contaminated.

7. Once the procedure is completed remove gloves (if worn) and wash hands.

   Standard Precautions.

● **Never** wear a lab coat to lunch, on breaks, or when leaving the lab to go home.
● **Never** wear any of the PPE items outside of their designated areas.
● **Never** pipette specimens or reagents by mouth.
● **Always** wear hair restrained back away from your face if shoulder length or longer.
● **Always** wear uniforms or work clothes that are neither form fitting nor floppy. Work clothes should **always** be neat and clean.
● **Always** wear a buttoned lab coat when working in the laboratory.
● **Always** wear closed-toed, leather or nonporous, nonskid-sole shoes. Sandals, slippers, or high heels are inappropriate.
● **Always** wear a face shield when performing specimen collections or processing specimens that might generate splashes or aerosol of body fluids.
● **Always** wear gloves for phlebotomy procedures and specimen processing.

Safety is also a consideration when the phlebotomist is working outside the laboratory such as in a patient's room or at an off-site collection. The following are general guidelines for safety outside the laboratory:

● Perform all activities using "Standard Precautions."
● *Never* recap contaminated needles. (There is an acceptable one-handed scoop method of recapping contaminated needles that will be presented in Chapter 10.)
● Properly dispose of all contaminated material in the appropriate biohazardous waste container.
● Properly dispose of all "sharps" in the appropriate puncture-resistant container.
● Replace bed rails of patient's bed after performing specimen collection.
● Report infiltrated IVs or any other concerns about a patient's IV.
● Report unresponsive patients to the nurse.
● Report unusual odors to the nurse.
● Report any spills or items dropped on the floor to the nurse or to housekeeping.
● Avoid running or yelling.
● Know what procedure to follow if a patient has fainted or is unconscious.
● Know basic lifesaver cardiopulmonary resuscitation.

LABORATORY HAZARDS
Biological Hazards

Biological hazards, or biohazards, are any materials that are dangerous to health. Most commonly, biohazards in the medical laboratory are any items that are contaminated by blood or body fluids containing blood, with the potential to contain blood-borne pathogens. All biohazardous material is identified by a special symbol called the biohazard symbol.

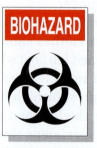

FIGURE 4-4: Biohazard symbol

Sharps

All health care workers should take precautions to prevent injuries caused by needles, glass slides, and other sharp instruments during procedures, cleaning used instruments, disposing of used needles, and handling sharp instruments. To prevent needle stick injuries, needles should not be recapped by hand, purposely bent or broken by hand, removed from disposable syringes, or otherwise manipulated by hand. After they are used, disposable syringes and needles, glass slides, and other sharps should be placed in puncture-resistant containers for disposal. The puncture-resistant containers should be located as close as practical to the area of use.

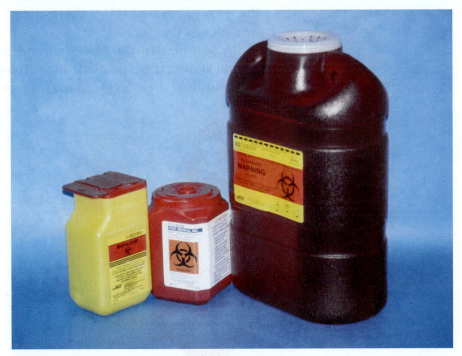

FIGURE 4-5: Puncture-resistant sharps containers

Chemical, Electrical, and Radioactive Hazards

Chemical Hazards

The phlebotomist may come in contact with chemical hazards when adding preservatives to a 24-hour urine collection, using cleaning solutions, or when assisting the medical laboratory technician in the lab.

Chemicals can be very dangerous, especially mixing the wrong chemicals together. For example, mixing bleach with other cleaning agents can create a dangerous gas, which can render a person unconscious and may compromise the respiratory system to the point of death.

In 1988, OSHA introduced the Hazard Communication Standard, also known as the "Right-to-know rule." These regulations were implemented to better inform organizations and individuals about the possible hazards of individual and combined chemicals.

OSHA requires chemical manufacturers to make available a Material Safety Data Sheet (MSDS) for each hazardous chemical they manufacture or import. The MSDS contains more information than is listed on the label of the product. The MSDS provides detailed information regarding special conditions for safe handling and properties of the chemical. It is important that the phlebotomist takes the time to read all MSDS sheets that apply to chemicals he might be exposed to.

In addition to the MSDS all containers containing hazardous chemicals must be labeled, identifying the hazard (for example, poisons and corrosives) (Figures 4-6 and 4-7).

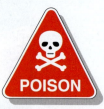

FIGURE 4-6: Poison label

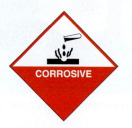

FIGURE 4-7: Corrosive label

ENVIRONMENTAL PROTECTION AGENCY (EPA)

The federal agency that regulates and monitors the inventory, storage, usage, techniques, and disposal of harmful substances to the environment.

Chemical spills require special chemical clean-up kits containing absorbant and neutralizer materials, which are used depending on the type of chemical spilled. An indicator supplied in the clean-up kit determines when the spill has been neutralized. Disposal of chemicals is regulated by the **Environmental Protection Agency (EPA)**.

As a safety measure in the treatment of chemical spills, every laboratory should have a safety shower and eye wash station. The phlebotomist must be instructed as to their location and use at the time of employment. The eyes or body parts affected by a chemical spill or chemical splash should be flushed with water for a minimum of 15 minutes, followed by a visit to the emergency room for evaluation.

Electrical Hazards

The phlebotomist is at risk of electrical hazards whenever using electrical equipment, such as a centrifuge. Following basic safety guidelines helps reduce the risk of injuries from electrical hazards. When working with electrical equipment:
● Periodically inspect cords and plugs for fraying or breakage.
● Do not attempt to repair electrical equipment or do routine maintenance if you are not trained to do so. (All equipment in a health care facility must be equipped with a three-prong plug to allow for grounding of the equipment.)
● Do not handle electrical equipment with wet hands or while standing on a wet floor.
● Report any damaged or malfunctioning equipment to a supervisor immediately.
● Avoid the use of extension cords.
● Do not touch electrical equipment in a patient's room, especially during a blood draw. Electrical current can travel through the phlebotomist to the patient.

If an electrical accident does occur, shut off the source of electricity immediately. If this is impossible, move the electrical hazard away from the injured person. Use a substance that does not conduct electricity to do so, such as something made of glass or wood, like a glass beaker or a broom handle. Call for medical assistance. Start cardiopulmonary resuscitation (CPR) if necessary and keep the victim warm.

Radioactive Hazards

Safety procedures surrounding radioactive hazards depend on the level of possible exposure. The amount of radiation, how far the phlebotomist is from the source of radiation, and the length of time exposed will determine what precautions must be taken.

Radiation hazard signs must be posted in areas where exposure will be likely. This includes refrigerators or cabinets where radioactive material is stored (Figure 4-8).

The phlebotomist may be exposed to radiation risks while collecting specimens from patients who have been injected with radioactive dyes, delivering specimens to areas of the laboratory where testing with radioactive materials is done, or collecting specimens from patients in the radiology department or nuclear medicine.

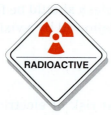

FIGURE 4-8: Radioactive hazard sign

Precautions include wearing lead aprons and lead-lined gloves. Phlebotomists who are or may be pregnant should refrain from collecting specimens from patients who may present a radioactive hazard and should avoid areas labeled with radioactive hazard signs.

Fire/Explosion Hazards

Every Policy and Procedure Manual should contain a section on fire safety, and every employee of any institution should be aware of the procedures to follow in case of fire. Employees should know where to locate a fire extinguisher and how to use it.

Box 4-4: How to Operate a Fire Extinguisher

To effectively operate a fire extinguisher, think **PASS**:

P—Pull the pin
A—Aim the hose at the base of the fire
S—Squeeze the handle
S—Sweep the hose back and forth

There are four classifications of fire and four classifications of fire extinguishers that correspond with each class of fire:

● Class A: Ordinary combustibles such as wood, paper, or clothing. Class A fires require extinguishers of water or water-based solutions.

● Class B: Flammable liquids and vapors such as paint, oil, grease, or gasoline. Class B fires require extinguishers that can block the source of oxygen, such as foam, dry chemical, or carbon dioxide materials.

● Class C: Electrical equipment fires. Class C fires require extinguishers of nonconductible agents such as dry chemical, carbon dioxide, or halon.

● Class D: Combustible or reactive metals such as sodium, potassium, magnesium, uranium, powdered aluminum, and lithium. Class D fires require extinguishers of dry powder agents or sand. These are the most difficult fires to control and most often lead to explosions.

- Class ABC (Multipurpose) extinguishers: Use dry chemical reagents to smother the fire. They can be used on Class A, B, or C fires. This eliminates some of the confusion of finding the right extinguisher when it is needed. Multipurpose extinguishers are the kind most often found in health care facilities.

In case of a fire remember to follow these basic guidelines:

- Pull the nearest fire alarm.
- Call 911 or activate the fire department and EMS.
- Attempt to extinguish a small fire.
- Smother a clothing fire by wrapping the victim in a fire blanket or having the victim "Stop, Drop, and Roll." In other words, have the victim lie on the floor and roll to smother the fire. Allowing a victim to continuing walking or running only fuels the fire.
- Stay low: Crawl to the nearest exit when heavy smoke is present.
- Do not panic, run, abandon a patient, nor block entrances.
- Use the stairs.

There are a variety of fire hazard signs. One thing they all have in common is the classic symbol of flames (Figure 4-9).

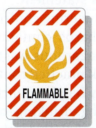

FIGURE 4-9: Flammable hazard sign

BLOOD-BORNE PATHOGENS—OSHA REGULATIONS

All health care professionals are at risk of occupational exposure to blood-borne pathogens, including hepatitis B (HBV), hepatitis C (HCV), and human immunodeficiency virus (HIV). Understanding the precautions that reduce the risk of exposure, and knowing what protocols to follow if exposed, greatly improves the chance of disease prevention.

The most common exposure is caused by contaminated needle sticks, cuts from other sharp contaminated items such as glass slides or pipettes, or from direct contact of an infected patient's blood or body fluids. The risk of infection depends largely on the type of exposure, the pathogen involved, the amount of blood involved in the exposure, and the amount of virus in the patient's blood at the time of exposure.

Prevention of Occupational Exposure

The majority of contaminated needle sticks and other punctures or lacerations can be prevented by using safer techniques, such as not recapping needles by hand, disposing of used needles in the appropriate sharps containers, and using medical devices with safety features designed to prevent injuries. Using the appropriate barrier precautions, such as gloves, face shields, protective eyewear, or gowns, can prevent exposure to the eyes, nose, mouth, and hands.

Personal Exposure Control Plan

What should you do if you are exposed to the blood of a patient? In order to be in compliance with OSHA standards, employers must have a written exposure control plan. Therefore, every medical facility will have its own Exposure Control Plan documented in its Policy and Procedures Manual. The written plan must include the following areas:

● List of all job classifications in which occupational exposure may occur.
● Standard Precautions statement.
● Identification of engineering controls, such as accessible hand-washing facilities, sharps containers, self-sheathing needles, autoclaves, and biohazardous waste symbols.
● Identification of work practice controls, such as prohibiting recapping of needles by hand, requiring handwashing after glove removal, and no eating, drinking, or smoking in the laboratory.
● Requirements of personal protective equipment.
● Housekeeping standards, such as decontamination of surfaces and blood spill clean-up.

Box 4-5: Decontamination of Surfaces and How to Clean Up Blood Spills

OSHA requires that surfaces, such as phlebotomy draw stations, tables, and countertops, be decontaminated at the end of every shift, whenever the surface is visibly contaminated, and between patients. The Environmental Protection Agency (EPA) recommends the use of a 1:10 bleach solution or other EPA-approved disinfectant. Bleach solutions should be prepared daily.

Gloves should be worn when cleaning up spills. Spills of no more than a few drops can be absorbed into a paper towel and then properly disinfected. Large blood or body fluid spills can be cleaned up using special clay or chlorine-based powder that absorbs or gels the liquid and allows it to be scooped or swept up for disposal in a biohazardous waste container. The area is then wiped with a disinfectant. Dried spill should be moistened with disinfectant before cleaning up. This avoids having to scrape the dried blood or body fluids, which could generate particles into the air. Spills involving broken glass should be cleaned up while wearing heavy-duty utility gloves. Avoid handling broken glass with your hands. Sweep or scoop up the glass and dispose of it in a puncture-proof sharps container. All disposable materials, such as paper towels, should be discarded in the appropriate biohazardous waste container. Reusable materials should be properly disinfected.

Hepatitis B vaccinations must be offered free of charge to employees within 10 days of assignment to duties of occupational exposure risk. The employee has the right to decline the vaccine series. A signed and dated statement of refusal must be retained in the employee's personnel file.

Warning labels and signs must be affixed to appropriate biohazardous waste containers. Labels must be fluorescent orange or orange-red, with the words "Biohazardous Waste" printed on the label. Training, in regards to blood-borne pathogens, must be provided to all employees at risk for occupational exposure, free of charge. Employers who hire employees at risk for occupational exposure must maintain confidential medical records as well as records documenting all training sessions.

The following are basic guidelines that are approved by OSHA and recommended by the CDC, for the Post-Exposure Action Plan maintained at every facility.

Immediately following an exposure:
● Wash needle sticks, punctures, or lacerations with soap and water.
● Flush splashes to the nose, mouth, or skin with water.
● Irrigate eyes with clean water, saline, or sterile irrigants.

No scientific evidence shows that using antiseptics or squeezing the wound will reduce the risk of transmission of blood-borne pathogens. Using a caustic agent such as bleach is not recommended.

Following any exposure, you should report the incident to the appropriate personnel that manage exposures. Prompt reporting is imperative because in some cases, postexposure treatment may be recommended and should be started as soon as possible.

All health care professionals who have a reasonable risk of being exposed to blood or body fluids should receive the hepatitis B vaccine. The ideal time to be vaccinated is during the health care professional's training period. The hepatitis B vaccine is a series of three vaccinations: the first dose is given initially with the second dose following at 1 month, and the third dose is given 5 months later. After completion of the vaccination series, the health care professional should be tested to make sure the vaccination has provided immunity to HBV. Approximately 87% of those who take the series develop immunity after the second dose; 96% develop immunity after the third dose. Hepatitis B immune globulin (HBIG) is effective in preventing HBV infection after an exposure.

There is not a vaccine for hepatitis C and no treatment after an exposure that will prevent infection. Immune globulin is not recommended. For this reason alone, following recommended infection control practices is essential. There is also no vaccine for HIV. However results from a small number of studies suggest that the use of zidovudine after certain occupational exposures may reduce the chance of HIV transmission. Postexposure treatment is not recommended for all occupational exposures to HIV. Many types of exposures will not lead to an HIV infection and the medications may have serious side effects.

In 1996, the CDC recommended the preventive treatment of AZT and other drugs in combination after a possible occupational exposure to HIV. It is believed that the action of AZT prevents the virus from entering the cell. However, to be most effective, **chemoprophylaxis** must begin immediately within a 1 to 2 hour window after exposure.

CHEMOPROPHYLAXIS

The use of a drug or chemical to prevent a disease (e.g., the taking of an appropriate medicine to prevent malaria).

Follow-Up Treatment

● HBV: The CDC does not recommend follow-up treatment because postexposure treatment is highly effective in preventing HBV. However, any symptoms suggesting hepatitis, such as yellow eyes or skin, loss of appetite, nausea, vomiting, fever, stomach or joint pain, and extreme tiredness, should be reported to your health care provider.

● HCV: You should have an antibody test for the hepatitis C virus and a liver enzyme test as soon as possible after the exposure. This creates a baseline and at 4 to 6 months another test should be performed. Report any symptoms suggesting hepatitis to your health care provider.

● HIV: You should be tested for HIV antibody as soon as possible after exposure for a baseline, and periodically for at least 6 months after exposure. The recommended sequence of testing is at 6 weeks, 12 weeks, and then again at 6 months.

Precautions Taken During Follow-Up Period

If you are exposed to HBV and treated postexposure, it is unlikely you will become infected. Therefore, no treatment is recommended. The risk of becoming infected and passing the infection on to others is very low, and no precautions are recommended after exposure to HCV. During the first 6 to 12 weeks of postexposure to HIV you should follow the recommendations for preventing transmission of HIV. These include not donating blood, semen, or organs and not having sexual intercourse. If you do choose to have sexual intercourse, using a condom consistently and correctly may reduce the risk of HIV transmission. HIV may also be transmitted through breast milk. Breast-feeding should be discontinued.

Box 4-6: Hepatitis B—Get Vaccinated—It's Preventable

- Who is at risk?
  Hepatitis B can affect anyone. Each year in the United States, more than 200,000 people of all ages get hepatitis B and close to 5,000 die of sickness caused by HBV. If you have had other forms of hepatitis, you can still get hepatitis B.

- How great is your risk for hepatitis B?
  One out of 20 people in the United States will get hepatitis B some time during their lives. Your risk is higher if you:
  - Have sex with someone infected with HBV
  - Have sex with more than one partner
  - Are a man and have sex with a man
  - Live in the same house with someone who has lifelong HBV infection
  - Have a job that involves contact with human blood
  - Shoot drugs
  - Are a patient or work in a home for the developmentally disabled
  - Have hemophilia
  - Travel to areas where hepatitis B is common

  Your risk is also higher if your parents were born in Southeast Asia, Africa, the Amazon Basin in South America, the Pacific Islands, or the Middle East.

  If you are at risk for HBV infection, ask your health care provider about hepatitis B vaccine.

- How do you get hepatitis B?
  You get hepatitis B by direct contact with the blood or body fluids of an infected person. For example, you can become infected by having sex or sharing needles with an infected person. A baby can get hepatitis B from an infected mother during childbirth.

  Hepatitis B is not spread through food or water or by casual contact.

(continues)

Box 4-6: Hepatitis B—Get Vaccinated— It's Preventable *(continued)*

● Who is a carrier of hepatitis B virus?

Sometimes, people who are infected with HBV never recover fully from the infection; they carry the virus and can infect others for the rest of their lives. In the United States, about one million people carry HBV.

● How do you know if you have hepatitis B?

You may have hepatitis B (and be spreading the disease) and not know it. Sometimes a person with HBV infection has no symptoms at all.

If you have symptoms:

- Your eyes or skin may turn yellow.
- You may lose your appetite.
- You may have nausea, vomiting, fever, or stomach or joint pain.
- You may feel extremely tired and not be able to work for weeks or months.

● Is there a cure for hepatitis B?

There is no cure for hepatitis B; this is why prevention is so important. Hepatitis B vaccine is the best protection against HBV. Three doses are needed for complete protection.

● If you are pregnant, should you worry about hepatitis B?

If you have HBV in your blood, you can give hepatitis B to your baby. Babies who get HBV at birth may have the virus for the rest of their lives, can spread the disease, and can get cirrhosis of the liver or liver cancer.

All pregnant women should be tested for HBV early in their pregnancy. If the blood test is positive, the baby should receive vaccine along with another shot, hepatitis B immune globulin, at birth. The vaccine series should be completed during the first 6 months of life.

● Who should get vaccinated?

- All babies, at birth
- All children 11 to 12 years of age who have not been vaccinated
- Persons of any age whose behavior puts them at high risk for HBV infection
- Persons whose jobs expose them to human blood

(Courtesy of the Centers for Disease Control and Prevention)

SUMMARY

The phlebotomist plays an integral role in preventing the spread of infection and disease in the health care setting. Understanding the infection cycle and how pathogens are transmitted is the first step in this process, and routine handwashing is the second. The conscientious use of Standard Precautions reduces the risk of contracting communicable infections. Implementing and maintaining the integrity of correct isolation techniques aids in the reduction of nosocomial infections. Practicing aseptic techniques ensures that both the phlebotomist and the patient are safeguarded against pathogens.

STUDY AND REVIEW EXERCISES

Defining Key Terms

Write the definition for each of the following key terms.

1) blood-borne pathogen _____

2) carrier _____

3) causative organism _____

4) chain of infection _____

5) chemoprophylaxis _____

6) Environmental Protection Agency (EPA) _____

_____

7) fomites _____

8) infection _____

9) invasive procedure _____

10) means of exit _____

11) means of transmission _____

12) microbe _____

13) microorganism _____

14) nonpathogenic _____

15) nosocomial _____

16) pathogen _____

17) pathogenic _____

18) reservoir host _____

19) strike through _____

Reviewing Key Points

1) List the links in the chain of infection and briefly describe each link.

2) List the ten general laboratory safety rules.

3) List the seven types of isolation techniques. Give an example of conditions or diseases requiring each type listed.

4) Identify the personal protective equipment that a phlebotomist will use.

5) Describe the difference between Universal Precautions and Standard Precautions.

Sentence Completion

1) _____ can be classified as bacteria, virus, fungi, or protozoa.

2) A causative organism will take up residence in the _____, who may or may not display symptoms of an infection.

3) _____, _____, _____, and _____ all assist hospitals and laboratories to maintain up-to-date isolation practices and to establish guidelines and enforce regulations governing infection control.

4) In 1990, the CDC stated that surgical masks may not be effective in preventing the inhalation of droplet nuclei (i.e., tuberculosis) and recommended the use of _____ certified by the CDC as an acceptable alternative.

5) _____ is a condition free from germs, infection, and any form of life.

6) All items used for _____ must remain sterile.

7) _____ are any materials that are dangerous to health.

8) The phlebotomist may come in contact with _____ when adding preservatives to a 24-hour urine collection.

9) Disposal of chemicals is regulated by _____.

10) _____ must be offered free of charge to employees within 10 days of assignment to duties that would place the employee at risk for occupational exposure.

Multiple Choice

1) You should be tested for HIV antibody as soon as possible after an exposure, for a baseline and periodically for at least _____ after exposure.
   A. 2 weeks
   B. 6 weeks
   C. 2 months
   D. 6 months

2) All the following are a part of an Exposure Control Plan *except*:
   A. Identification on engineering controls
   B. Standard Precautions statement
   C. Documentation of BSI training
   D. List of all job classifications in which occupational exposure might occur

3) Wearing a lead apron and gloves are precautions for which one of the following laboratory hazards?
   A. electrical hazards
   B. radioactive hazards
   C. chemical hazards
   D. fire hazards

4) If an electrical accident should occur, you should:
   A. shut off the source of electricity immediately
   B. activate EMS
   C. start CPR, if necessary
   D. all of the above

5) OSHA requires that manufacturers of chemicals make a(n) _____ available to consumers.
   A. Operating Manual (OM)
   B. Material Safety Data Sheet (MSDS)
   C. Occupational Standard Hazard Sheet (OSHS)
   D. Laboratory Chemical Component Sheet (LCCS)

6) All of the following are examples of biohazardous waste except:
   A. Wet paper towels
   B. Used gloves
   C. Used 2 X 2 gauze squares
   D. All the above are examples

7) Of the following, which one is not a sterile pack a phlebotomist is likely to be required to open?
   A. Sterile gloves
   B. Sterile needles
   C. Sterile syringes
   D. Sterile surgical instruments

8) To maintain medical asepsis, hands and wrists are washed for a minimum of:
   A. 1 to 2 minutes
   B. 3 to 4 minutes
   C. 5 to 6 minutes
   D. 10 minutes

9) When entering an AFB isolation room you must have all the following supplies before entering except:
   A. specimen collection supplies
   B. isolation bags
   C. HEPA respirator
   D. all the above

10) A substance that adheres to and transmits infectious material is called a:
    A. fomite
    B. reservoir host
    C. susceptible host
    D. parasite

Critical Thinking

1) You have lab orders to draw a CBC and Chem Panel on the patient in room 314, Mr. O'Toole. When you arrive on the unit, you discover that Mr. O'Toole is in an AFB isolation room. You were not notified, nor is it written on the lab request. What supplies will you need to take into the room with you? What supplies should already be in the patient's room?

2) What precautions will you take before entering room 314 to draw Mr. O'Toole's labs? What precautions will you take while drawing the patient's blood? When removing the needle from Mr. O'Toole's arm, he accidentally bumps your hand and you stick yourself with the contaminated needle. What should you do now?

Documentation

OBJECTIVES

Upon completion of this chapter the student should be able to:

- Describe how tests are ordered, how requisitions forms are generated, and the pertinent information that must be supplied on each request.
- Describe accession numbers, their use, and how they are generated.
- List the ways laboratory requisition forms are transferred to the laboratory.
- Describe the importance of documentation.
- Explain how laboratory reports are filed in a patient's chart.
- List the methods by which a health care provider is paid for services rendered.
- Define third-party payer.
- Explain premiums, copayments, deductibles, and explanation of benefits.
- Describe how usual and customary fees are derived.
- Explain the basic principle behind health maintenance organizations (HMOs) and preferred provider organizations (PPOs).
- Identify the main components of a computer.
- Define common computer terms.
- Describe a Laboratory Information Management System (LIMS).

❙ INTRODUCTION

The accuracy of documenting a patient's care is critical. The phlebotomist shares this responsibility with every health care provider who interacts with the patient. Learning the correct procedure for each aspect of laboratory documentation is as important an undertaking as learning to correctly obtain specimens and performing diagnostic testing. Accurate documentation for the phlebotomist begins when a laboratory test is ordered.

❙ LABORATORY REQUISITION FORMS

A laboratory requisition form is generated either manually on preprinted paper forms or automatically by computer. If the laboratory is hospital-based, a health unit coordinator or nurse writes the request or enters the patient information into the computer. If the laboratory is nonhospital-based, the phlebotomist or ordering physician writes the request manually or enters the information into the computer. If the laboratory test is ordered for an outpatient from a physician's office, the physician, nurse, or medical assistant calls the laboratory with the order, or the patient may arrive at the laboratory with the order in hand.

Computer Requisition Forms

Computer requisition forms are typically preprinted, with self-adhesive labels attached. The labels can be peeled off and placed directly on the collection tube once the specimen has been collected. Computer requisition forms are not only preprinted with pertinent patient information, they may be printed with special considerations such as "anticoagulant therapy" or "no venipuncture on left arm."

There are many advantages to computer-generated requisition forms. The computer-generated requisition forms list the specific test, the required specimen, and the specimen requirements. The **software** program used to print the forms has the capability to sort tests by patient, generate requisitions by draw times, and record test results in addition to printing numerous other laboratory reports (Figure 5-1).

SOFTWARE

Coded instructions (programs) required to make hardware perform a specific function.

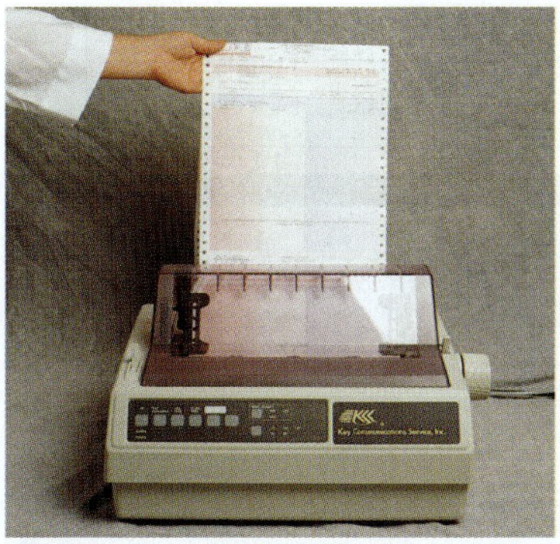

```
                        Service Laboratories
                           734 Dunlap Street
                           Chicago, IL 60171
                        Telephone: 312-824-6925
                           Fax: 312-824-5829


Patient:        Samuels, Annette (ID #ICH 041309)
                Female, Age 22


Referred by:    Inner City Health Care
                Susan Rice
                #10004086


SAMP COLL: 04/24/__ 10:40 AM      SAMP RECD: 04/24/__ 12:10 PM


===============================================================
     TEST            RESULTS          REFERENCE RANGE       UNITS        *
===============================================================

CBC
 Col: 04/26/  11:30                                                     (1)
   WBC             5.3                5.0-16.0             X10-3
   RBC             4.5                3.9-5.3              X10-6
   HGB             12.8               11.5-13.5            G/DL
   HCT             37.2               34.0-40.0            %
   MCV             83                 79-99                FL
   MCH             28                 27-32                PG
   MCHC            34                 32-37                G/DL
   RDW             13                 11-15                %
   PLT             290                130-400              X10-3
   MPV             7                  7-11                 FL


AUTO DIFF
 Col: 04/26/  11:30                                                     (1)

DIFFERENTIAL (MAN)
 Col: 04/26/  11:30                                                     (1)
   SEGS            34      L          41-85                %
   LYMPHS          56      H          15-48                %
   MONOS           9                  2-15                 %
   EOS             1                  0-55                 %
   RBC MORPH       RBC NORM

URINALYSIS (ROUTINE)
 Col: 04/26/  11:31                                                     (1)
   SP GRVTY        1.025              1.003-1.030
   PH              6.5                5.0-8.0
   PROTEIN         NEGATIVE           <= TRACE
   GLUCOSE         NEGATIVE           NEGATIVE
   KETONES         NEGATIVE           NEGATIVE
   BILIRUBIN       NEGATIVE           NEGATIVE
   UROBILINOGEN    0.2 E.U./dL        0.2-1.0
   BLOOD/HGB       NEGATIVE           NEGATIVE
   NITRITE         NEGATIVE           NEGATIVE
   LEUKOCYTES      NEGATIVE           NEGATIVE
```

FIGURE 5-1: Computerized laboratory reports

Manual Requisition Forms

There are a variety of manual requisition form styles. Many facilities color code their manual requisition forms by department so that it is easy to recognize which department is responsible for the specimen. Some manual requisition forms use NCR carbonless paper, providing three copies of the requisition: one copy for the laboratory request, one copy for billing purposes, and one copy as the report. Manual requisition forms typically are *not* preprinted. Self-adhesive identification labels are *not* attached and the phlebotomist must manually label each collection tube.

Manual requisition forms are generally $3\frac{1}{4}$ inches wide by $7\frac{1}{2}$ inches long and are easily attached to $8\frac{1}{2}$ by 11 inch courier paper, which is the traditional format for maintaining laboratory reports in a patient chart. The requisition form is divided into several sections. One section records patient information, one records test requests, and another records test results. The information in each section is always arranged in the same order to create consistency and maintain standardization between departments. Some institutions use one $8\frac{1}{2}$ by 11 inch form that is divided into separate sections, with one section for each department (e.g., microbiology, hematology, chemistry, etc.).

Manual requisition forms (Figure 5-2) are either handwritten or imprinted using an addressograph plate that prints the patient's name, identification number, physician, and room number. The addressograph plate is similar to a credit card plate.

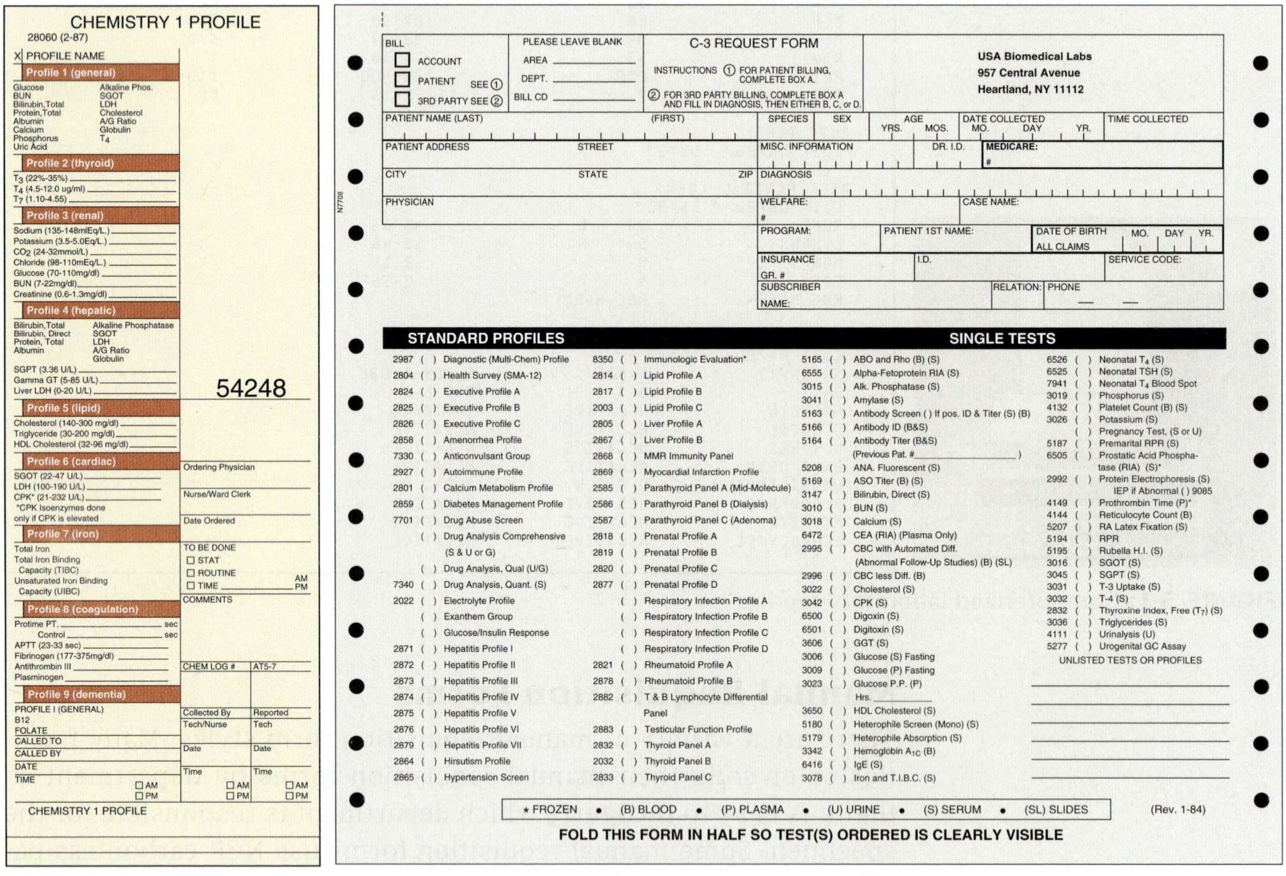

FIGURE 5-2: Manual requisition forms

Generalities of Laboratory Requisition Forms

Both types of requisition forms can contain barcodes. A barcode is a series of black and white bands of varying widths and lengths. Each band corresponds to specific numbers and letters. Bands are grouped together in specific sequences. The sequence represents patient information, such as name, date of birth, identification numbers, or laboratory test requested. The barcodes are then scanned into a computer using a special device that interprets the information and stores it in the computer. When the test requisition is generated, the sequence of bands is printed on the form as the appropriate numbers and letters (i.e., patient name, ID number, etc.). Barcodes are fast and accurate. They accelerate specimen processing and have proven to reduce laboratory errors caused by clerical errors.

Regardless of the type of requisition form, the information must be detailed and easy to follow. The design and format of the request form or computer screen must be as streamlined as possible. Forms must be generated that are easy to handle, are inexpensive, and produce legible copies. The following specific information must be included:

● Patient's full name
● Patient's identification number
● Patient's date of birth
● Room number and bed (if applicable)
● Physician's name requesting the test
● Date of test
● Test requested
● Test status (timed, fasting, priority)
● Billing information (optional)
● Special precautions (optional)

The following information must be handwritten onto the specimen tube label *after* the collection of the specimen:

● Time of test
● Initials of the phlebotomist who obtained the specimen
● Accession number

ACCESSION NUMBER

A unique number given to each test request.

Accession numbers (Figure 5-3) are alpha/numerical numbers that are assigned to each request for a laboratory specimen. This number is used to identify all paperwork and supplies associated with each patient. A computerized requisition form generates the accession number when the specimen request is ordered in the computer. The numbers and/or letters are unique to that specimen and are used in tracking the specimen, entering test results, and/or checking on patient test results.

Manual requisition forms are a more common source of errors. Manual requisition forms may be misplaced, lost, or misfiled. Tests may be overlooked, or wrong specimens may be collected. A few guidelines to help minimize these errors are to: 1) specify a desig-

\#	File Name
800	CARRERA, Jaime
801	AU, Rhoda
802	TREMONT, Sheilia
803	
804	
805	
806	
807	

ACCESSION LOGBOOK

FIGURE 5-3: Accession record or log sequentially lists numbers to be used to assign to numeric records. The next number available in this system is 803.

nated location in the laboratory where all requisition forms are processed; 2) file a copy of the test request in the patient's file and/or file one copy with the blood collection log kept in the laboratory. The log can be used to verify that a test was ordered, when the specimen was collected, and any comments of the phlebotomist regarding the collection can be recorded directly into the logbook. The blood collection logbook serves as an excellent means of communication between the laboratory and the patient's other health care providers. It also serves as another means of documentation. Remember, if it is not documented, it has not been done.

Computerized requisition forms are the most accurate. Laboratory software programs are able to perform automatic checks and balances. The computer is programmed not to accept a request for any test that is not in its database. It will not allow a plasma sample to be entered for a test requiring serum. The program automatically creates and updates the "blood collection logbook." Specimens are logged into the computer database when the specimen accession number is scanned. It also allows the phlebotomist to access the most up-to-date information regarding the requested test such as revised specimen collection requirements, delivery instructions, **assay** techniques, reference ranges, and fees.

Occasionally, in an emergency situation, a test may be requested verbally. The request is to be documented on a laboratory requisition form prior to collection of the specimen. In emergency situations it is important that test requests be executed quickly.

ASSAY

The analysis of a substance or mixture to determine the components and relative proportion of each.

Failing to document the requested procedure correctly costs precious time when verification of test results cannot be matched to the correct patient, and treatment is delayed until specimens are collected again for accuracy.

Transmission of Laboratory Requisition Forms

Laboratory tests ordered by computer can be either E-mailed or transmitted through the hospital's electronic communications system. The physician orders tests for a patient from a computer, and the laboratory requisition form is printed at a computer terminal at the phlebotomist station in the laboratory. Manual requisition forms are dispatched to the laboratory by either a **pneumatic tube system**, by courier, or are collected during "**sweeps**" by the phlebotomist. A phlebotomist then sorts through the requisitions and prioritizes them by date, time, and priority of collection.

CLIENT/PATIENT CHARTING

Manually generated laboratory reports are filed chronologically in the patient's paper chart. The laboratory reports are **shingled**, with the most recent report on top (Figure 5-4). The laboratory reports are typically color coded, with like test reports shingled on the same **courier sheet**. For example, urinalysis reports are color-coded yellow. All yellow urinalysis report forms are chronologically attached to a yellow courier sheet. Hematology reports are color-coded red, and are filed on a red courier sheet.

PNEUMATIC TUBE SYSTEM

A unidirectional, continuously operating vacuum system that transfers specimens in plexiglass carriers from the patient units to the laboratory.

SWEEPS

Hospital rounds (visiting each department or patient of the hospital) which occur at regular intervals throughout the day.

SHINGLED

Attaching a report to a courier sheet in a layered fashion (like shingles on a roof), with the most recently dated report on top.

COURIER SHEET

A blank sheet of paper used to attach laboratory reports chronologically, in a shingled fashion.

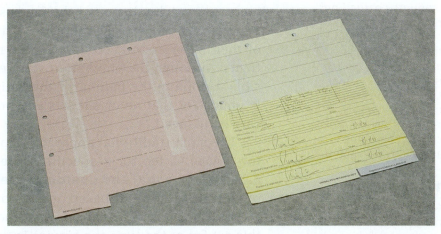

FIGURE 5-4: Shingled lab reports: (Left) shingling base form with sticky tape for attaching lab forms; (Right) shingled lab forms attached to base

Computerized laboratory software programs have automated the "filing" of the laboratory reports. Each patient has a section on their computer patient file labeled "laboratory tests." When the physician orders tests, the information is entered into the computer by either manually typing in the information, or by scanning barcodes. The laboratory requisition form is thus created and stored in the patient's computer file. When test results are completed, they are entered into the patient's computer file in the previously created requisition form, again either manually typed or scanned by barcode, depending on the facility's computer system. This information can be printed and delivered to the physician, phoned to the physician followed by a "**hard copy**" of the report, or the test results can be E-mailed or faxed to the physician. Some physicians have computers and software that connect directly to the hospital's or laboratory's computer system, providing them with immediate test results for their patients.

Computerization of laboratory test results requires a minimal amount of computer storage space, allowing test results to be maintained and accessed for months or years. Reports can be retrieved and printed as needed for comparison to current results and for documentation of charges billed to insurance companies, thereby adding another advantage to computerized laboratory requisition forms.

INSURANCE BILLING/PRIVATE PAY

Health care costs have increased dramatically over the years. The increase in technology and the increase in liability insurance premiums have required health care institutions to increase the cost of their services to keep up with the rising cost of caring for patients. Although the phlebotomist is generally not directly responsible for billing the patient or the patient's insurance company, it is important that he or she has an understanding of how medical care is financed.

The most traditional approach to paying for health care is fee-for-service. A fee for a specific procedure or test is determined based on the **usual and customary fee** within that community. In other words, the fee is based on what other laboratories in the area are charging for the service. The laboratory charges the patient this set fee at the time the service is provided.

Patients can also pay for health care services by using health insurance. This type of insurance is considered a third-party payer, as is medical coverage through government agencies, such as Medicare, Medicaid, and **Tricare**. Third-party payers pay all or part

HARD COPY

A printed paper copy of a computer-generated report.

USUAL AND CUSTOMARY FEE

A method used by insurance companies to establish their fee schedules (specific amounts charged per procedure). It employs a complex system in which three fees are considered in calculating payment: the fee that is usually charged, the fee that is customarily charged by similar practices in the same geographic location, and the reasonable fee.

TRICARE

A managed health care program offered to spouses and dependents of military service personnel. Benefits and fees are uniformly implemented nationwide by the federal government.

INSURED

Individual or organization covered for protection and loss under the specific terms of an insurance policy.

PRE-EXISTING CONDITION

Any illness that began before the insurance policy was written.

PREMIUM

A monthly fee that enrollees pay for medical insurance.

COPAYMENT

A specific dollar amount that the patient must pay the provider for each encounter; also called copay.

DEDUCTIBLE

Specific dollar amount that must be paid by the insured before a medical insurance plan or government program begins covering health care costs.

CLAIM

A billing sent to an insurance carrier.

EXPLANATION OF BENEFITS

An explanation of services periodically issued to recipients or providers on whose behalf claims have been paid.

of the cost of health care services on behalf of the patient. It is a contract between the insurance company and the patient or eligible family member.

There are numerous insurance companies offering health/medical insurance coverage. Each company sets its own requirements for eligibility and determines all aspects of the coverage. Before a policy is issued, the insurance company decides whether it will enter into a contract with the applicant. An application is filled out and submitted to the insurance carrier for determination of eligibility. These applications generally have two sections: the first section asks for basic information about the **insured**, the second section asks for specific medical history. The insurance company, as stipulated by the company's specific guidelines, has the right to limit or restrict portions of a policy based on this information. For example, an insurance company may delay certain coverage for an applicant if another carrier has not covered the person for some types of **pre-existing conditions**.

The insured is required to pay a **premium** to the insurance company every month. Because some policies only partially pay for services provided, the patient is required to make an additional payment at the time services are rendered. This payment is a predetermined amount that is paid regardless of the treatment. This is called a **copayment** and is typically $5 to $10. The patient may also be required to meet a **deductible** prior to the insurance company paying its portion. A deductible is a predetermined amount that the patient must pay directly for health care services prior to receiving insurance benefits. For example, a patient or policyholder (i.e., family member) may have insurance coverage with a $250.00 per year deductible with a monthly premium of $376.00. Another patient or policyholder may have a $500.00 deductible per year with a monthly premium of $234.00. Generally, the higher the deductible, the lower the monthly premium. If the patient or policyholder has not met the deductible when a **claim** is submitted, the insurance company will send the health care provider an **explanation of benefits** stating that the patient has not met the deductible and that the insurance company is not responsible to pay the provider the full amount of the charges (Figure 5-5). The insurance company also sends the patient and/or policyholder a statement of services covered and portions or amounts paid.

A

XYZ Insurance Company

P.O. Box 1234
Anywhere USA 00000-0000
(800) 555-1234
(800) 555-1235 TTY

EXPLANATION OF BENEFITS

Insured: Dee Post
Member ID #: 123456789
Group ID #: 1001

PATIENT: Dee Post
1 Main St
Alfred NY 14802

10-15-2000

PATIENT: Dee Post   **CLAIM:** 89562462-00   **PROVIDER:** Joy Small, MD   **PAYEE:** Joy Small, MD

For Services From To	Type of Service	CPT Code	Total Charges	Disallowed Charges	Deductible (-)	Remaining Covered Charges	Co-Pay	Total Benefit	Patient Responsibility	Comments
0730 073000	Xray	73510	65.00	31.65	.00	0.00	0.00	33.35	0.00	P1
0730 073000	E&M	99203	90.00	.00	.00	0.00	15.00	75.00	15.00	P3
	TOTALS		155.00	31.65	.00	0.00	15.00	108.35	15.00	P2

COMMENTS:

P1   PREFERRED PROVIDER ORGANIZATION DISCOUNT OF $31.65 PROVIDED, PATIENT NOT RESPONSIBLE.
P2   PAYMENT IN THE AMOUNT $108.35 WAS MADE TO JOY SMALL MD ON 10/15/00.
P3   PATIENT IS RESPONSIBLE FOR PAYMENT OF $15.00 TO PROVIDER.

DEE POST   HAS MET $200.00 OF THE $200.00 PATIENT DEDUCTIBLE FOR THE 2000 BENEFIT YEAR.
HAS MET $ 0.00 OF THE OUT-OF-POCKET MAXIMUM FOR THE 2000 BENEFIT YEAR.

THIS IS NOT A BILL. PLEASE SAVE THIS COPY FOR YOUR RECORDS.

B

Explanation of Benefits

XYZ INSURANCE COMPANY   10-15-2000

Provider ID	Provider Name	Date of Service	Patient Name	Member ID	CPT Code	Total Charge	CoPay Amount	Amount Paid	Total
001	Small, Joy	07/30/00	Dael, Tim	125627	29888	2,400.00	0.00	0.00	0.00
001	Small, Joy	07/30/00	Post, Dee	236594	73510	65.00	0.00	0.00	0.00
001	Small, Joy	07/30/00	Post, Dee	236594	99203	90.00	15.00	75.00	90.00
					Practice Total	2555.00	15.00	75.00	90.00

FIGURE 5-5: (A) Explanation of Benefits form sent to patients. (B) Computer-generated Explanation of Benefits sent to providers.

Payment for Services Rendered

Once the laboratory has provided services to the patient, the laboratory has two options for receiving payment:

1. The patient pays for the services at the time the service is rendered and then personally submits the claim to their insurance company. The insurance company determines the usual and customary fee appropriate for the service and reimburses the patient based on the policy benefits. For example: The patient

has a thyroid profile performed. The laboratory charges $210.00 for this test. The patient writes a check for $210.00 and receives a copy of the statement showing the procedure performed, the amount of the procedure, and the payment made. The patient then fills out an insurance claim form, attaches a copy of the statement, and mails it to the insurance company. The insurance company determines that the usual and customary fee for a thyroid profile is $195.00. The patient's policy states that the insurance company will pay 80% of approved charges and the patient is responsible for 20%. The insurance company then sends a check in the amount of $156.00 (80% of the $195.00) as reimbursement.

2. The laboratory bills the insurance company. A claim form is filled out and signed by the patient. The laboratory can either keep this originally signed claim form on file and submit the claim electronically by computer, or they can type out the original claim form with the correct information and submit it to the insurance company. If the patient submits the paper claim form, then the patient must complete a new claim form for every visit to the laboratory. The process then proceeds as if the patient submitted the claim. The insurance company issues the check to the patient. The patient is responsible to pay the laboratory directly.

ASSIGNMENT OF BENEFITS

The transfer of one's right to collect an amount payable under an insurance company contract.

REASONABLE FEE

A charge is considered reasonable if it is deemed acceptable after peer review, even though it does not meet the customary or prevailing criteria. Reasonable fees include unusual circumstances or complications requiring additional time, skill, or experience in connection with a particular service or procedure.

COINSURANCE

A cost-sharing requirement specified in a health insurance policy, provided that the insured will assume a percentage of the costs for covered services.

Some laboratories and health care providers accept **assignment of benefits**. If the laboratory or health care provider accepts assignment of benefits, the laboratory has the patient sign a release of information and assignment of benefits form. Many insurance forms including the universal Health Insurance Claim form (HCFA-1500) contain boxes for the patient's signature with authorization for release of information and assignment of benefits.

When a patient agrees and has signed the box for assignment of benefits, it indicates that the insurance company is to pay the provider rendering the services. The check is sent to the laboratory or health care provider rather than to the patient. When the laboratory or health care provider receives the payment of $156.00, the laboratory bills the patient the difference of $54.00.

Health care services and procedures covered by Medicare, Medicaid, or Tricare require the health care provider to accept the "**reasonable fee**" criteria as 100% payment of the charges. These programs pay 75% to 80% of reasonable charges. This sharing of cost is called **coinsurance**, which is a requirement under some health insurance programs.

CAPITATION

A system of payment used by managed care plans in which physicians and hospitals are paid a fixed, per capita amount for each patient enrolled, regardless of the number of services provided over a specific period of time.

HEALTH MAINTENANCE ORGANIZATION (HMO)

A type of health care program in which enrollees receive benefits for services from authorized and preselected providers, usually a primary care physician. Generally, enrollees do not receive coverage, except for emergency services or for the services of providers who are not in the HMO network.

PREFERRED PROVIDER ORGANIZATION (PPO)

A type of health benefit program in which enrollees receive the highest level of benefits when they obtain services from a physician, hospital, or other health provider designated by their program as a "preferred provider."

Health care providers are paid in one of three ways: fee-for-service, **capitation**, or salary. Fee-for-service has been previously discussed. Capitation is a method of reimbursement where the provider is paid an established fee for each patient in a group of assigned patients, called a panel. Under capitation, the fee is not tied to the services performed, but rather to the number of patients in the assigned group. Therefore, the provider's fee is the same regardless of the amount of time or supplies that are used per patient. This type of payment is the underlying philosophy of managed care. The third type is salaried reimbursement. This method is used by governmental facilities and some managed care organizations. The provider is paid a fixed salary. The salary is not dependent on the number of patients or the quantity of procedures.

Health Care Revisions

The health care industry is continuously in revision in an attempt to contain costs, provide better health care to more people, and keep up with new technology. The American Medical Association originally designed the prospective payment system (PPS) in 1983. This plan sets a schedule of reimbursement to hospitals for each patient procedure, using established disease categories called diagnostic related groups (DRGs). DRGs were originally created as a means to hold down rising health care costs. DRGs are a classification system categorizing patient procedures using like diagnosis and treatment. There are approximately 500 DRGs. When a patient is admitted to the hospital, he or she is assigned a DRG. The DRG defines the amount of reimbursement the facility will receive for that particular admission. The patient is responsible for any additional charges not covered.

Another alternative developed to help keep the cost of health care down is the prepaid health plan. **Health maintenance organizations (HMOs)** are group practices where members pay a fixed periodic payment in advance for all eligible services of participating providers who render these services. Patients are required to obtain all their health care needs with the participating HMO providers. Unless pre-authorized, services obtained from a nonparticipating provider will not be reimbursed and must be paid for by the patient.

Preferred provider organizations (PPOs) are a variation on the HMO theme. Like an HMO, PPOs contract with a group of independent providers, each designated as a "preferred provider" to deliver care to its members. Unlike HMO members, PPO members have the freedom to choose any physician or hospital for services.

However, when a patient selects a preferred provider they receive a higher level of benefits.

HMOs and PPOs were the precursor for managed care systems. The idea of managed care evolved because the act of prepayment basically changed the relationships between the patient and the health care provider. Managed care places the financial risk on the health care provider rather than the insurer. With the implementation of managed care, concepts were developed to provide a better relationship between health care provider and patient. One of these concepts is the primary care physician. The primary care physician's responsibility is to advise and coordinate the patient's health care needs and serve in the role of **gatekeeper**. Provider networks were established when managed care organizations contracted with local providers to establish a complete network of services. For example, the network would contract with specialty physicians in pediatrics, Ob-Gyn, orthopedics, ophthalmology, and so forth. The organization would also contract with laboratories and hospitals. The goal is to reduce the total cost of health care while maintaining patient satisfaction. The providers are paid by capitation. The primary care physician must refer the patient to the appropriate specialist in order to receive the maximum benefits of the plan.

Billing the Insurance Company

In order for a third-party payer to reimburse the medical facility, an insurance claim form must be submitted. The universal Health Insurance Claim Form (HCFA-1500) is a standard form accepted by most insurance companies (Figure 5-6).

This claim form can be filled out by hand, typewritten, or processed using a computer. The form can then either be mailed to the insurance company, or sent electronically by computer.

When completing claim forms, diagnostic and procedure codes are used to specifically classify the patient's diagnosis and the procedures used to treat the patient. The *International Classification of Diseases 9th Revision Clinical Modification* (ICD-9-CM) is the reference used to code diagnoses. It has three volumes. Volume 1 is Diseases: Tabular (numerical) List. Volume 2 is Diseases: Alphabetic Index. Volume 3 is Procedures: Tabular List and Alphabetic Index. Volume 3 is used primarily in the hospital setting. Volumes 1 and 2 are used in physicians' offices to complete insurance claim forms. The Current Procedure Terminology (CPT) is the reference used to code procedures. For example, collection of a blood sample would require a CPT code on an insurance claim form.

GATEKEEPER

Primary care physician responsible for advising and coordinating the patient's health care needs.

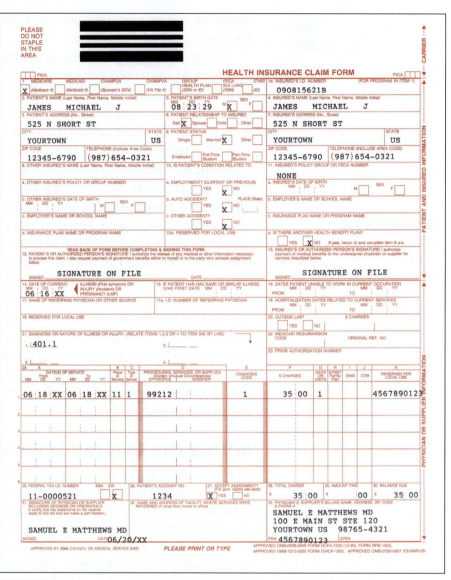

FIGURE 5-6: Completed HCFA-1500 health insurance claim form.

LABORATORY COMPUTER

The computer has become an important tool in every medical facility. What was once laboriously done by hand is now mostly automated. In the medical laboratory, the computer is used to manage data, analyze specimens, and as a diagnostic tool (Figure 5-7). The computer has increased productivity, increased accuracy, and has created a more user-friendly system of managing laboratory reports.

The laboratory computer has the capability to perform many functions. Based on the specific software program the facility is using, the computer can be used to perform one or all of the following:

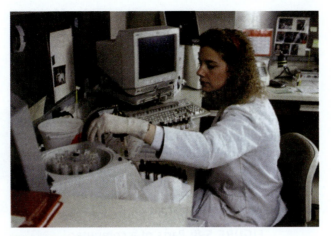

FIGURE 5-7: Laboratory computer

● Data entry: Entering all of the required patient information into a **database**.

● Test requisitions: Test requests are ordered for a patient by entering the request into the computer.

● Printing of test request forms, labels, and accession numbers: Once the patient data are entered and a test is ordered, the computer can be instructed to print a hard copy of the request with the appropriate labels and accession numbers attached.

● Printing schedules and collection lists: The computer is instructed to generate a detailed list of all laboratory tests ordered for a specific date and time.

● Entering test results: Once the specimens are collected and the tests are completed, test results are entered either manually (data entry) or electronically (barcodes).

● Maintenance of medical records: The patient's laboratory test results are stored in a computer patient file indefinitely.

● Transferring of information: Laboratory test results and other laboratory reports are sent immediately via E-mail from the laboratory's computer system to the nurse's station, to the billing department, or to the physician's office.

Computers, although extremely complex, are really very easy to learn and to use—even with no previous exposure or experience. The computer essentially has three basic components.

1. Input: data processed into the machine for internal storage from peripheral equipment such as the keyboard, floppy or compact disk, light pen, scanner, and modem, for internal storage.

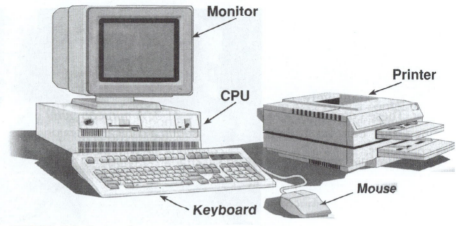

FIGURE 5-8: Parts of a computer

HARDWARE

Equipment used to process data (i.e., keyboard, disk drive, monitor, and printer).

SERVER

A computer in a network shared by multiple users, which serves as a central repository of data and programs. The term may apply to both the hardware and software, or just the software that performs the service.

NETWORK

A group of microcomputers that are linked for the purpose of sharing resources and providing internal communication.

2. Processing: Once information is input into the computer, it is processed by the hardware and/or computer software. The **hardware** refers to the hard disk drive, the CPU (central processing unit), the monitor, and the keyboard. Software is the program(s) containing instructions to the computer that enable it to perform tasks. A computer is useless without the software instructions for accessing and entering data. The central processing unit oversees the processing of each task required by the operator. The arithmetic and logic unit (ALU) performs mathematical processes and makes decisions based on logical comparison of input data. As part of the processing function, the computer is capable of retaining vast amounts of information in its memory banks. There are two types of memory: random access memory (RAM) and read-only memory (ROM). RAM is for temporary storage of data and is lost if the computer is shut off. Information that needs to be saved for later use must be stored either in the computer's main storage unit, called the hard drive, or saved on a disk. Computer systems that are networked with a facility may store information on the network **server**. The computer's hard drive can store enormous amounts of information, which can be retrieved almost immediately.

3. Output: the information the computer produces after recorded information is processed, revised, and printed. A printed laboratory requisition form is an example of output.

Laboratory computers are often **networked** to other computers. This can be an interoffice network, such as the systems in hospitals, or it can be much larger and more complicated, where computers are linked not only to other companies within the same city, but are linked to other states and countries. This is the case when a computer has access to the Internet. Networking has many advantages, such as access to unlimited information world wide, greater efficiency in sending and receiving communications, and cost-efficiency. Facilities with several workstations, individual computers, or terminals, can be networked with a service or mainframe computer. This central unit contains the software programs and the data banks of information to be shared in the office. Each terminal can access information to be shared throughout the facility. Each terminal can access information from the central computer, thereby freeing up hard drive space at each workstation. A properly networked system permits input and updating of records from all stations and allows the information to be accessed from all stations.

Computer software capabilities are virtually limitless. Software companies are continually designing programs, making it possible to direct a computer to produce differently prescribed outcomes. It often takes 12 to 24 months to research, write, and test a comprehensive software program. When the project is begun, the latest and greatest technology is used. By the time the project is completed and fully tested, the software may be two years old. It is important to keep current with the software programs that the laboratory computer uses. Take advantage of training programs offered to keep up with the current trends.

Box 5-1 contains common computer terms that should be committed to memory.

Box 5-1: Common Computer Terms

Backup—duplicate of data files made to protect information. Records should be backed up daily. Some experts recommend twice daily.

Batch—an accumulation of data to be processed.

Boot—to start up a computer.

Bug—an error in a program.

Catalog—a list of files on the storage media.

CD-ROM—compact disk read-only memory. The term indicates the computer is capable of playing compact disks.

Characters per second—term used to measure printer output.

(continues)

Box 5-1: Common Computer Terms *(continued)*

CPU—central processing unit, or the brain of the system. The memory is made up of bits. A bit is a single **BI**nary digi**T**. Binary refers to a situation in which there are only two choices: for example, yes/no, on/off, and pass/fail. Digit refers to a single number. A bit is either 0 or 1. A **byte** is the fundamental groups of bits that a computer will treat as a word. A byte consists of 8 bits. A 16-bit processor is twice as fast as an 8-bit processor. One K is equal to 1,024 bytes. A 64-K computer can handle 65,536 bytes. The greater the number of bytes, the greater the memory.

Cursor—a marker on the screen that shows where the next letter, number, or symbol will be placed (may be an underline dash or a blinking rectangle or square).

Data—information that can be processed or produced by a computer.

Debugging—finding errors and correcting them in computer programs.

Disk—a magnetic storage device made of rigid material or flexible plastic.

Disk drive—the device used to get information on and off a disk.

DOS—(Disk Operating System) a program that tells the computer how to use the disk drive.

Downtime—a period of lost work time during which a computer is not operating or is malfunctioning because of machine failure.

Electronic mail—(E-mail) the transmission of letters, messages, or memos from one computer to another over telephone or cable lines.

External memory—recording on disks.

File—a single, stored unit of information that is given a file name so it can be accessed.

Font—a family or assortment of characters of a given size or style.

GB—gigabyte, approximately one billion bytes (1,073,741,824 bytes, to be exact).

Hard copy—the readable paper copy or printout of information.

Hardware—the electronic, magnetic, and electromechanical equipment of a computer system (keyboard, disk drive, monitor, and printer).

Initialize—to prepare a disk to receive data. This is usually referred to as "formatting" a disk.

Input—data processed from peripheral equipment into the machine via the keyboard or disk for internal storage.

Interface—the hardware and software that enable individual computers and components to interact.

K—computer shorthand for 1,024 bytes; a term used to measure computer memory capacity.

Keyboard—an input device resembling a typewriter keyboard that converts keystrokes into electrical signals which are displayed on the screen as words or symbols.

Kilobyte—one thousand bytes.

Log on—signing on to a computer system by entering a username and a password.

Main memory—the internal memory of the computer.

Megabyte—approximately one million bytes.

Memory—data held in storage.

Menu—a display of available machine functions for selection by the operator.

Microcomputer—a self-contained computer system that uses a microprocessor as the central processing unit (often called a desktop or personal computer, or PC). Has limited capacity for internal memory.

Microprocessor—a single chip where the computer computes.

Minicomputer—a computer significantly smaller in size, capacity, and software capability than its larger mainframe counterparts.

Modem—**MO**dulator/**DEM**odulator. A peripheral device that enables a computer to communicate with other computers or terminals over normal telephone or cable lines.

Monitor—visual display unit with a screen called a cathode-ray tube (CRT).

Mouse—a hand-held computer input device, separate from a keyboard, used to control cursor position on a VDT (video display terminal).

On-line—making a system operational, or being on the Internet.

Output—what the computer produces after recorded information is processed, revised, and printed.

Peripheral—anything you plug into a computer; for example, a printer, disk drive, scanner, or CRT terminal.

Printer—a device that produces hard copy. It may be dot matrix, letter quality, or laser.

(continues)

Box 5-1: Common Computer Terms *(continued)*

Program—a set of instructions written in computer language.

Prompting—messages issued to a user requesting information necessary to continue processing.

RAM—acronym for **R**andom **A**ccess **M**emory. This is temporary, or programmable memory. You can put new information into RAM. When you turn off the computer this memory is deleted.

ROM—acronym for **R**ead **O**nly **M**emory. This is permanent memory. You cannot put new information into ROM. It has been predetermined by the computer manufacturer.

Scrolling—moving the cursor up, down, right, or left through information on a computer display to view information otherwise not visible.

Security code—a code the operator must enter into the computer before a procedure may be completed. Used to prevent unauthorized access to data in a system.

Software—computer programs necessary to direct the hardware of a computer system to perform specific tasks.

Terminal—a device used to communicate with a computer, usually a keyboard and monitor. Terminals depend on the main (host) computer for their abilities. A hospital may have several terminals and a host computer physically removed from any of them.

Write-protect—process or code that prevents overwriting of data or programs on a disk.

Laboratory Information Management Systems (LIMS)

The LIMS were designed to manage patient data and interface with automated analyzers and main hospital information systems. Several companies produce software for laboratories and extensive research is done by the facility to determine which software program is best suited for their laboratory needs. Considerations in this decision process are the ease of inputting and retrieving information, the format of output, and the cost-effectiveness of the program. Once the system is brought on-line, the hospital management information system (MIS) specialist oversees the system's daily operations, trains laboratory personnel, and updates the system as necessary. Most hospital LIMS are fully integrated through networking. This means that all patient data can be shared from department to department. The patient has an "electronic chart" that every department working with the patient can use to enter information. Someday medicine may be a totally paperless profession.

When facilities are networked it is often necessary to assign each employee using the system a user name and password. Each time the employee logs onto the computer to perform a task, the user name and password must be entered to identify which employee is entering data into the system. Passwords are confidential and are not shared with fellow employees. Some facilities assign levels of access to the computer by user name and password. For example, a phlebotomist is given access to the laboratory section of the system, but not the financial management section.

Computer technology is continuously improving. Voice-activated systems and hand-held scanners and barcode label systems are becoming the norm rather than the exception. Medical laboratories continue to become more efficient both in cost of service and productivity.

SUMMARY

Documentation of laboratory procedures is critical. Understanding the process of how tests are ordered, how requisition forms are generated, and how data is input into the computer is a vital part of the phlebotomist's job description. Not only must documentation be accurate, it must be completed in a timely manner and as cost-effectively as possible. Remember, if it is not documented, it was not done.

STUDY AND REVIEW EXERCISES

Defining Key Terms

Write the definition for each of the following key terms.

1) accession number _____

2) assay _____

3) assignment of benefits _____

4) capitation _____

5) claim _____

6) coinsurance _____

7) copayment _____

8) courier sheet _____

9) database _____

10) deductible _____

11) explanation of benefits_____

12) gatekeeper _____

13) hard copy _____

14) hardware_____

15) health maintenance organization (HMO)_____
_____

16) insured _____

17) network_____

18) pneumatic tube system _____

19) pre-existing condition_____

20) preferred provider organization (PPO)_____
_____

21) premium _____

22) reasonable fee _____

23) server_____

24) shingled _____

25) software _____

26) sweeps_____

27) Tricare _____

28) usual and customary fee _____

Reviewing Key Points

1) List the pertinent information that is required on all laboratory requisition forms.

2) Describe the term "third-party payer."

3) Describe how usual and customary fees are derived.

4) Describe the importance of documentation.

5) Identify the main components of a computer.

Sentence Completion

1) A computer generates a _____ either manually on preprinted paper forms or automatically.

2) Many facilities _____ their manual requisition forms by department so that it is easy to recognize which department is responsible for the specimen.

3) Manual requisition forms are either handwritten or imprinted using a(n) _____ that prints the patient's name, identification number, physician, and room number.

4) A _____ is a series of black and white bands of varying widths and lengths, representing patient information.

5) _____ are alpha/numeric numbers that are assigned to each request for a laboratory specimen.

6) Manual requisition forms are dispatched to the laboratory by either a _____, by courier, or are collected during _____ by the phlebotomist.

7) The most traditional approach to paying for health care is _____.

8) _____ pay all or part of the cost of health care services on behalf of the patient.

9) Health care providers are paid one of three ways: fee-for-service, _____, or salary.

10) _____ are group practices where members pay a fixed periodic payment in advance for all eligible services of participating providers who render these services.

Multiple Choice

1) The primary care physician's responsibility is to advise and co-ordinate the patient's health care needs and serve in the role of _____.
   A. sentinel
   B. gatekeeper
   C. watchdog
   D. guardian

2) In order for a third-party payer to reimburse the medical facil-ity, an insurance claim form must be submitted. The universal claim form accepted by the majority of third-party payer is called a(n):
   A. HCFA-1000
   B. UHCF-1500
   C. HCFA-1500
   D. UHCF-1000

3) The _____ is the reference used to code diagnosis.
   A. Current Procedural Terminology—CPT
   B. Diagnostic Related Groups—DRG
   C. National Disease Classification 6th Edition—NDC 6
   D. International Classification of Disease 9th Revision Clini-cal Modification (ICD-9-CM)

4) The laboratory computer has the capability to perform many functions. Which one of the following is not a function per-formed by a laboratory computer?
   A. Test requisitions
   B. Data entry
   C. Entering test results
   D. The laboratory computer is capable of performing all the above functions

5) Which one of the following is not one of the three basic com-ponents of a computer?
   A. Service
   B. Input
   C. Processing
   D. Output

6) The type of computer memory that stores data temporarily and is lost if the computer is shut off is:
   A. RAM
   B. ROM
   C. DOS
   D. CPU

7) To start up a computer is to:
   A. backup
   B. boot
   C. hard copy
   D. log on

8) A display of available machine functions for selection by the operator is called a:
   A. font
   B. cursor
   C. program
   D. menu

9) Computer programs necessary to direct the hardware of a computer system to perform specific tasks are called:
   A. RAM
   B. CD-ROMs
   C. software
   D. hardware

10) Anything you plug into the computer—for example, a printer, disk drive, scanner, or CRT terminal—is called a computer
    _____.
    A. peripheral
    B. program
    C. microprocessor
    D. hardware

Critical Thinking

1) Grace Spencer, a 78-year-old female patient, is in the lab today to have a series of blood tests done. Mrs. Spencer has Medicare to help pay for the charges, but she is unsure of what Medicare will pay and what she will have to pay. The total charges for today are $745.00. You know that Medicare will pay 80% of the allowable charge. For the tests that were performed on Mrs. Spencer, Medicare considers $498.00 as the allowable charge. Your laboratory is a participating provider and accepts assignment, which means Mrs. Spencer is responsible for paying 20% of the allowable charge. How much will Medicare pay for today's charges? How much will Mrs. Spencer be required to pay?

2) Your laboratory has a new computer system. Dr. Sarah Wilcox has ordered a Protime and CBC on Mr. Garrison to be drawn this morning, using her office computer. Describe the process of preparing the paperwork for these tests.

Vital Signs

OBJECTIVES

Upon completion of this chapter the student should be able to:

- Define and correctly spell each of the key terms.
- List the four vital signs and describe the body functions they monitor.
- Describe what causes a pulse and identify where a pulse can be located.
- Locate the three major pulse points and describe their common uses.
- Identify the normal pulse range for a healthy adult.
- List and define the three characteristics used to describe a pulse.
- Identify the normal rate of respirations and describe the associated characteristics.
- Describe how the body regulates temperature.
- Describe the methods used to obtain body temperature.
- Identify the phases of blood pressure and relate them to the actions of the heart.
- Identify and describe the equipment used to obtain a patient's blood pressure.
- Demonstrate how a patient's vital signs are recorded in a patient's chart.
- Demonstrate the ability to accurately measure a patient's vital signs, including TPR (temperature, pulse, and respiration) and blood pressure.

VITAL SIGNS

The traditional signs of life (i.e., heartbeat, body temperature, respiration, and blood pressure).

PULSE

Rate, rhythm, and condition of arterial walls.

PALPATE

To examine by touch; to feel.

RADIAL

1) Radiating out from a given center. 2) Pertaining to the radius. 3) Pulse palpated over the radial artery of the arm.

BRACHIAL

Pertaining to the arm.

ANTECUBITAL

Triangular area lying anterior to and below the elbow.

AUSCULTATE

To examine by auscultation. To listen for sounds within the body.

CAROTID

Pertaining to the right and left common carotid arteries, which comprise the principal blood supply to the head and neck.

❚ INTRODUCTION

Vital signs are measurements of an individual's essential life-sustaining functions. As a phlebotomy technician you may be asked to perform these skills as part of your routine duties, or you may only perform them in an emergency situation. Regardless, it is every allied health professional's responsibility to know these skills and be able to perform each step in the process of taking vital signs and recording the measurements with a high degree of accuracy. Remember that vital sign measurements are never to be estimated. Results are always recorded immediately following the procedure.

Vital signs are the primary indicators of a patient's overall health. The four vital signs are temperature, pulse, respiration, and blood pressure, also known as TPRs and BP.

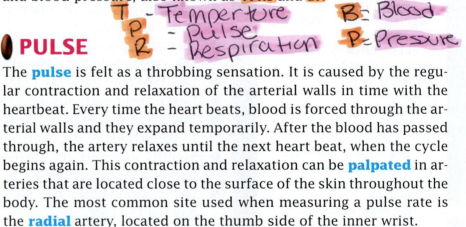

❚ PULSE

The **pulse** is felt as a throbbing sensation. It is caused by the regular contraction and relaxation of the arterial walls in time with the heartbeat. Every time the heart beats, blood is forced through the arterial walls and they expand temporarily. After the blood has passed through, the artery relaxes until the next heart beat, when the cycle begins again. This contraction and relaxation can be **palpated** in arteries that are located close to the surface of the skin throughout the body. The most common site used when measuring a pulse rate is the **radial** artery, located on the thumb side of the inner wrist.

The **brachial** pulse is located on the inner medial surface of the elbow at the **antecubital** space. This pulse point is used to palpate and **auscultate** blood pressure. The **carotid** pulse is located when pressure is applied with the fingertips to either side of the trachea. This pulse point is most commonly used when palpating for a pulse during cardiopulmonary resuscitation (CPR). See Table 6-1 for a description of pulse points.

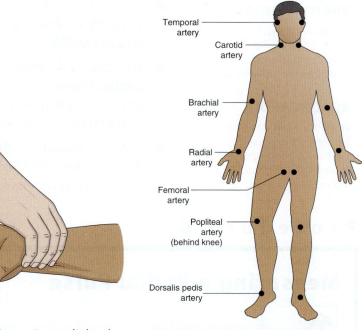

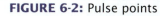

FIGURE 6-1: Measuring radial pulse   **FIGURE 6-2:** Pulse points

Table 6-1: Pulse Points

The pulse can be felt throughout the body in several locations. The following is a list of these locations:

Radial: Thumb side of the inner surface of the wrist, lying over the radius bone. The radial pulse point is used most frequently when measuring the pulse rate.

Brachial: Inner medial surface of the elbow, at the antecubital space (crease of elbow). This point is used to palpate and auscultate blood pressure.

Carotid: Carotid artery of the neck at either side of the trachea. This pulse point is used during cardiopulmonary resuscitation.

Femoral: Midway in the groin where the artery begins its descent down the femur. This pulse point is used to establish and evaluate circulation of the lower extremities.

Popliteal: Behind the knee. This pulse point is used to evaluate circulation of the lower extremities below the knee.

Dorsalis pedis: Instep of foot. This pulse point is used to evaluate circulation below the ankle.

A pulse is recorded as beats per minute preceded by a capital P (for example, P 72). Writing BPM after the pulse is unnecessary, as trained medical personnel know this is how it is measured. The normal pulse range for a healthy adult is 60 to 100 beats per minute. It is important to keep in mind three key pulse characteristics when checking a patient's pulse: rate, rhythm, and quality.

● Rate: The number of beats per minute. Two associated terms used to describe a patient's pulse rate are **tachycardia** and **bradycardia**.

● Rhythm: The rhythm of a pulse refers to its regularity. An **arrhythmia** is an irregular heart beat. It may have intermittent beats, or unequally spaced beats. When the pulse pattern is consistent it is defined as regular.

● Quality: Quality is determined by the amount of blood that is flowing through the artery. Weak, strong, thready, and bounding are all terms used to describe the quality of blood.

Procedure 6-1

Measuring a Radial Pulse

Equipment/Supplies

● Watch with a second hand
● Pen
● Patient's chart

Method/*Rationale*

1. Assemble equipment and supplies.

   Ensures everything is available to perform the procedure.

2. Wash hands.

   Thorough handwashing aids in controlling the spread of infections.

3. Identify the patient.

   Ensures procedure is performed on the correct patient.

4. Explain the procedure.

   Helps relieve patient anxiety.

5. Position your patient either by sitting the patient in a comfortable position or having the patient lie down.

   If the patient is not comfortable or is exerting excess energy, the pulse rate may be falsely increased.

6. Extend the patient's arm at a level equal to or lower than the heart.

   If the arm is raised higher than the heart level, the pulse may be falsely increased.

7. Physically support the arm on a table or bed, palm of hand facing down (Figure 6-3).

   If not supported, the pulse rate may be affected.

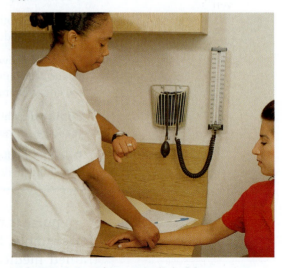

FIGURE 6-3: Taking a radial pulse

◖ RESPIRATIONS

Respiration is defined as the act of breathing, in which the lungs take in oxygen on inhalation and give off carbon dioxide on exhalation. One respiration equals one inhalation and one exhalation.

Respirations are counted as part of the patient's total vital signs. The respiration rate indicates how well a patient's body is providing oxygen to tissues. Pulse and respirations go hand in hand, as the circulatory and respiratory systems work together. As discussed in Chapter 3, the circulatory system carries blood throughout the body. The blood cells carry oxygen from the lungs to the tissues and carbon dioxide from the tissues back to the

8. Place the fingertips of your first and second finger over the patient's radial pulse, on the thumb side of the wrist.

   It is important to use only the fingertips as they are more sensitive than other parts of the finger. Never use your thumb; the thumb has a slight pulse of its own and you may be counting your own pulse instead of the patient's.

9. Depress the tissue directly over the radial artery. Press firmly enough to feel the pulse but lightly enough that you do not obliterate it.

   Too much pressure exerted on the artery will compress it and obliterate the pulse. If you exert too little pressure, you will be unable to feel the pulse.

10. Observe the quality of the pulse before counting the beats per minute (BPM). Determine if the pulse is weak or strong, regular or thready. A thready pulse is a fine, scarcely perceptible pulse.

    Concentrating on the qualities of the pulse allows for a more accurate determination.

11. Begin counting the pulse by watching the second hand on your watch. If the pulse is regular and strong, count the pulse for 30 seconds and multiply by two to determine the beats per minute. If the pulse is weak or thready, count the pulse for one full minute.

    Because of the irregularities, counting a weak or thready pulse for less than a full minute will give inaccurate results. Be careful not to count the seconds ticking on your watch. It is helpful to look at the watch when you start counting, then look away and check the time every few seconds.

12. Record the results in the patient's chart. Record the BPM and the quality of the pulse.

    Record the results as quickly as possible to reduce the risk of errors. Procedures not recorded are considered not performed. Record pulse with the following format:

    ● *P—72 regular*
    ● *P—120 bounding*

13. Wash hands.

    Wash your hands before and after every patient to reduce the risk of infection.

lungs. Generally, if the pulse rate is high or low, the respirations will also be high or low. A normal pulse/respiration ratio is about 4:1 (four pulse beats to one respiration).

Because a patient can control his or her breathing to some degree, it is important that the patient not know you are counting respirations. To accomplish this, respirations are generally counted immediately after counting the patient's pulse, while still holding your fingers over the radial artery. The patient will assume you are still taking the pulse.

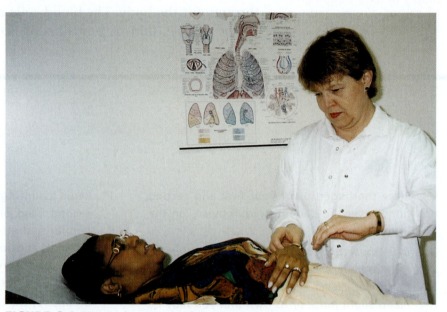

FIGURE 6-4: Measuring respirations

Characteristics of Respiration

The characteristics of respiration are rate, volume, and rhythm.

● The number of respirations per minute is the rate. The rate for an average healthy adult is 16 to 20 respirations per minute. **Bradypnea** (respirations below 16 per minute), **tachypnea** (more than 20 breaths per minute), and **apnea** (the absence of breathing), are all terms used to describe respiration rates. Respirations can be counted by watching the patient's chest, back, stomach, or shoulders rise and fall. If visualization of respirations is difficult, alternative methods for counting should be employed. One alternative is to place your hand on the patient's back, enabling you to feel the patient's chest rise and fall. Another alternative is to use a stethoscope. Place the stethoscope on one side of the patient's spine in the middle of the back and listen for inhalation and expiration.

BRADYPNEA

Abnormally slow breathing.

TACHYPNEA

Abnormal rapidity of respiration.

APNEA

Temporary cessation of breathing.

● Volume is the amount of air being inhaled and exhaled. Three terms are used to describe this characteristic: normal, shallow, or deep. Volume is determined by observing the chest rise and fall. A patient with normal respiration volume is breathing easily through the nose, with the chest gently rising and falling. Shallow respirations are more difficult to visualize. Alternative methods of counting respirations are used when shallow breathing is present. Deep respirations often require the use of the accessory respiratory muscles of the rib cage, neck, shoulders, and back. Deep respirations are often labored, with the patient having difficulty breathing. The patient may be breathing through the mouth rather than the nose.

● Rhythm is a specific pattern and is determined by the period of time between each respiration. The amount of time or pattern is equal in normal respirations and is documented as regular. Abnormal patterns are documented as irregular. Examples of abnormal or irregular breathing patterns include:

  • Dyspnea: difficult or labored breathing
  • Apnea: no respirations
  • Hyperpnea: abnormally deep, gasping breaths
  • Hyperventilation: a respiratory rate that greatly exceeds the oxygen demand
  • Hypopnea: shallow respirations
  • Orthopnea: inability to breathe or difficulty breathing in a supine or prone positions; the patient must be upright to breathe
  • Cheyne-Stokes: begins with slow, shallow breathing, escalates to deep, rapid breathing, and then decreases to slow, shallow breathing, followed by a period of apnea. The pattern continues until the apnea is permanent and death occurs.

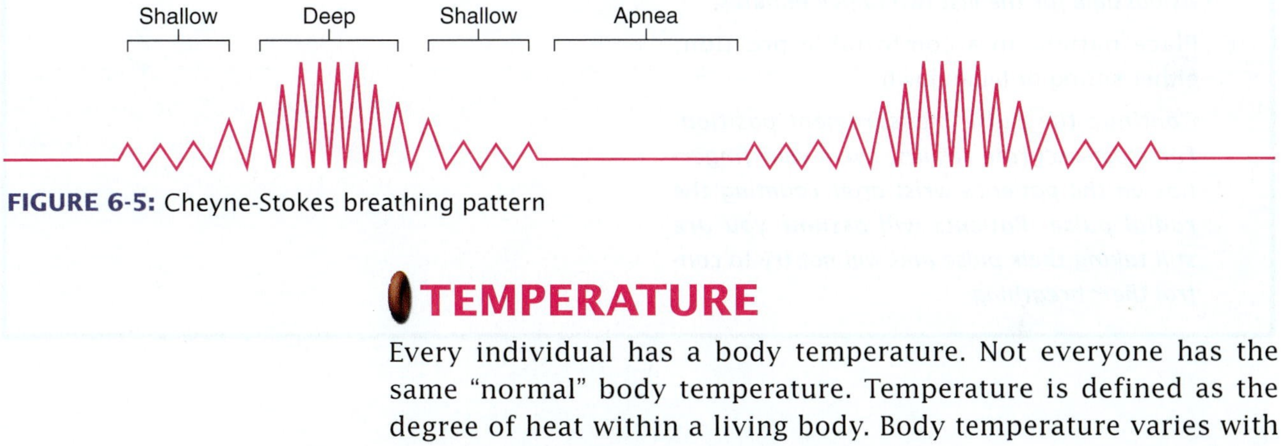

FIGURE 6-5: Cheyne-Stokes breathing pattern

TEMPERATURE

Every individual has a body temperature. Not everyone has the same "normal" body temperature. Temperature is defined as the degree of heat within a living body. Body temperature varies with the time of day, amount of exertion, and the site of measurement.

Procedure 6-2

Measuring a Respiration

Equipment/Supplies

- Watch with a second hand
- Pen
- Patient's chart

Method/*Rationale*

1. Assemble equipment and supplies.

   Ensures everything is available to perform the procedure.

2. Wash hands.

   Thorough handwashing aids in controlling the spread of infections.

3. Identify the patient.

   Ensures the procedure is performed on the correct patient.

4. Generally explain the procedure.

   This is a procedure better not explained in detail, as patients can control their breathing, resulting in inaccurate measurements.

5. Ask the patient about recent activities.

   In order to obtain accurate results, the patient should have been as inactive and calm as possible for the last two to five minutes.

6. Place patient in a comfortable position, either sitting or lying down.

   Continue the pulse measurement position. For most accurate results, leave your fingertips on the patient's wrist after counting the radial pulse. Patients will assume you are still taking their pulse and will not try to control their breathing.

7. Assess the quality of the respirations.

   Do this before you start counting. Remember to check for volume and rhythm before counting the respiration rate.

8. Count respirations (Note: One rise and fall of the chest equals one respiration).

   If the quality of the respirations seems normal, count for thirty seconds and multiply by two. If the quality seems irregular, count for a full minute.

9. Record results.

   To reduce the risk of errors, record the results as quickly as possible. The presence or absence of the respiration's characteristics is very significant in some conditions or diseased states. When recording respirations, use the following format:

   - *R—12 shallow*
   - *R—18 regular*

10. Wash hands.

    Wash your hands before and after every procedure to reduce the risk of infection.

Oral temperatures are usually 97.5° to 99.5° F (36° to 38° C). Rectal temperatures are generally 0.5°to 1° F (0.28° to 0.56° C) higher than oral temperatures. Axillary (armpit) temperatures are generally 1° F lower than oral temperatures.

Body temperature is regulated by thermoregulatory centers in the hypothalamus that balance heat production and heat loss. This process can be compared to the thermostat that turns the furnace in your home on and off. The hypothalamic thermostat is very effective. When receptors sense the body is too warm, they send a message to the brain, which in turn activates the sweat glands of the skin to produce moisture (sweat). The moisture evaporates from the skin's surface and cools the body. At the same time, nerve impulses are sent to the skin's surface blood vessels to dilate, which brings more blood in contact with the surface of the skin. The blood gives up heat, which cools the blood within the vessels and, therefore, cools the body. When the body senses coolness, the opposite activities occur.

Elevation of temperature above normal is called fever and the patient is said to be **febrile**. The patient with a normal body temperature is said to be **afebrile**. Temperatures below normal are called subnormal temperatures, or **hypothermia**. When the body's temperature falls below 96.0° F, a person may collapse into coma. If the body's temperature remains at 93.0° F or below for an extended period of time, death will occur. Temperatures above 106° F in adults for extended periods will also cause death.

Thermometers

A thermometer is a device used to obtain a temperature. There are several types of thermometers. The phlebotomy technician uses one of the following types of thermometers:

Glass Mercury

There are three types of glass mercury thermometers (Figure 6-6):

1. Oral thermometer with a long slender bulb which is placed under the tongue

2. Rectal thermometer with a fat rounded bulb which is stronger and safer to insert into the rectum

3. Safety or security thermometer with a rounded "stubby" bulb which is used for oral or axillary measurements

These three thermometer types are further identified by a color-coded dot on the end of the stem. A red dot indicates a rectal thermometer, a blue dot an oral thermometer, and a white dot

FEBRILE

Feverish; pertaining to a fever. Abnormal elevation of temperature.

AFEBRILE

Without fever.

HYPOTHERMIA

The state in which an individual's body temperature is reduced below normal range: <96.0° F.

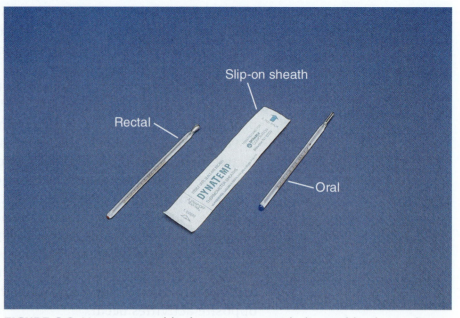

FIGURE 6-6: Mercury reusable thermometers with disposable plastic slip-on sheath

or no dot indicates a safety thermometer. It is very important that the specifically identified thermometer only be used for its intended purpose and site(s). For example, a rectal thermometer is never used for an oral measurement nor is an oral thermometer used for a rectal measurement; the oral thermometer bulb could perforate the delicate tissue of the rectum.

Reading a Glass Thermometer

Glass thermometers are cylindrical tubes made of glass with a hollow cavity from the bulb to the tip of the stem. The cavity is filled with mercury. The stem of a Fahrenheit thermometer is calibrated in even tenths of degrees (Figure 6-7). The whole degrees are marked by long lines and numbers, the tenths by shorter lines. Only the even tenths are labeled with numbers, 0.2, 0.4, 0.6, 0.8. An even longer line, or a red arrow, indicates the normal average oral temperature of 98.6 degrees.

To read a glass thermometer, hold it by the stem in your right hand, at eye level, between the thumb and index finger. View it with the lines at the top and the numbers at the bottom. Rotate the stem slowly back and forth until you see the silver of the mercury in the middle of the column. The point where the mercury stops is read and recorded as the temperature (Figure 6-8). If the mercury stops between tenths, the next highest two-tenths of a degree is recorded.

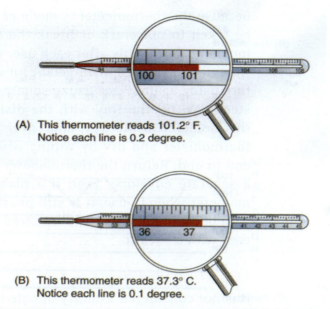

(A) This thermometer reads 101.2° F.
Notice each line is 0.2 degree.

(B) This thermometer reads 37.3° C.
Notice each line is 0.1 degree.

FIGURE 6-7: (A) Fahrenheit thermometer. (B) Celsius thermometer.

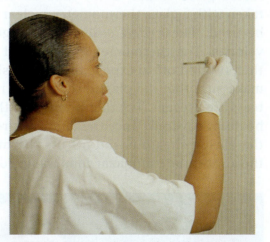

FIGURE 6-8: Reading a glass thermometer

Box 6-1: Universal/Standard Precautions

Taking an oral temperature requires contact with mucous membranes of the mouth or rectum. It is extremely important to practice Universal/Standard Precautions as described in Chapter 4 during this procedure. Wash hands, wear gloves, and dispose of items that come in contact with body fluids into the appropriate biohazardous container. Wash hands again. Remember that every patient should be considered infectious.

Care of Glass Thermometers

Because the thermometer is made of glass, it is fragile. Care must be taken to not crack or break the thermometer. Wash the thermometer thoroughly after each use. Wash with lukewarm, running water, and soak in a disinfectant for a minimum of 20 minutes before using again. Place gauze squares in the bottom of a stainless steel tray, fill the tray with the disinfectant, carefully place the thermometer in the tray, and cover with the tray's lid. Rinse the thermometer and dry by wiping with a clean gauze square from end to end. Return the thermometer to its original plastic case or a separate envelope. Even if a plastic sheath covered the thermometer when in use, it is still possible that it was contaminated with body fluid and should be cared for as if it had not been covered with a sheath.

Protective Sheaths

It is not considered sanitary or safe to take a temperature with an unsheathed thermometer, even if it has been cleaned and disinfected prior to use. Every time an oral or rectal temperature is taken with a glass thermometer, a clear plastic slip-on sheath must be used. These covers are prepackaged in individual paper envelopes. The thermometer is inserted into one end; the paper is then twisted off to expose the plastic sheath (Figure 6-9). Check to make sure that the plastic sheath has remained intact and that no tears are present. The thermometer is then used exactly as it would be if not covered. Once the temperature of the patient is obtained, the plastic sheath is slid off the thermometer and discarded into the appropriate biohazardous waste container.

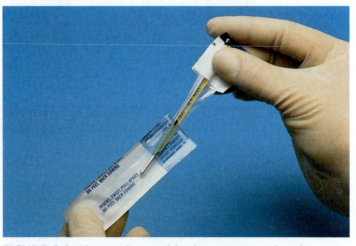

FIGURE 6-9: Slip-on disposable thermometer sheath

Box 6-2: Mercury

Mercury is a metallic element with an abbreviation of Hg. It is insoluble in ordinary solvents but soluble in hydrochloric acid on boiling. It is a silvery liquid at room temperature. When heated or placed under pressure within confined spaces, such as within the chamber of an oral thermometer or mercury sphygmomanometer, mercury expands. When the mercury expands, it is forced to rise up the chamber. Thus, it provides a visual record of the body's temperature and/or blood pressure. The possibility of mercury poisoning from swallowing mercury in a broken thermometer is remote, but possible. To prevent this, care should be taken so that a patient does not bite down on an oral thermometer.

Measuring an Oral Temperature

Oral temperatures are used frequently because they are convenient, quick, and accurate. Once sheathed, the thermometer is placed **sublinguially** (under the tongue) for a minimum of 3 minutes. Caution the patient not to bite down on the thermometer but to gently cradle it under the tongue, using the lips to secure it in place. A broken thermometer is a serious hazard; swallowing glass fragments or mercury can cause serious problems. If a thermometer does break while in a patient's mouth, carefully remove the broken glass and any mercury (remember to wear gloves) and notify the physician immediately. Temperature results will be inaccurate if the patient talks, coughs, or sneezes during the procedure. The results will also be inaccurate if the patient has had something hot or cold to eat or drink or has smoked within 10 minutes prior to the procedure. If any of these situations occur, the procedure must be repeated later.

There are some instances when taking an oral temperature is contraindicated. In these cases the temperature must be measured in another way, such as the tympanic (ear), rectal, or axillary methods. These methods are preferred for infants, small children, patients who are confused or disoriented, have respiratory complications requiring them to breathe through the mouth, are on oxygen, have oral injuries, or have had recent oral surgery, and patients with facial paralysis.

SUBLINGUAL

Beneath or concerning the area beneath the tongue.

Procedure 6-3

Measuring an Oral Temperature with a Glass Mercury Thermometer

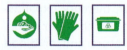

Equipment/Supplies

● Oral thermometer (blue dot on stem)
● Thermometer sheath
● Latex gloves
● Biohazardous waste container
● Watch or timer
● Pen
● Patient chart

Method/*Rationale*

1. Assemble equipment and supplies.

   Ensures everything is available to perform the procedure.

2. Wash hands/put on gloves.

   Thorough handwashing aids in controlling the spread of infections. Remember that you must comply with Standard Precautions whenever you may come in contact with body fluids or blood.

3. Identify the patient.

   Ensures the procedure is performed on the correct patient.

4. Explain the procedure.

   Helps ensure you will have the cooperation of the patient.

5. Ask the patient about recent activities.

   If the patient has had something hot or cold to drink or has smoked within the last 10 minutes, the results will be inaccurate. If so, allow 10 minutes before measuring.

6. Position your patient either by sitting the patient in a comfortable position or having the patient lie down.

   If the patient is not comfortable or is exerting excess energy, the temperature rate may be falsely increased.

7. Remove the thermometer from case or envelope.

   Avoid touching the end of the bulb.

8. Inspect the thermometer.

   Discard if chipped or cracked.

9. Shake down the thermometer to 96° F or lower.

   Thermometers that have been previously used with a recorded higher temperature will not measure accurately. For example, if the last temperature taken with the thermometer was 101.2° F and the thermometer was not shaken down, and the next patient's temperature is actually less than 101.2° F, the temperature will still read 101.2° F, even though it is actually lower. The patient may be treated for a fever he or she does not have.

10. Place plastic sheath on the thermometer and check to make sure it is intact.

    The plastic sheath prevents cross-contamination.

11. Place the bulb of the thermometer sublingually in patient's mouth.

    The large number of blood vessels located under the tongue creates an ideal environment for accurate measurement of the body temperature.

12. Explain to the patient how to keep the thermometer in the proper position.

    Advise the patient to keep the thermometer under the tongue, with lips closed, not to talk, and not to bite down.

13. Time the procedure for a minimum of 3 minutes.

    Use a watch or timer.

14. Remove the thermometer and read the results.

    If the temperature is 97° F or lower, reinsert the thermometer for an additional minute.

15. Remove the plastic sheath and discard in the appropriate biohazardous container.

    Hold the thermometer by the end of the stem, pull the plastic sheath off, and discard.

16. Rinse the thermometer and place in the disinfectant.

    Remember: The thermometer must remain in the disinfectant for a minimum of 20 minutes before rinsing and storing in the appropriate container.

17. Remove gloves and discard in appropriate biohazardous waste container.

    Per Standard Precautions.

18. Wash hands.

    Washing your hands reduces the risk of infection.

19. Record results in patient chart.

    Record the results as quickly as possible to reduce the risk of errors. Record results using the following format:

    T—P.O. (by mouth) 103.2° F.

Measuring a Rectal or Axillary Temperature—Glass Thermometer

Phlebotomy technicians will rarely, if ever, be required to take a rectal temperature on a patient. Tympanic temperatures have routinely replaced axillary temperatures in most laboratory and hospital settings. Therefore, these procedures are only briefly discussed in this text. The rectal temperature procedure is performed with the same steps as the oral temperature procedure with these exceptions:

● Rectal thermometer (red dot on stem) is selected.
● KY Jelly is required.
● Position the patient lying face down on exam table or bed. The patient pulls his left leg up towards the chest. Expose the rectal area. Protect the patient's modesty.
● Apply KY Jelly to the sheathed rectal thermometer.
● Insert the thermometer into the rectum, just past the anal sphincter. (Sometimes asking the patient to bear down makes insertion easier.)
● Hold the thermometer physically in place for a minimum of 2 minutes.

The procedure for an axillary temperature follows the same steps as the oral temperature procedure, with the following exceptions:

● Safety/security thermometer is used.
● Insert the thermometer into either the right or left axillary space.
● Have the patient support the thermometer by holding it between the arm and the body. Leave the thermometer in place for a minimum of 10 minutes.

Measuring an Oral Temperature with a Disposable Thermometer

Disposable thermometers may be used in some hospital emergency rooms, smaller clinical laboratories, and some blood banking facilities. Disposable thermometers have several advantages. They are used only once and then discarded, eliminating the risk of cross-contamination. They are also time-efficient, and require no additional equipment.

Disposable thermometers are made of a thin piece of plastic with temperature-sensitive dots on the wider end. The dots react to the temperature inside the patient's mouth (Figure 6-10).

The thermometer is inserted into the mouth and is positioned under the tongue as far back as possible into the heat pockets (located in the back corners of the sublingual area), with the tongue pressed against it and the mouth closed (Figure 6-11). It does not make any difference if the dots are face up or down. Leave the thermometer in place for 60 seconds, and then remove. Allow the dots to stabilize for 10 seconds, then read and record the temperature. The dots are read by looking at the last dot to change color within a degree grouping. Discard the thermometer in the appropriate biohazardous waste container. Disposable thermometers are not as accurate as other thermometers, so when working with a patient with a sensitive medical condition in which an accurate temperature reading is required (for example, an infant with possible spinal meningitis), choose a glass or tympanic thermometer.

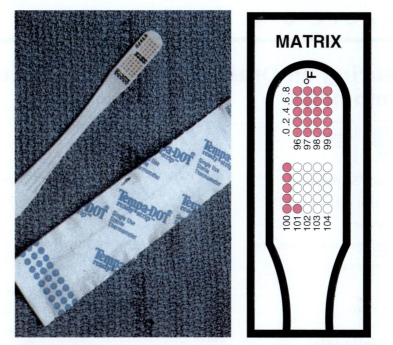

FIGURE 6-10: Disposable thermometer (Courtesy 3M Health Care)

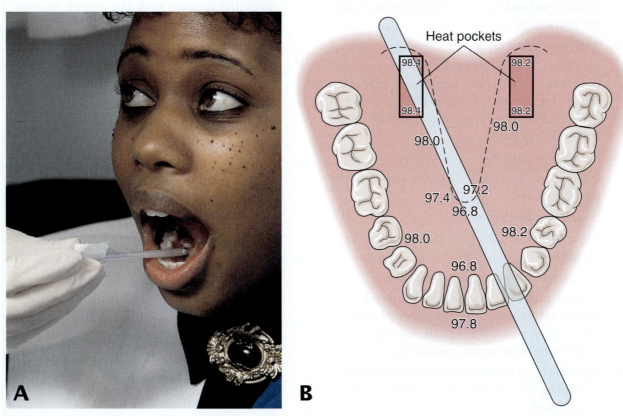

FIGURE 6-11: (A) Place oral thermometer sublingually into a heat pocket; (B) Dot matrix portion of disposable thermometer must be placed sublingually into a heat pocket. (Courtesy 3M Health Care)

Procedure 6-4

Measuring an Oral Temperature with a Disposable Thermometer

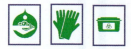

Equipment/Supplies

- Disposable thermometer
- Latex gloves
- Biohazardous waste container
- Watch or timer
- Pen
- Patient chart

Method/*Rationale*

1. Assemble equipment and supplies.

   Ensures everything is available to perform the procedure.

2. Wash hands/put on gloves.

   Thorough handwashing aids in controlling the spread of infections. Remember that you must comply with Standard Precautions whenever you may come in contact with body fluids or blood.

3. Identify the patient.

   Ensures the procedure is performed on the correct patient.

4. Explain the procedure.

   Helps ensure you will have the cooperation of the patient.

5. Ask the patient about recent activities.

   In order to obtain accurate results the patient should not have had something hot or cold to eat or drink within the last 10 minutes. If so, allow 10 minutes before measuring.

6. Open package by peeling back the protective wrapping to expose the handle of the thermometer.

   Grasp the handle and remove from the wrapper. Avoid touching the end of the thermometer displaying the dots. Touching the dots may interfere with the chemical reaction of the dots.

7. Insert thermometer sublingually in patient's mouth.

   Put it as far back as possible into one of the heat pockets to get the most accurate reading.

8. Explain to the patient how to keep the thermometer in the proper position.

   Advise patient to keep the thermometer under the tongue, with the tongue pressed firmly against the thermometer and lips closed, not to talk, and not to bite down.

9. Time the procedure for 60 seconds.

   Use a watch or timer.

10. Remove the thermometer and wait for 10 seconds for the dots to stabilize.

11. Read the results.

12. Discard the thermometer in the appropriate biohazardous waste container.

13. Remove gloves and discard in the appropriate biohazardous waste container.

    Per Standard Precautions.

14. Wash hands.

    Washing your hands helps to reduce the risk of infection.

15. Record results in patient's chart.

    Record the results as quickly as possible to reduce the risk of errors. Record results using the following format:

    T—P.O. (by mouth) 102.6° F

    Chart in the same manner as for an oral temperature taken with a glass thermometer.

Electronic Thermometers

The use of electronic thermometers is widely practiced in hospital and laboratory settings. Each unit is battery-operated, portable, easy to read, sanitary, and does not require cleaning (Figure 6-12). The electronic thermometer is equipped with a metal probe that is color-coded—blue for oral and red for rectal—just like the glass mercury thermometers. A cord attaches the probe to the battery unit. Prior to taking an oral temperature, the probe is inserted into a rigid plastic disposable sheath and then inserted into the patient's mouth exactly like the glass thermometer. However, it needs to be held in place by the phlebotomy technician because the probe with the attached cord is too heavy for the patient to hold in the mouth without support. When the patient's true temperature has been reached, usually in just a matter of a few seconds, the unit beeps and the temperature is displayed in the digital readout area of the device. When not in use, the unit must be returned to its charger to maintain adequate battery levels.

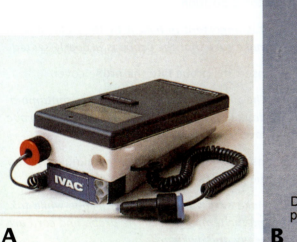

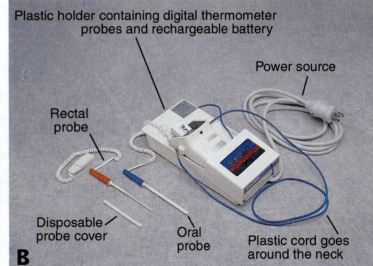

Plastic holder containing digital thermometer probes and rechargeable battery

Power source

Rectal probe

Disposable probe cover

Oral probe

Plastic cord goes around the neck

A

B

FIGURE 6-12: (A) Electronic thermometer; (B) Digital thermometers have interchangeable oral and rectal probes attached to a battery-operated portable unit.

Aural/Tympanic Membrane Thermometers

The most recent development in measuring temperatures is the tympanic membrane, or aural thermometer (Figure 6-13). These thermometers measure the body's core temperature by measuring the infrared heat waves generated by the tympanic membrane in the ear. Because the tympanic membrane shares the same blood supply as the hypothalamus located in the brain, it makes it an ideal site for obtaining an accurate assessment of the body's core tempera-

Procedure 6-5

Measuring an Oral Temperature with an Electronic Thermometer

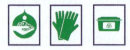

Equipment/Supplies

- Electronic oral thermometer (blue)
- Thermometer charger
- Thermometer probe cover
- Latex gloves
- Biohazardous waste container
- Watch or timer
- Pen
- Patient chart

Method/*Rationale*

1. Assemble equipment and supplies.

   Ensures everything is available to perform the procedure.

2. Wash hands/put on gloves.

   Thorough handwashing aids in controlling the spread of infections. Remember that you must comply with Standard Precautions whenever you may come in contact with body fluids or blood.

3. Identify the patient.

   Ensures the procedure is performed on the correct patient.

4. Explain the procedure.

   Helps ensure you will have the cooperation of the patient.

5. Ask the patient about recent activities.

   If the patient has had something hot or cold to drink or has smoked within the last 10 minutes, the results will be inaccurate. If so, allow 10 minutes before measuring.

6. Remove the appropriate probe from the stored position.

   It is important to hold it by the collar and to make sure that the probe is properly seated.

7. Insert the probe into the probe cover.

   The probe cover prevents cross-contamination. Press firmly to make sure the probe cover is properly seated.

8. Insert the covered probe sublingually into the patient's mouth.

   Make sure you support the probe while taking the temperature. The probe and cord are heavy and awkward.

ture. The tympanic thermometer is very easy to use and the results are obtained in seconds. The site is more accessible, and it does not require the health care worker to come in contact with mucous membranes. The patient does not even need to be conscious. The readings are also not affected by eating or drinking hot or cold foods or liquids, or by smoking, so the process is more time efficient.

A lightweight plastic probe cover is placed over the end of the device and is fully inserted into the patient's ear. The ear canal must be sealed completely with the probe or the results will be inaccu-

9. Keep the thermometer in place until the patient's temperature registers and the unit beeps.

   This is usually just a matter of seconds.

10. Remove the probe and read the results.

    The results will display in the digital readout window.

11. Remove the plastic probe cover by pressing the eject button, and discard in the appropriate biohazardous waste container.

    Press the eject button while holding the probe over the biohazardous waste container. Complies with Standard Precautions.

12. Return the probe to the storage position and return the unit to the charger.

    The thermometer will zero out and then shut off. Returning the unit to the charger will ensure that the battery will always be charged.

13. Remove gloves and discard in the appropriate biohazardous container.

    Per Standard Precautions.

14. Wash hands.

    Washing your hands helps to reduce the risk of infection.

15. Record results in patient's chart.

    Record the results as quickly as possible to reduce the risk of errors. Record results using the following format:

    T—P.O. (by mouth) 99.6° F

    Charting is the same as for a glass thermometer. No change in charting procedure is necessary because the thermometer is disposable.

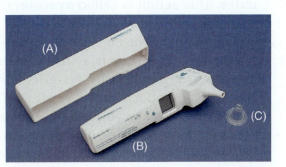

FIGURE 6-13: Tympanic thermometer: (A) Holder; (B) Tympanic thermometer; (C) Disposable speculum or cover

rate. You may need to straighten the ear canal by gently pulling the ear lobe down and back for an adult, or down and forward for a child (Figure 6-14). The scan button is pressed to activate the thermometer. The infrared beam then measures the heat waves of the tympanic membrane, and seconds later the patient's temperature is displayed in the digital readout window of the device. The release button is pressed and the probe cover ejects. Ten seconds later the device is ready to be used on another patient. The device operates on three AAA alkaline batteries and will measure thousands of temperatures before new batteries are needed. Most hospital and clinical laboratories use the tympanic thermometer.

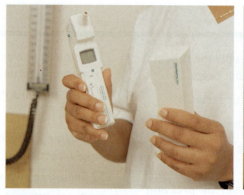

FIGURE 6-14 (A): Attach the disposable speculum or cover to the tympanic thermometer to prevent spread of microorganisms between patients.

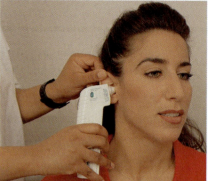

FIGURE 6-14 (B): Pull up on the ear to straighten the auditory canal for an accurate reading.

⬤ BLOOD PRESSURE

Blood pressure is the tension exerted by blood against the arterial walls as the heart alternately contracts and relaxes. After the heart contracts, blood is pumped out of the ventricles into the body's arteries. This action is called **systole**, the phase when the heart is at work. When the heart contracts it then relaxes and the ventricles fill with blood from the body's veins. This action is called **diastole**, the phase when the heart is at rest. Taking a patient's blood pressure measures the heart's activity, reflecting the condition of the heart at work and at rest. It also measures the condition of the arteries, and, to some degree, the volume and viscosity (stickiness) of the blood.

Learning to measure blood pressure requires understanding the process, learning the correct technique, and paying attention to details. Measuring blood pressure is a noninvasive procedure and relatively easy to master. It requires the use of a stethoscope and a **sphygmomanometer** (blood pressure cuff). There are two basic types of sphygmomanometers: the aneroid, which has a dial for reading, and the mercury, which has a calibrated mercury-filled tube, much like the mercury thermometer, for readings (Figures 6-15 and 6-16). The mercury sphygmomanometer is considered to be the most accurate. Both types measure the blood pressure in millimeters of mercury, which is abbreviated "mm Hg." Both sphygmomanometers are attached by tubing to a rubber bladder called the "cuff." A second rubber tube is attached to a hand pump with a screw valve. This hand pump is used to inflate the bladder in the cuff, which creates pressure on the arteries of the arm.

SYSTOLE

Contractions of the chambers of the heart, in which blood is pumped from the chamber.

DIASTOLE

The normal "rest period" in the heart cycle, during which the muscle fibers lengthen, the heart dilates, and the cavities fill with blood.

SPHYGMO-MANOMETER

An instrument for indirectly determining arterial blood pressure. The two types are aneroid and mercury.

Procedure 6-6

Measuring Core Body Temperature with a Tympanic Thermometer

Equipment/Supplies

- Tympanic thermometer
- Tympanic thermometer probe cover
- Waste container
- Pen
- Patient chart

Method/*Rationale*

1. Assemble equipment and supplies.

   Ensures everything is available to perform the procedure.

2. Wash hands.

   Thorough handwashing aids in controlling the spread of infections. Remember that you must comply with Standard Precautions whenever you may come in contact with body fluids or blood. It is not required to wear gloves for this procedure as you will not come in contact with mucous membranes or body fluids.

3. Identify the patient.

   Ensures the procedure is performed on the correct patient.

4. Explain the procedure.

   Helps ensure you will have the cooperation of the patient.

5. Remove thermometer from base.

6. Attach probe cover.

   The probe cover prevents cross-contamination. Press firmly to make sure the probe cover is properly seated.

7. The display window should read "ready."

8. Insert the covered probe into the patient's ear canal.

   Make sure you have the area sealed by inserting fully.

9. Press the scan button to activate the thermometer.

   This usually takes just a matter of seconds.

10. Withdraw the thermometer.

    The results will display in the digital readout window.

11. Remove the plastic probe cover by pressing the eject button, and discard in the appropriate waste container.

    Press the eject button while holding the probe over the waste container. Complies with Standard Precautions.

12. Wash hands.

    Washing your hands helps reduce the risk of infection.

13. Record results in patient's chart.

    Record the results as quickly as possible to reduce the risk of errors. Record results using the following format:

    T—T or Tc (tympanic) 99.6˚ F

    The tympanic thermometer can be set to correlate with an oral or rectal reading. Generally the oral mode is used and a temperature of 98.6˚ F is considered normal.

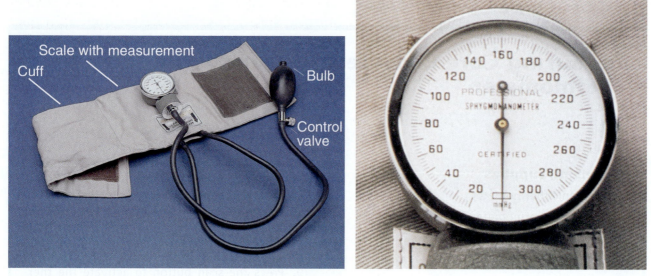

FIGURE 6-15: Aneroid sphygmomanometer

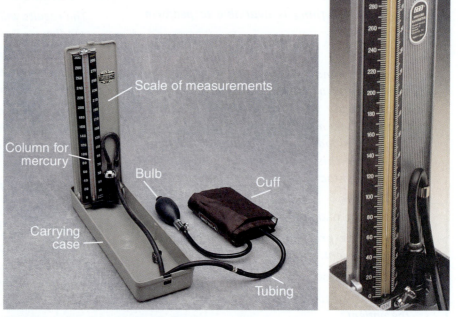

FIGURE 6-16: (A) Mercury sphygmomanometer with cuff; (B) Mercury sphygmomanometer scale.

Every time you use an aneroid or mercury sphygmomanometer you must check to see that it is correctly calibrated. The aneroid recording needle on the dial must rest within the small square at the bottom of the dial. With the mercury sphygmomanometer, check to see that the column of mercury at the **meniscus** rests at zero when viewed at eye level. Quality control procedures require these two in-

MENISCUS

The curved upper surface of a liquid in a container.

struments to be calibrated every 6 months by the manufacturer or a medical repair company. Not routinely calibrating your sphygmomanometers increases the risk of recording inaccurate results that could lead to the patient being incorrectly diagnosed. The patient could then be treated for a condition she does not have.

A third type of blood pressure device is the electronic sphygmomanometer (Figure 6-17). Although easier to use and an excellent method for individuals to use at home, most medical facilities prefer the aneroid or mercury sphygmomanometers because they are more accurate.

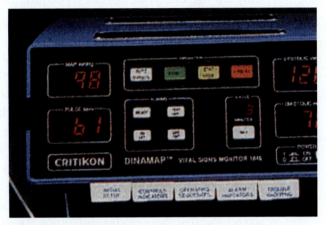

FIGURE 6-17: Electronic sphygmomanometer

A stethoscope is the second piece of blood pressure measuring equipment. Once the cuff has been inflated, the bell of the stethoscope is placed over the brachial artery, allowing the phlebotomy technician to listen to the first and last heartbeats as the cuff is slowly deflated.

Box 6-3: Sphygmomanometer and Stethoscope

In 1816, Rene Laennec invented the stethoscope. It is still one of the physician's most valuable diagnostic tools.

In 1896, an Italian physician, Scipinoi Riva-Rocci, invented the sphygmomanometer. He used a mercury column for measurement of external arterial blood pressure.

An average adult blood pressure is 120 systolic and 80 diastolic. The normal adult ranges are 90 to 140 mm Hg systolic and 60 to 90 mm Hg diastolic. Blood pressure is recorded as a fraction with the systolic pressure as the numerator (top) and the diastolic pressure as the denominator (bottom) (i.e., 120/80 mm Hg).

HYPERTENSION

A condition in which the patient has a higher than normal blood pressure. For adults, this usually means a BP >140/90.

HYPOTENSION

A decrease of the systolic and diastolic blood pressure value, which are significantly lower than normal.

Medications and various conditions, such as diabetes and shock, can cause the blood pressure to increase or decrease above or below the normal ranges. Blood pressure consistently measured at 140/90 mm Hg or higher is defined as **hypertension**, or high blood pressure. Hypertension is called the "silent killer," because it often has no symptoms. Also, if undiagnosed or untreated, it is the leading cause of heart attacks. A blood pressure consistently measured at 90/60 mm Hg or lower is defined as **hypotension**, or low blood pressure. Slightly lower blood pressure is not uncommon in healthy adults. Shock, heart failure, severe burns, and excessive bleeding may be the cause of severe hypotension.

Measuring Blood Pressure

The first step in taking a blood pressure is choosing the cuff size that is most appropriate for the patient. Blood pressure cuffs are available in a variety of sizes: neonate, child, adult, obese adult, and adult thigh (Figure 6-18). Using the correct size is critical in measuring the patient's blood pressure accurately. If the cuff is too small, the reading will be falsely high, and if too large, falsely low. The cuff should be approximately 20% wider than the arm and/or approximately 3/4 of the length of the upper arm.

To measure a patient's blood pressure, wrap the cuff around the patient's arm, approximately two finger widths above the bend of the arm or brachial artery. Either arm may be used. However, if there has been an injury to one arm, or if the patient has had a mastectomy or some other surgery on one side, then the blood pressure must be taken on the opposite arm. If a patient has had double mastectomies or double amputations of the arms, the blood pressure may be taken on the thigh, using a thigh cuff.

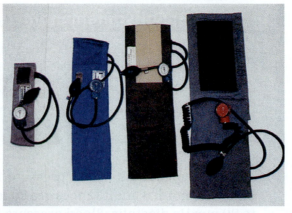

FIGURE 6-18: Blood pressure cuffs in sizes to fit the arm of a small child to an adult thigh. It is important to have the correct size to obtain an accurate reading.

After selecting the appropriate site, the cuff is inflated. The stethoscope (Figure 6-19) is placed over the brachial artery, and the air is released slowly, 2 mm Hg per second. To ensure that the air is released slowly from the cuff, place the hand pump bulb in your dominant hand and turn the screw counterclockwise until the dial of the aneroid cuff or the mercury in the column of the mercury cuff is slowly moving downward (Figure 6-20). As you listen through the stethoscope you should hear only silence at first. If you hear a heartbeat, you have not inflated the cuff to a high enough level—deflate and reinflate. The first vascular sounds you hear are called Korotkoff's sounds. The expansion and relaxation of the arterial walls as blood pulses through produces these vascular, or Kortokoff's, sounds. Record the first sound you hear as the systolic pressure. The sound will change to a softer muffled sound as the pressure in the sphygmomanometer continues to fall. The last sound you hear is recorded as the diastolic pressure.

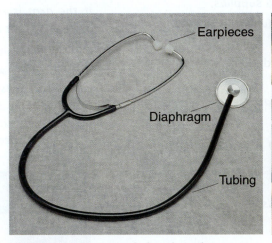

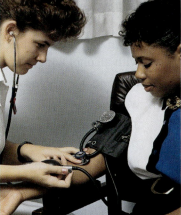

FIGURE 6-19: A single-head stethoscope. Used with a sphygmomanometer to measure blood pressure.

FIGURE 6-20: Measuring blood pressure

Box 6-4: Blood Pressure

If your patient is anxious, nervous, agitated, or in pain prior to measuring blood pressure, the pressure may be falsely elevated. Talk to your patient calmly and explain that you are going to have him or her wait quietly for 10 minutes. Have your patient take a few deep breaths in through the nose and out through the mouth. Retake the blood pressure. If the pressure is still elevated, have the patient contact the physician for follow-up care or, if the patient is hospitalized, notify the nurse or physician.

Procedure 6-7

Measuring a Blood Pressure

Equipment/Supplies

- Stethoscope
- Mercury or aneroid manometer
- Alcohol wipe
- Pen
- Patient chart

Method/*Rationale*

1. Assemble equipment and supplies.

   Ensures everything is available to perform the procedure.

2. Clean earpieces and head of the stethoscope with alcohol wipes.

   Prevents the spread of pathogens.

3. Wash hands.

   Thorough handwashing aids in controlling the spread of infections.

4. Identify the patient.

   Ensures the procedure is performed on the correct patient.

5. Explain the procedure.

   Helps ensure you will have the cooperation of the patient.

6. Have your patient either sitting in a comfortable position or lying down.

   If the patient is not comfortable or is exerting excess energy, the blood pressure may be falsely increased.

7. Position the blood pressure cuff either on a level surface for the mercury cuff, or near the patient for the aneroid cuff.

The mercury cuff may be mounted on a wall at eye level, on a portable cart, which is easy to move from room to room, or placed on a counter or tabletop. The aneroid cuff should be placed within easy reach. A clip may attach the dial to the cuff or the dial may be placed on the table or bed for easy viewing.

8. Extend the patient's arm at a level less than or equal to the patient's heart, palm up.

   If the arm is raised higher than the heart level, the pulse may be falsely increased.

9. Expose the patient's arm well past the elbow.

   It is best if the arm is bare. However, an accurate blood pressure can be taken over light clothing. Make sure that nothing is constricting the arm, such as the sleeve of a shirt that has been pushed up to expose the arm.

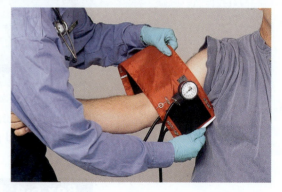

10. Support the arm, palm of hand facing up.

    The arm should be relaxed but well supported, with the elbow slightly bent.

11. With the valve of the inflation bulb open, squeeze all the air from the bladder. Fold the cuff to identify the center and place the bottom of the cuff edge 1 to 2 inches above the bend of the elbow. Wrap the cuff smoothly and snugly around the arm.

    It is important that all air is removed from the bladder prior to placing the cuff on the patient's arm. Residual air in the bladder will cause the results to be inaccurate.

12. With one hand, close the valve on the bulb, clockwise.

    Do not close the valve too tightly as it will be difficult to loosen when releasing the air from the bladder.

13. Place the fingertips of your other hand on the radial pulse.

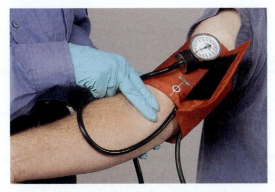

14. While watching the sphygmomanometer, inflate the cuff to 30 mm Hg above the level where the pulse disappears.

15. Open the valve, slowly releasing air until the radial pulse is detected once again.

    This will provide you with a palpatory systolic pressure. The result is recorded, using the format B/P 120 (P).

16. Deflate cuff completely. Squeeze any remaining air from the cuff.

    The bladder must be completely empty between inflations to obtain accurate results. Allow a minimum of 30 seconds before reinflating the cuff. Thirty seconds is the average amount of time necessary for the blood flowing through the arteries to return to normal.

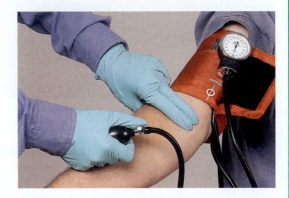

17. Position earpieces of stethoscope in your ears with openings entering your ear canal.

18. Palpate the brachial artery at the medial antecubital space with your fingertips.

19. Place the head of the stethoscope directly over the palpated pulse.

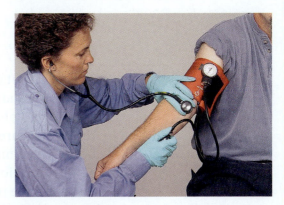

20. Close the valve of the bulb and quickly inflate the cuff to 30 mm Hg above the palpated systolic pressure.

(continues)

Procedure 6-7 *(continued)*

21. Open the valve and slowly deflate the cuff.

    Pressure should drop between 2 to 3 mm Hg per second.

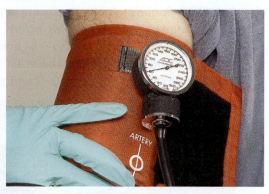

22. Note the reading either on the aneroid dial or at the meniscus of the mercury column.

    The first sound you hear is the systolic pressure. It must be a minimum of two consecutive beats.

23. Allow the pressure to steadily lower until you note a change in sound.

    The sound will continue as a soft muffled beat, until you can no longer hear a beat. Note, the last beat you hear is the diastolic pressure.

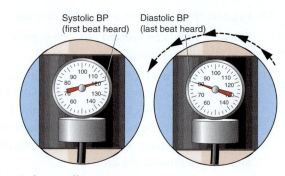

Systolic BP (first beat heard)   Diastolic BP (last beat heard)

24. Release all remaining air.
25. Re-evaluate if necessary after a minimum of 30 seconds.
26. Remove stethoscope from ears.
27. Remove the cuff from the patient's arm.
28. Record systolic and diastolic pressure in patient's chart.

    Example: B/P 124/86 mm Hg

29. Clean tips of stethoscope with alcohol wipes.
30. Return equipment to storage area.
31. Wash hands.

    Washing your hands before and after every patient reduces the risk of infection.

❙ SUMMARY

A patient's vital signs are measurements of essential life-sustaining functions and are the primary indicators of a patient's overall health. As a phlebotomy technician you may be required to perform these measurements as part of your routine duties. Other phlebotomy technicians may only perform these functions occasionally as the situation demands. Regardless, these important diagnostic tests provide the patient's physician with valuable information. It is your responsibility to maintain proficiency with these skills.

COMPETENCY CHECK-OFF SHEETS
Respiration Competency Check

Given all the equipment and supplies, the student will be required to perform, within 3 minutes, a respiration rate.

A "0" in more than two areas or an overall percent of less than 80 will require the procedure to be repeated for competency.

Points to Be Awarded:	5 pts	2.5 pts	1 pt	0 pt	total pts
1. Assemble equipment and supplies					
2. Wash hands					
3. Identify patient					
4. Explain procedure					
5. Ask the patient about recent activities					
6. Position patient					
7. Assess the quality of the respirations					
8. Count respirations					
9. Record results in patient chart					
10. Wash hands					

Total points possible: _____ Total points earned: _____

Start time: _____ End time: _____

Instructor signature: _____ Date: _____

Student signature: _____ Date: _____

Radial Pulse Competency Check

Given all the equipment and supplies, the student will be required to perform, within 3 minutes, a radial pulse.

A "0" in more than two areas or an overall percent of less than 80 will require the procedure to be repeated for competency.

Points to Be Awarded:	5 pts	2.5 pts	1 pt	0 pt	total pts
1. Assemble equipment and supplies					
2. Wash hands					
3. Identify patient					
4. Explain procedure					
5. Position patient					
6. Locate radial pulse					
7. Observe quality of pulse					
8. Count beats per minute—30 seconds × 2					
9. Record results in patient chart					
10. Wash hands					

Total points possible: _____ Total points earned: _____

Start time: _____ End time: _____

Instructor signature: _____ Date: _____

Student signature: _____ Date: _____

Oral Temperature—Glass Mercury Thermometer Competency Check

Given all the equipment and supplies, the student will be required to perform, within 6 minutes, an oral temperature.

A "0" in more than two areas or an overall percent of less than 80 will require the procedure to be repeated for competency.

Points to Be Awarded:	5 pts	2.5 pts	1 pt	0 pt	total pts
1. Assemble equipment and supplies					
2. Wash hands/glove					
3. Identify patient					
4. Explain procedure					
5. Ask the patient about recent activities					
6. Remove thermometer from case or envelope					
7. Inspect the thermometer					
8. Shake down thermometer below 96° F					
9. Sheath thermometer/insert sublingually					
10. Explain proper positioning to patient					
11. Time procedure for a minimum of 3 minutes					
12. Remove thermometer/read results					
13. Remove and discard sheath in biohazard waste					
14. Rinse thermometer and disinfect					
15. Remove gloves/discard in biohazard waste					
16. Wash hands					
17. Record results in patient chart					

Total points possible: _____ Total points earned: _____

Start time: _____ End time: _____

Instructor signature: _____ Date: _____

Student signature: _____ Date: _____

Oral Temperature—Disposable Thermometer Competency Check

Given all the equipment and supplies, the student will be required to perform, within 3 minutes, an oral temperature.

A "0" in more than two areas or an overall percent of less than 80 will require the procedure to be repeated for competency.

Points to Be Awarded:	5 pts	2.5 pts	1 pt	0 pt	total pts
1. Assemble equipment and supplies					
2. Wash hands/glove					
3. Identify patient					
4. Explain procedure					
5. Ask the patient about recent activities					
6. Open disposable thermometer package					
7. Insert thermometer sublingually					
8. Explain proper positioning to patient					
9. Time procedure for a minimum of 60 seconds					
10. Remove thermometer/read results					
11. Discard in biohazard waste					
12. Remove gloves/discard in biohazard waste					
13. Wash hands					
14. Record results in patient chart					

Total points possible: _____ Total points earned: _____

Start time: _____ End time: _____

Instructor signature: _____ Date: _____

Student signature: _____ Date: _____

Oral Temperature—Electronic Thermometer Competency Check

Given all the equipment and supplies, the student will be required to perform, within 3 minutes, an oral temperature.

A "0" in more than two areas or an overall percent of less than 80 will require the procedure to be repeated for competency.

Points to Be Awarded:	5 pts	2.5 pts	1 pt	0 pt	total pts
1. Assemble equipment and supplies					
2. Wash hands/glove					
3. Identify patient					
4. Explain procedure					
5. Ask the patient about recent activities					
6. Remove appropriate probe from stored position					
7. Insert probe into the probe cover					
8. Insert covered probe sublingually					
9. Hold thermometer in patient's mouth					
10. Unit beeps/temperature registers					
11. Remove probe/read results					
12. Remove probe cover and discard in biohazard waste					
13. Return probe to storage position/charger					
14. Remove gloves/discard in biohazard waste					
15. Wash hands					

Total points possible: _____ Total points earned: _____

Start time: _____ End time: _____

Instructor signature: _____ Date: _____

Student signature: _____ Date: _____

Measuring Body Temperature—Tympanic Thermometer Competency Check

Given all the equipment and supplies, the student will be required to perform, within 3 minutes, a tympanic temperature.

A "0" in more than two areas or an overall percent of less than 80 will require the procedure to be repeated for competency.

Points to Be Awarded:	5 pts	2.5 pts	1 pt	0 pt	total pts
1. Assemble equipment and supplies					
2. Wash hands					
3. Identify patient					
4. Explain procedure					
5. Remove thermometer from base					
6. Attach probe cover					
7. Check display window for "ready" signal					
8. Insert probe into ear canal and check the seal					
9. Press scan button to activate					
10. Withdraw thermometer					
11. Remove probe cover and discard in biohazard waste					
12. Return thermometer to base					
13. Wash hands					
14. Record results in patient chart					

Total points possible: _____   Total points earned: _____

Start time: _____   End time: _____

Instructor signature: _____   Date: _____

Student signature: _____   Date: _____

Measuring Blood Pressure Competency Check

Given all the equipment and supplies, the student will be required to perform, within 8 minutes, a blood pressure.

A "0" in more than two areas or an overall percent of less than 80 will require the procedure to be repeated for competency.

Points to Be Awarded:	5 pts	2.5 pts	1 pt	0 pt	total pts
1. Assemble equipment and supplies					
2. Clean earpieces and head of stethoscope					
3. Wash hands					
4. Identify patient					
5. Explain procedure					
6. Position patient					
7. Expose patient's arm					
8. Squeeze all air from bladder of cuff					
9. Close valve					
10. Locate radial pulse					
11. Inflate cuff 30 mm Hg above disappearance of radial pulse					
12. Release air/deflate cuff completely					
13. Palpate brachial artery					
14. Position stethoscope					
15. Inflate cuff to 30 mm Hg above palpated pulse					
16. Open valve slowly—deflate cuff					
17. Note first sound heard as systolic pressure					
18. Note last sound heard as diastolic pressure					
19. Release remaining air					
20. Re-evaluate if necessary after 30 seconds					
21. Remove stethoscope and cuff from patient's arm					
22. Clean equipment/return to storage					

Points to Be Awarded:	5 pts	2.5 pts	1 pt	0 pt	total pts
23. Wash hands					
24. Record results in patient chart					

Total points possible: _____ Total points earned: _____

Start time: _____ End time: _____

Instructor signature: _____ Date: _____

Student signature: _____ Date: _____

STUDY AND REVIEW EXERCISES
Defining Key Terms
Write the definition for each of the following key terms.

1) afebrile _____

2) antecubital _____

3) apnea _____

4) arrhythmia _____

5) auscultate _____

6) brachial _____

7) bradycardia _____

8) bradypnea _____

9) carotid _____

10) diastole _____

11) febrile _____

12) hypertension _____

13) hypotension _____

14) hypothermia _____

15) meniscus _____

16) palpate _____

17) pulse _____

18) radial _____

19) respiration _____

20) sphygmomanometer _____

21) sublingual _____

22) systole _____

23) tachycardia _____

24) tachypnea _____

25) vital signs _____

Reviewing Key Points

1) List the four vital signs and describe the body functions they monitor.

2) Describe what causes a pulse and identify where a pulse can be located.

3) Identify the normal rate of respirations and describe the associated characteristics.

4) Describe how the body regulates temperature.

5) Identify the phases of blood pressure, and compare them to the actions of the heart.

Sentence Completion

1) _____ are a measurement of essential life-sustaining functions.

2) The _____ is felt as a throbbing sensation caused by the regular contraction and relaxation of the arterial walls.

3) The _____ pulse is located on the inner medial surface of the elbow at the _____ space.

4) A pulse that lacks a regular rhythm is an _____.

5) The _____ rate indicates how well a patient's body is providing oxygen to tissues.

6) Body temperature is regulated by thermoregulatory centers in the _____.

7) The cavity of a glass thermometer is filled with _____.

8) _____ is the tension exerted by blood against the arterial walls as the heart alternately contracts and relaxes.

9) Every time you use a sphygmomanometer you must make sure that it has been correctly _____.

10) When taking a patient's blood pressure with a mercury sphygmomanometer you will read the column of mercury at the _____ when viewed at eye level.

Multiple Choice

1) All the following are vital signs except:
   A. respiration
   B. blood pressure
   C. reflex
   D. pulse

2) The _____ pulse can be felt behind the knee.
   A. radial
   B. carotid
   C. femoral
   D. popliteal

3) The _____ pulse can be felt on the thumb side of the inner surface of the wrist.
   A. radial
   B. dorsalis pedis
   C. brachial
   D. popliteal

4) The amount of blood that flows through an artery is the pulse _____.
   A. rate
   B. rhythm
   C. volume
   D. capacity

5) Because a patient can control this vital sign to some degree, it is important that the patient not know you are measuring it.
   A. Temperature
   B. Reflex
   C. Pulse
   D. Respiration

6) The terms weak and thready describe which vital sign?
   A. Temperature
   B. Pulse
   C. Respiration
   D. Blood pressure

7) Oral temperatures of average healthy adults range from:
   A. 97.5° F to 99.5° F
   B. 98.6° F to 99.6° F
   C. 95.6° F to 98.4° F
   D. 96.8° F to 98.6° F

8) When the heart contracts and blood is pumped out of the ventricles into the body's arteries it is called:
   A. palpation
   B. systole
   C. diastole
   D. auscultation

9) The average healthy adult blood pressure is:
   A. 110/90
   B. 120/80
   C. 140/90
   D. 90/60

10) Shock, heart failure, severe burns, and excessive bleeding can cause:
   A. hypertension
   B. hyperthermia
   C. hypotension
   D. hypothermia

Critical Thinking

1) Your patient in Room 312 needs to have her temperature taken. The nurse asks you if you would mind taking it before you draw your labs. You introduce yourself to Mrs. Thompson and identify her by her hospital identification band. You wash your hands and start to assemble your equipment. You can only find a glass mercury thermometer with a red dot on the stem. You are pretty sure that Mrs. Thompson will not require a rectal temperature. She is coherent with no visual injuries of the face or mouth. What would you do?

2) Mr. Goldberg rushes into your outpatient laboratory to have his blood drawn before going to work this morning. He is agitated and yells at the laboratory clerk that he does not have time to wait. Your laboratory requires you to obtain a patient's blood pressure before drawing any labs. Mr. Goldberg's blood pressure is 152/102. What is your next step?

Electrocardiography

KEY TERMS

apex
arrhythmia (ah-**RITH**-mee-ah)
artifact
atria (plural); atrium (singular)
atrioventricular (AV) node
bipolar
bundle of His
cardiac cycle
complexes
coronary circulation
dermis (**DUR**-mis)
depolarization
diaphoretic (**dye**-ah-for-**ET**-ik)
electrocardiogram (ECG)
electrodes
endocardium
   (**en**-do-**KAR**-dee-um)
epicardium
   (**ep**-ih-**KAR**-dee-um)
epidermis (**ep**-ih-**DUR**-mis)
galvanometer
   (**gal**-van-**OM**-et-er)
intervals
ischemia (ih-**SKEE**-me-ah)
mediastinum
   (**mee**-dee-as-**TIH**-num)
myocardium
   (**MY**-oh-**kar**-dee-um)
P wave
polarized
P-R interval
precordial leads
   (pre-**KOR**-dee-al leeds)
pulmonary circulation
Purkinje fibers (pur-**KIN**-gee)

(continues)

OBJECTIVES

Upon completion of this chapter the student should be able to:

- Describe the structures of the heart.
- Distinguish between systemic, pulmonary, and coronary circulation.
- List the components of the electrical conduction system of the heart and the sequence of impulse origination.
- State the four properties of cardiac cells.
- Identify the basic electrophysiology of the heart, including polarization, depolarization, and repolarization.
- Describe the components of a 12-lead ECG and the lead wire orientation.
- Differentiate between ECG waves, segments, intervals, and complexes.
- Describe how the electrical impulse produces a predictable wave pattern as it moves through the heart.
- Describe the method used to detect and record electrical impulse wave patterns by an ECG machine.
- Describe the function and graph of ECG paper.
- Describe Einthoven's triangle and how it measures the electrical polarity of the heart.
- Differentiate between unipolar, bipolar, and precordial leads.
- Demonstrate the correct placement of limb leads and chest leads.
- Demonstrate the correct use of ECG equipment.
- Perform simple maintenance of, and troubleshoot, ECG equipment.

(continues)

- Perform an accurate ECG tracing in various situations for interpretation by a physician.
- Understand the importance of patient preparation for an ECG.
- Describe the effects of proper patient positioning for an ECG.
- Understand how the electrical impulse originating in the heart can be detected through the patient's skin.
- Demonstrate proper skin preparation and lead placement.
- Recognize artifacts on an ECG tracing and ways to prevent them.
- Describe special circumstances requiring special consideration when performing an ECG.
- Identify basic cardiac rhythms, including normal sinus rhythm, various other sinus rhythms, atrial arrhythmias, and ventricular arrhythmias.

OUTLINE

- Introduction
- History of Electrocardiography
- Review of the Anatomy and Physiology of the Heart
- Electrical Conduction of the Heart
- 12-Lead ECG Machine
- ECG Tracings
- The Lead System
- Performing an ECG
- Identifying Cardiac Rhythms

INTRODUCTION

The health care industry is continuously evolving and expanding. Part of this evolving process has been the expansion of duties and the development of the multiskilled allied health care provider. Phlebotomists, who once only collected laboratory specimens, are now performing expanded duties such as point-of-care testing and electrocardiography. With the addition of these skills comes added responsibility, a higher level of commitment, and increased job satisfaction. This chapter focuses on the phlebotomist's role in performing 12-lead ECGs. Basic anatomy and physiology of the circulatory system are reviewed. The principles of the heart's electrical conduction, the normal **cardiac cycle**, and the normal ECG complex are also presented. The phlebotomist must have an understanding of how the ECG machine works, how to prepare the patient for the procedure, proper placement of ECG leads, and how to identify a normal ECG rhythm. Identifying **artifacts** and trou-

CARDIAC CYCLE

A single rhythmic repetition of the mechanical and electrical events that constitute the heartbeat.

ARTIFACT

The appearance of a false signal not consistent with results expected from the signal being studied; may be produced by a defective machine, patient movement, or loose electrodes.

bleshooting interference is imperative in order to present a quality ECG tracing for interpretation by a physician. Upon completion of this chapter, the phlebotomist will also be able to recognize basic **arrhythmias**.

ARRHYTHMIA

An abnormal heart rhythm.

ELECTROCARDIO-GRAM (ECG)

A record of the electrical activity of the heart.

HISTORY OF ELECTROCARDIOGRAPHY

Since the invention of the **electrocardiogram (ECG)** in 1901, great advances have occurred in the understanding and treatment of diseases and conditions of the heart. Prior to this time, the heart was only observed by direct contact through an open chest.

Today, ECGs are a common diagnostic procedure performed routinely in medical facilities. However, the development of the modern ECG has quite a lengthy history, dating back to the 17th and 18th centuries. During the 1600s, scholars, scientists, physicians, and lay people were experimenting with harnessing electricity. William Gilbert, physician to Queen Elizabeth I and president of the Royal College of Surgeons, is credited with actually introducing the term "electric," which he applied to objects that held static electricity. The word is derived from the Greek word for amber, "electra."

With the ability to harness electricity, the next step was to discover what it could do. Early experiments were performed on frogs and chickens. It was soon discovered that if you applied an electrical current to the head of a chicken, it would die. However, if you applied the electrical current to the chest of the dead chicken it would come back to life, and even though it might not eat for a day or two, eventually it would lay eggs again. Soon, this technology was applied to the resuscitation of humans. In 1774, a 3-year-old girl fell to the ground from a first-story window and was determined to be dead. The young girl's parents rushed her across the street to the apothecary, where a Mr. Squires was working. With the girl's parents' permission, Mr. Squires tried the effects of electricity on the child, shocking her in various parts of her body without success. However, after sending several "shocks" through the thorax, the child sighed, and began to breathe. Although she remained in a stupor for days, she was eventually restored to perfect health. In 1791, Galvani discovered that electrical stimulation of a frog's heart results in cardiac muscle contraction. This led to further enthusiasm in the study of the use of electricity, and in 1792, attempts were made at reanimating the dead, with experiments on criminals put to death by hanging.

It was in the early 1800s that instruments were designed that were sensitive enough to detect the small electrical currents of the heart. Johann Schweigger invented the first galvanometer, the device that allows the recording of an electrical current on a graph. In 1842, Carlo Matteucci, a professor of physics at the University of Pisa, showed that an electrical current accompanies each heartbeat. In 1850, Ludwig M. Hoffa demonstrated that a single electrical impulse caused ventricular fibrillation in cats and dogs, and in 1887, the British physiologist Augustus D. Waller of St. Mary's Medical School in London, published the first electrocardiogram. Two years later in 1889, Willem Einthoven, a Dutch physiologist, observed Waller demonstrate the electrocardiogram on his dog "Jimmy," who stood patiently with his paws in a glass jar of saline through the procedure. In 1893, Einthoven introduced the term "electrocardiogram." In 1895, he improved the electrometer, distinguished five deflections, developed criteria for the normal ECG, and named the **waves** PQRS and T, which are based on a mathematical convention, using letters from the second half of the alphabet. Einthoven also established the positions for **electrode** placement on the body.

At this point, attention was paid to developing the ECG as a clinical tool, and refinements of the "tracings" occurred. In 1901, Einthoven invented a silver-coated fine quartz string galvanometer that was thousands of times more sensitive than previous models, and in 1903, he discussed commercial production of his string galvanometer after winning the Nobel prize for the invention of the electrocardiograph machine. In 1905, Einthoven transmitted an ECG from the hospital to his office via telephone, the first "telecardiogram." In 1906, the first fetal ECG was performed from the abdominal surface of a pregnant woman, and Einthoven published the first organized presentation of normal and abnormal electrocardiograms. The abnormalities included right and left atrial and ventricular hypertrophy, premature ventricular beats, ventricular bigeminy, atrial flutter, and the complete heart block. He also noted the U wave for the first time.

In 1908, the first string galvanometer was purchased by Edward Schafer for the University of Edinburgh. In 1912, Einthoven described an equilateral triangle formed by his standard leads I, II, and III. This was later called Einthoven's triangle and is still in use today. For the next several years, clinical observation and documentation of the size and shape of the PQRST waves and complexes took place during various cardiac situations. Heart blocks were also classified. In 1928, Ernstine and Levine reported the use of vacuum tubes to amplify the electrocardiogram instead of the mechanical amplification of the string galvanometer. During this year, the table model ECG machine became portable, weighing 50 pounds and powered by a 6-volt automobile battery. In 1932, Charles Wolferth and Francis Wood described the clinical use of chest leads, and in 1934, Frank Wilson defined unipolar limb leads VR, VL, and VF. In 1938, the American Heart Association and the Cardiac Society of Great Briton defined the standard positions and wiring of chest leads V_1 to V_6. Emanuel Goldberger increased the voltage of Wilson's unipolar leads by 50%, and in 1942, created the augmented limb leads aVR, aVL, and aVF. When added to Einthoven's three limb leads and the six chest leads, this resulted in the 12-lead ECG we use today.

REVIEW OF THE ANATOMY AND PHYSIOLOGY OF THE HEART

Remember from Chapter 3 that the heart is a hollow muscular organ that pumps blood (Figure 7-1). The heart is located between the lungs, in the middle of the chest, in the area referred to as the **mediastinum**. The heart is bordered anteriorly by the sternum and posteriorly by the spine. It consists of four chambers; the upper two chambers are called **atria** and function in a receiving or collecting capacity. The two lower chambers are called **ventricles** and are the pumping chambers of the heart. The chambers are separated into right and left halves by a wall of cartilage called the **septum**. The right atrium receives deoxygenated blood from the body via the superior and inferior vena cava. As the atria contract, blood is pushed through the tricuspid valve into the right ventricle. When the ventricles contract, the right ventricle pumps the blood through the pulmonary semilunar valve into the pulmonary artery and into the lungs, where the blood is oxygenated. The blood is then returned to the heart, into the left atrium. From there, the blood is pumped through the bicuspid (mitral) valve and into the left ventricle. The walls of the left ventricle are the thickest and strongest, because the greatest amount of exertion is required to pump the blood through the aorta and aortic valve into the body. The oxygenated blood is carried to the tissues through arteries. The arteries become smaller and smaller arterioles, which branch into the microscopic capillaries. In the capillaries, oxygen and nutrients are given to the tissues in exchange for waste products. The blood, now depleted of its supply of oxygen and nutrients, returns to the heart through the veins. The largest veins are the superior and inferior vena cava. The superior and inferior vena cava return the deoxygenated blood back to the right atrium and the process starts again. This entire process takes place every time the heart beats.

MEDIASTINUM

Region of the thoracic cavity containing the heart and blood vessels, lying between the sternum and vertebral column and between the lungs.

ATRIA (PLURAL) ATRIUM (SINGULAR)

Upper, collecting chambers of the heart.

VENTRICLES

Lower pumping chambers of the heart.

SEPTUM

A dividing wall between parts of the body. In the heart, the septum is located between the atria and also between the ventricles.

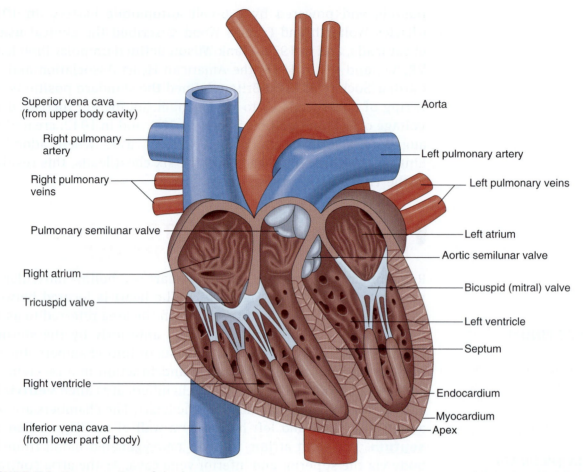

Superior vena cava
(from upper body cavity)

Right pulmonary
artery

Right pulmonary
veins

Pulmonary semilunar valve

Right atrium

Tricuspid valve

Right ventricle

Inferior vena cava
(from lower part of body)

Aorta

Left pulmonary artery

Left pulmonary veins

Left atrium

Aortic semilunar valve

Bicuspid (mitral) valve

Left ventricle

Septum

Endocardium

Myocardium

Apex

FIGURE 7-1: Cross-section of the heart

ENDOCARDIUM

Inner layer of the heart.

MYOCARDIUM

Middle layer of heart
muscle, responsible for
pumping action.

EPICARDIUM

External layer of the heart
and part of pericardial sac.

PURKINJE FIBERS

Modified myocardial cells
found in distal areas of the
bundle branches. They
conduct electricity from
the bundle of His through
the ventricles.

The heart is composed of three layers of cardiac muscle. Cardiac muscle is unique in that it is both striated (striped; marked by streaks) for strength like skeletal muscles, but at the same time, is an involuntary muscle like the smooth muscles of the stomach. The three layers of the heart muscle are the **endocardium**, **myocardium**, and **epicardium**. The endocardium is a smooth layer of cells lining the inside of the heart. It consists of a membrane composed of connective tissue and specialized cardiac fibers called **Purkinje fibers**. The Purkinje fibers play a vital role in the electrical conduction system of the heart. The middle layer is the myocardium, composed of cardiac muscle. These muscle cells are responsible for the contraction of the heart and the ultimate pumping of the blood. The myocardium is relatively thin in the atria, thicker in the right ventricle, and thickest in the left ventricle. The epicardium is the fatty outer layer of the heart. It forms a protective coating around the heart and consists of two layers. The outermost layer is the called the pericardium, which is a double layer of fibrous tissue. Between the two pericardial layers is a space filled with a lubricating fluid called pericardial fluid. This fluid prevents the two layers from rubbing against each other and creating friction.

Types of Circulation

The heart provides the body with three types of circulatory pathways.

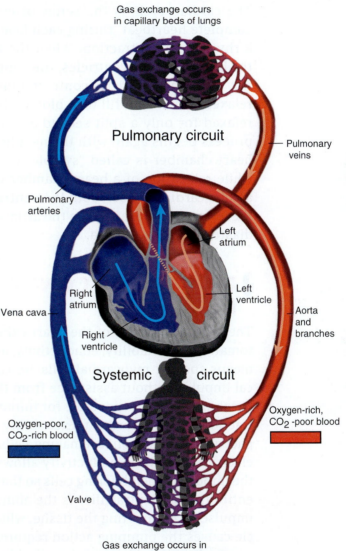

Gas exchange occurs
in capillary beds of lungs

Pulmonary circuit

Pulmonary veins

Pulmonary arteries

Left atrium

Right atrium

Left ventricle

Vena cava

Right ventricle

Aorta and branches

Systemic circuit

Oxygen-poor, CO_2-rich blood

Oxygen-rich, CO_2-poor blood

Valve

Gas exchange occurs in capillary beds of all body tissues

FIGURE 7-2: Systemic and pulmonary circulation

SYSTEMIC CIRCULATION

Flow of oxygen-rich blood to all body tissue and organs from the left ventricle via the arteries and the return of oxygen-depleted blood to the right atrium via the veins.

PULMONARY CIRCULATION

Flow of blood from right ventricle through the lungs, and back to the left atrium.

Systemic circulation consists of the blood vessels that provide oxygenated blood from the heart to all parts of the body and the return of deoxygenated blood back to the heart. **Pulmonary circulation** is the path deoxygenated blood follows from the right ventricle of the heart to the lungs and the path of oxygenated blood from the lungs back to the left atrium of the heart (Figure 7-2). The heart has its own circulatory system, called **coronary circulation**. The right and left coronary arteries are branches of the aorta. They supply the heart muscle and tissues with oxygen and nutrients.

The Cardiac Cycle

The cardiac cycle is the series of events that occurs during one complete heartbeat. During each heartbeat the heart goes through a rhythmical contraction. When the atria walls contract, pushing the blood into the ventricles, the ventricles are relaxed and able to fill. When the ventricles contract, pumping blood out, the atria are relaxed and able to fill with blood. The atria and ventricles remain relaxed for only a split second at the end of the cycle before the process begins again with the next heartbeat. The contraction of a heart chamber is called "systole" or the "systolic cardiac phase," while relaxation of a heart chamber is called "diastole" or the "diastolic cardiac phase." Both the ventricles and the atria go through these cardiac phases. When the atria are systolic, the ventricles are diastolic, and vice versa.

ELECTRICAL CONDUCTION OF THE HEART

The myocardial cells of the heart exhibit four unique qualities: automaticity, excitability, conductivity, and contractility. Automaticity means specific myocardial cells are capable of initiating an electrical impulse without assistance from the nervous system. This electrical impulse is responsible for initiating and maintaining the contraction of each heartbeat. Excitability is the inherent ability of both pacemaking and nonpacemaking cells to respond to a stimulus or electrical impulse. Conductivity allows the myocardial cells to pass the impulse to neighboring cells so that it can spread throughout the entire tissue. Contractility is the ability to respond to an electrical impulse by contracting the tissue, which in the case of cardiac muscle causes the pumping action required to circulate the blood.

Cardiac cells that are not capable of contracting work to initiate the electrical impulse that causes the heart to contract. The first group of these specialized cells is located in the right atrium. This tiny bundle of nerve tissue is called the **sinoatrial (SA) node**. The SA node begins the electrical impulse that spreads throughout the heart and eventually results in contraction of the ventricles. The SA node is known as the body's natural pacemaker. The electrical impulse that is generated from the SA node spreads in wave-like motion across the atria at a rate of 60 to 100 times per minute.

Once the atria have been stimulated, the electrical impulse travels to another mass of specialized tissue called the **atrioventricular (AV) node**. The AV node is located at the bottom of the right atrium near the atrial septum. The fibers of the AV node are smaller than the SA node so there is a slight delay (1/10 of a second) in the conduction of the impulse. The AV node can serve as the heart's pacemaker, should the SA node fail, and can initiate impulses at a rate of 40 to 60 times per minute. The AV node also protects the ventricles from excessively fast heart rates that may be initiated in the atria.

From the AV node, the impulse passes through the **bundle of His**, or AV bundle. The bundle of His is continuous with the AV node, and as the bundle tracts reach the interventricular septum, the bundle of His branches into right and left bundle branches. The right bundle branch extends along the right side of the septum until it reaches the bottom of the right ventricle, where it divides into a network supplying a continued pathway to the myocardium of the right ventricle. The left bundle branch extends along the left side of the septum and divides further into an anterior and posterior segment. The anterior division delivers an electrical current to the upper part of the left ventricle and the posterior division supplies the lower portion of the left ventricle.

Approximately halfway down the septum the right bundle branch and both segments of the left bundle branch converge into larger Purkinje fibers. This complex network of Purkinje fibers spreads extensively along the septum and continues downward to the **apex** of the heart. There, the Purkinje fibers curve around the ventricles and spread upward over the lateral ventricular walls. The bundle of His, the bundle branches, and Purkinje fibers are responsible for the contraction of the ventricles. The ventricles themselves can initiate a heart rate of 20 to 40 beats per minute and can be used as a backup system to initiate a heartbeat, if necessary.

Electrophysiology of the Heart

In order for the heart muscles to contract and circulate blood, a sequence of events must occur (Figure 7-3). Cardiac cells with the potential to generate excitability undergo a series of chemical reactions to initiate the electrical impulse; this reaction is called the action potential. When the cardiac cell is in a resting or **polarized** state, the cell has a positive ionic charge on the outside of the

ATRIOVENTRICULAR (AV) NODE

Pacemaking cells found in the right atrium on the interatrial septum.

BUNDLE OF HIS

Nerve fibers within the interventricular septum that carry impulses to the bundle branches located in the right and left ventricles.

APEX

Distal tip of the heart, located between the fifth and sixth ribs, just below the left nipple.

POLARIZED

Resting state of cardiac cells.

DEPOLARIZATION

A reversal of charges at a cell membrane; an electrical change in an excitable cell in which the inside of the cell becomes positive in relation to the outside; opposite of polarization.

REPOLARIZATION

Re-establishment of a condition or state in which the inside of the cell is considerably more positive than the outside of the cell.

cell membrane and a negative ionic charge on the inside of the cell membrane. When the cell membrane is electrically activated, **depolarization** of the cell occurs. The positive ions on the outside of the cell membrane move to the inside of the cell and the negative ions on the inside of the cell move to the outside. This movement creates the electrical charge that travels through the heart, causing the atria and ventricles to contract. This electrical impulse is transmitted to the chest wall, where it is detected and recorded as an ECG. **Repolarization** occurs after contraction. It is a period of recovery and rest. During repolarization, the negative ions that moved to the outside of the cell now return to the inside of the cell and the positive ions move back to the outside of the cell. The cells then move back to their polarized state and start the process over again with the next heartbeat.

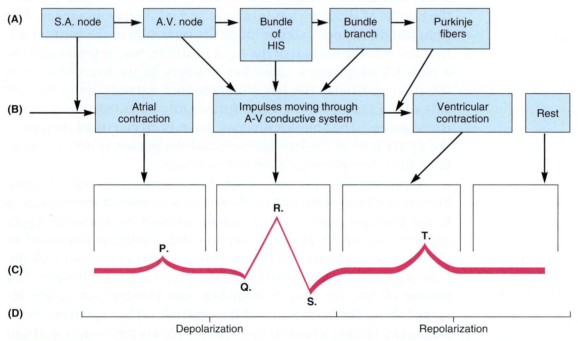

FIGURE 7-3: Diagrammatic representations of cardiac impulses on an ECG Tracing: (A) course of electrical impulses; (B) cardiac muscle reaction to impulses; (C) ECG tracing of impulse waves; (D) phases of cardiac cycle (Courtesy of Spacelabs Medical, Inc.)

COMPLEXES

Groups of related, recorded waves.

The electrical impulses that are measured when performing an ECG are the waves of depolarization and repolarization. The different waves, intervals, segments, and **complexes** recorded on an ECG tracing correspond to the depolarization and repolarization of the cardiac cells of the heart. With the invention of the ECG machine, Einthoven enabled the physician to monitor the electrical activity of the heart. Electrodes attached to wires that lead into the

ECG machine deflect the minute electrical impulses that travel to the surface of the patient's skin. By identifying and labeling which wave, interval, segment, or complex corresponds to specific electrical activity of the atria and ventricles, the physician can determine the condition of the patient's heart.

⬤ 12-LEAD ECG MACHINE

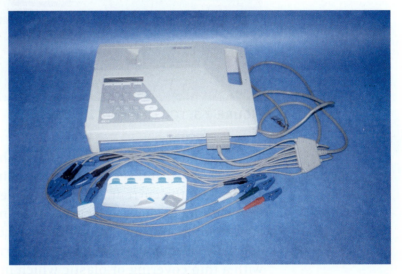

FIGURE 7-4: 12-lead ECG machine

GALVANOMETER

An instrument that measures electric current by electromagnetic action. The early ECG machine.

The ECG machine (Figure 7-4) is composed of a **galvanometer**, a heated stylus, lead wires, electrodes, and recording paper. A galvanometer is an instrument that measures electrical current by electromagnetic action. It is capable of detecting the heart's electrical activity through electrodes that are placed strategically on the patient's skin. The electrodes are small disposable tabs that come prepackaged and are saturated with conductive gel. Each lead wire is clipped onto a particularly designated electrode (Figure 7-5). The lead wires are color-coded and labeled to ensure proper placement.

Box 7-1: Color-Coded Lead Wires

- Right arm—Black
- Left arm—White
- Right leg—Green
- Left leg—Red
- Chest—Brown

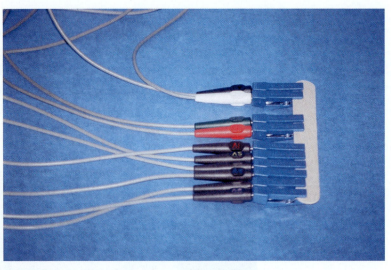

FIGURE 7-5: ECG electrodes and lead wires

The lead wires are connected to the ECG machine through an electrical port, and send the electrical impulse to the galvanometer to measure the current. The galvanometer is attached to the stylus or recording device. Deflections measured by the galvanometer are amplified enough for the stylus to record them. The ECG paper is specially designed graph paper (Figure 7-6). ECG paper is coated with a thin covering of plastic which melts when the heated stylus runs across it. The stylus is heated in order to melt the plastic on the ECG paper and produce an ECG tracing (electrocardiograph).

As a depolarization wave or **vector** moves toward a negative electrode, it produces a downward or negative deflection on the ECG tracing. When depolarization moves toward a positive electrode, it produces an upward or positive deflection. The magnitude of the current determines the amplitude of the deflection. If there is no electrical activity, or not enough electrical activity to move the stylus, the stylus records a straight line called an isoelectric line or baseline.

The ECG machine not only records the magnitude of the electrical impulses but also the time required for the electrical impulses to travel throughout the heart during each heartbeat. Each square on the graph paper is 1 millimeter long by 1 millimeter high. Darker lines mark every 5 squares and are thus 5 millimeters × 5 millimeters. Each millimeter square represents 0.1 millivolts (mV); each large square equals 5 × 0.1 mV = 5 mV. Time is measured horizontally. Each small square represents 0.04 seconds. Each large square represents 5 × 0.04 sec = 0.20 seconds. The duration of any part of the cardiac cycle can be determined by measuring along the hori-

VECTOR

Path or impulse representing the direction and magnitude of the heart's electrical current.

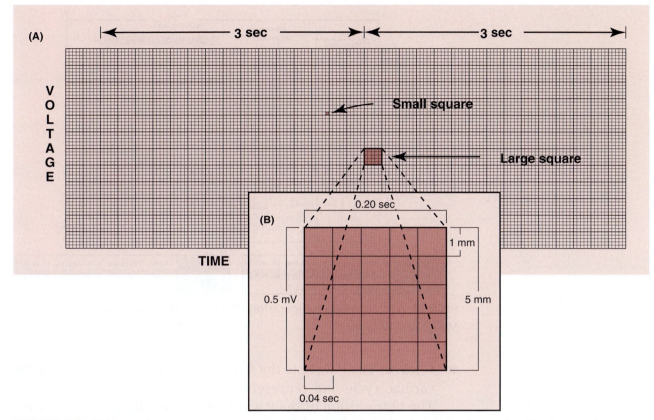

FIGURE 7-6: ECG graph paper measurements allow medical professionals to determine the time and voltage of heartbeats. (A) The small square is 1mm wide and 1mm high. One small square = 0.04 second. (B) The large square consists of 25 small squares and measures 5 mm wide and 5 mm high. One large square = 0.04 × 5 or 0.2 second.

zontal axis of the grid. A normal cardiac cycle is approximately 0.8 seconds long. ECG paper comes out of the ECG machine at a pre-set speed of 25 mm per second. This speed may be adjusted to 50 mm per second for pediatric patients who typically have faster heart rates. The paper scratches easily. Care must be taken when performing the ECG and also when mounting the ECG tracing for interpretation.

● ECG TRACINGS
Waves, Segments, Intervals, and Complexes

Deflections from the isoelectric line or baseline are called waves and are designated by the letters P, Q, R, S, and T. **Segments** are the straight lines that connect the waves. An **interval** is a wave in addition to a connecting straight line. Complexes are groups of related recorded waves (Figure 7-7).

SEGMENTS

The straight lines connecting waves.

INTERVALS

A wave in addition to a connecting straight line.

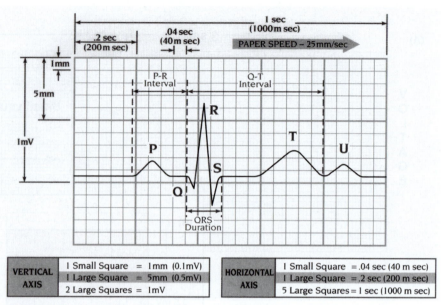

FIGURE 7-7: The ECG configuration (Copyright Marquette Electronics, Marquette, Wisconsin)

P WAVE

Records atrial depolarization and contraction.

● **P wave**: The P wave is the first initial upward deflection of the cardiac cycle and represents the depolarization of the atria. The first portion of the P wave represents the activation of the electrical impulse from the SA node and the depolarization of the right atrium. The last segment of the P wave represents the depolarization of the left atrium. The peak of the P wave represents the end of right atrial depolarization and the beginning of left atrial depolarization. Activation of the AV node occurs in the middle of the P wave as well. The wave representing depolarization of the ventricles obscures the wave representing atrial repolarization. Remember that the electrical impulse is delayed 1/10 of a second at the AV node. This delay allows the atria to empty before the ventricles contract. This delay is represented by the P-R interval.

P-R INTERVAL

Time for electrical impulse to conduct through atria and the AV node.

● **P-R interval**: The P-R interval is the line from the beginning of atrial depolarization to the beginning of ventricular depolarization, and is measured from the beginning of the P wave to the beginning of the QRS complex. It should be 0.12 to 0.20 seconds in duration. The P-R interval can vary in duration with age, physique, and heart rate. The greater the heart rate, the shorter the P-R Interval. The larger the heart, the larger the P-R interval.

QRS COMPLEX

Represents depolarization or contraction of the ventricles.

ST SEGMENT

Isoelectric line from the end of S wave to the beginning of T wave.

ISCHEMIA

Inadequate flow of blood to the heart, leading to angina pectoris and, if untreated, to myocardial infarction.

T WAVE

Represents repolarization (relaxation) of the ventricles.

QT INTERVAL

Measures from the beginning of ventricular depolarization to the end of ventricular repolarization.

U WAVE

Follows the T wave. Usually of low voltage; may become more prominent in some electrolyte imbalances, heart disease, or as an effect of medications.

● **QRS complex**: The QRS complex represents depolarization of the ventricles. The QRS complex is typically taller than the P wave because the ventricles are typically larger than the atria. The QRS complex can be broken down into waves. The Q wave is the first downward deflection, representing the electrical impulse traveling through the interventricular septum. Occasionally the Q wave may be absent or an upward deflection. The R wave is an upward deflection and is the largest portion of the complex. It represents the electrical impulse's progression through the bundle of His and the bundle branches of the right and left ventricles. The negative deflection following the R wave is called the S wave. S waves can only be negative and represent the completion of ventricular depolarization. The normal duration of the QRS complex is 0.04 to 0.10 seconds. Longer QRS complexes can indicate a block in the bundle branches. Shorter durations may indicate that depolarization may be occurring from within the ventricles themselves and not initiating from the SA node.

● **ST segment**: The ST segment begins at the end of the QRS complex and ends at the beginning of the T wave. The ST segment represents the window between ventricular depolarization and repolarization. The ST segment is normally at the baseline, or isoelectric. If there are injuries or **ischemia** within the heart, the ST segment may be either elevated or depressed. A normal ST segment may be elevated above the baseline for 1 to 2 mm. Elevation greater than 2 mm may indicate myocardial hypoxia, ischemia, or injury. A straight, horizontal ST segment above or below the baseline is highly likely to signify ischemia.

● **T wave**: The T wave represents repolarization of the ventricles. It may be a positive or negative deflection. It is usually about 0.5 mV in amplitude.

● **QT interval**: The QT interval represents total ventricular activity, depolarization (QRS) and repolarization (ST segment and T wave). The QT interval is proportionate to the heart rate. The faster the heart rate, the faster the repolarization and the shorter the QT interval. The slower the heart rate, the longer the QT interval. The normal QT interval measures 0.36 to 0.44 seconds and can vary between male and female and with age. Some cardiac drugs can also alter the QT interval.

● **U wave**: The U wave follows the T wave. It is usually of such low voltage that it is not seen. Its true origin and mechanism are unknown, but it does become more prominent in some electrolyte imbalances, heart diseases, and also with some medications.

Box 7-2: Waves, Segments, Intervals, Complexes

P wave: Atrial depolarization.

P-R interval: Time for electrical impulse to conduct through atria and the AV node.

Q wave: First negative deflection of QRS complex from impulse activation in the interventricular septum.

R wave: First upward deflection of QRS complex from impulse progression through the ventricles.

S wave: A negative deflection denoting completion of left ventricular activation.

QRS complex: Represents depolarization or contraction of the ventricles.

QT interval: Measures beginning of ventricular depolarization to end of ventricular repolarization.

ST segment: Isoelectric line from the end of S wave to the beginning of T wave.

T wave: Represents repolarization of ventricles.

U wave: Follows the T wave; usually of low voltage, may become more prominent in some electrolyte imbalances, heart disease, and with some medications.

Heart Rate Calculation

The heart rate is often displayed on newer ECG machines as an LED readout. However, the heart rate can also be calculated from the ECG tracing. Each P, QRS, T wave cycle represents one heartbeat. Time is measured on the horizontal axis of an ECG tracing. To calculate an approximate heart rate, count the number of large squares between R waves and divide 300 by this number. For example, 5 squares between R waves would indicate the heart rate is 300 ÷ 5, or 60 beats per minute. Special rate rulers for measuring the exact heart rate are also available.

● THE LEAD SYSTEM

An ECG traces the electrical impulses of the heart along 12 different pathways called "leads" or a "lead system." Each lead has a negative and a positive pole and measures the electrical differences between two or three electrodes. Einthoven used an equilateral triangle to represent this polarity (Figure 7-8).

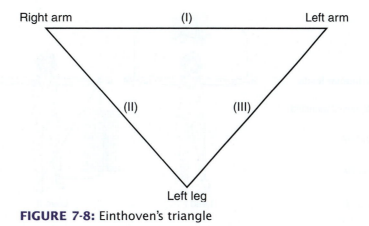

FIGURE 7-8: Einthoven's triangle

Leads I, II, and III are standard leads attached to the arms and legs and are commonly called limb leads (Figure 7-9). They measure the electrical activity on the frontal plane of the heart. They are **bipolar** leads, with one positive electrode and one negative electrode. A bipolar lead reflects the difference in electrical potential between the two connected limb electrodes. Lead I records the electrical activity between the left arm and the right arm. The positive electrode is placed on the left arm and records electrical activity on the left lateral surface of the heart.

Lead II records the electrical impulse between the right arm and the left leg. The positive electrode of lead II is on the left leg. Lead II records electrical activity on the left inferior and apical surfaces of the heart.

Lead III records the electrical impulse between the left arm and the left chest. Although the positive electrode is still on the left leg, it records activity of the inferior surface of the heart.

BIPOLAR

Composed of a negative and a positive pole; reflecting the difference in electrode potential between the two poles.

Box 7-3: Reciprocal Image

Leads I and III are mirror images of each other. This means that a positive deflection in lead I will be seen as a negative deflection in lead III, and a negative deflection in lead I will be seen as a positive deflection in lead III. The medical term for this is reciprocal image.

REMEMBER:

● In lead I and lead II the right arm is the negative pole, and the left leg is the positive. The electrode on the left arm is neutral.

● In lead III the left arm is the negative pole, the left leg is still the positive pole, and the electrode on the right arm is neutral.

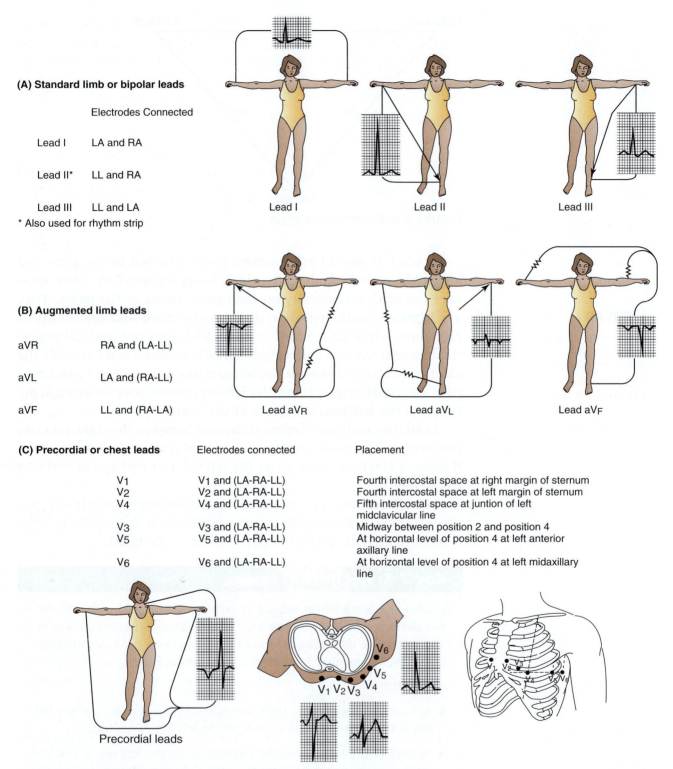

(A) Standard limb or bipolar leads

Electrodes Connected

Lead I — LA and RA

Lead II* — LL and RA

Lead III — LL and LA

* Also used for rhythm strip

Lead I — Lead II — Lead III

(B) Augmented limb leads

aVR — RA and (LA-LL)

aVL — LA and (RA-LL)

aVF — LL and (RA-LA)

Lead aV$_R$ — Lead aV$_L$ — Lead aV$_F$

(C) Precordial or chest leads — Electrodes connected — Placement

	Electrodes connected	Placement
V$_1$	V$_1$ and (LA-RA-LL)	Fourth intercostal space at right margin of sternum
V$_2$	V$_2$ and (LA-RA-LL)	Fourth intercostal space at left margin of sternum
V$_4$	V$_4$ and (LA-RA-LL)	Fifth intercostal space at juntion of left midclavicular line
V$_3$	V$_3$ and (LA-RA-LL)	Midway between position 2 and position 4
V$_5$	V$_5$ and (LA-RA-LL)	At horizontal level of position 4 at left anterior axillary line
V$_6$	V$_6$ and (LA-RA-LL)	At horizontal level of position 4 at left midaxillary line

Precordial leads

FIGURE 7-9: Lead types, connections, and placement: (A) Standard limb or bipolar leads; (B) augmented limb leads; (C) precordial or chest leads

UNIPOLAR LEAD

Measures absolute electrical force at the site of a positive electrode.

aVR, aVL, and aVF are **unipolar leads**. They are designed to record the electrical impulse from the center of the heart to the limb lead of the positive electrode. The amplitude in these leads must be increased about 50 percent, thus the term "augmented" is used. This is a programmed function within the ECG machine. Unipolar leads measure the absolute electrical force at the point of the positive electrode. The central terminal in the center of the heart has no electrical potential. VL is the lead designated from the central terminal to the left arm, VR is the lead to the right arm, and VF is the lead to the foot (left). The lead wire attached to the right foot serves as a ground.

PRECORDIAL LEADS

Leads situated on the chest directly overlying the heart.

Precordial leads, or chest leads, demonstrate electrical impulses transversing the heart from anterior to posterior. The chest leads are also unipolar leads, but do not need to be augmented because the precordial leads lie in close proximity to the heart. Each chest lead detects the electrical activity closest to it. The precordial leads are formed with the central terminal as the negative pole and each chest electrode as the positive pole.

Chest leads are numbered V_1 through V_6, and move from the right to the left side of the heart in successive steps. V_1 and V_2 are placed over the right ventricle; V_3 and V_4 are positioned over the interventricular septum, while V_5 and V_6 are arranged over the left ventricle. The chest leads are placed around the heart in its anatomic position within the chest.

Lead Placement

All ECG electrodes are placed on the patient using correct anatomic right and left. This means that right and left are relative to the position of the patient, not the health care provider (Figure 7-10).

RA and LA leads can be placed anywhere on the arm from the wrist to the shoulder. However, they are typically placed midway between the elbow and the shoulder to reduce the amount of interference. The upper arms usually have less hair, which allows better electrode contact. Less muscle contraction is also present in the upper arms. For example, when electrodes are placed closer to the wrist there is a greater chance for **somatic interference** caused by finger movement.

SOMATIC INTERFERENCE

An artifact on an ECG tracing caused by the patient (for example, talking, sneezing, muscle tremors).

RL and LL are typically positioned a few inches above the ankle on the calves of the legs. However, they may be positioned on the inside of the thigh to reduce artifact.

Even though there is a variety of acceptable limb lead placements, each health care facility generally recommends that all limb electrodes be consistently positioned using a particular placement.

LEAD ARRANGEMENT AND CODING

STANDARD LIMB LEADS

LEAD MARKING CODE	LEAD	ELECTRODES CONNECTED	COLOR CODE		
				BODY	INSERT
●	LEAD 1	LA and RA	RL	GREEN	GREEN
	LEAD 2	LL and RA	LL	RED	RED
			RA	WHITE	GRAY
	LEAD 3	LL and LA	LA	BLACK	GRAY

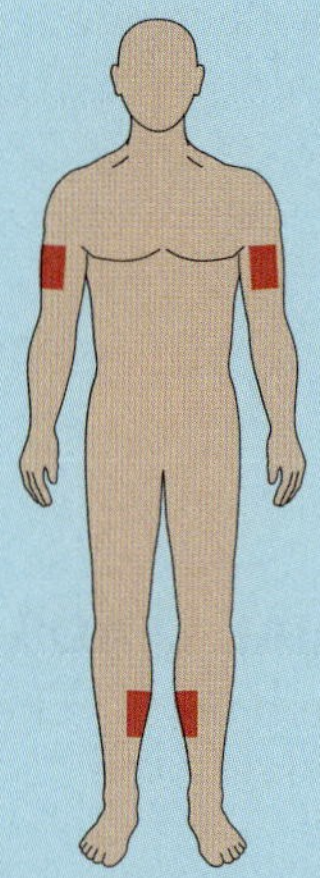

AUGMENTED LIMB LEADS

LEAD MARKING CODE	LEAD	ELECTRODES CONNECTED	COLOR CODE		
				BODY	INSERT
● ●	aVR	RA and (LA-LL)	RL	GREEN	GREEN
	aVL	LA and (RA-LL)	LL	RED	RED
			RA	WHITE	GRAY
	aVF	LL and (RA-LA)	LA	BLACK	GRAY

CHEST LEADS

LEAD MARKING CODE	LEAD	ELECTRODES CONNECTED	COLOR CODE		
				BODY	INSERT
● ● ●	V_1	V_1 and (LA-RA-LL)	V_1	BROWN	RED
	V_2	V_2 and (LA-RA-LL)	V_2	BROWN	YELLOW
	V_3	V_3 and (LA-RA-LL)	V_3	BROWN	GREEN
● ● ● ●	V_4	V_4 and (LA-RA-LL)	V_4	BROWN	BLUE
	V_5	V_5 and (LA-RA-LL)	V_5	BROWN	ORANGE
	V_6	V_6 and (LA-RA-LL)	V_6	BROWN	VIOLET

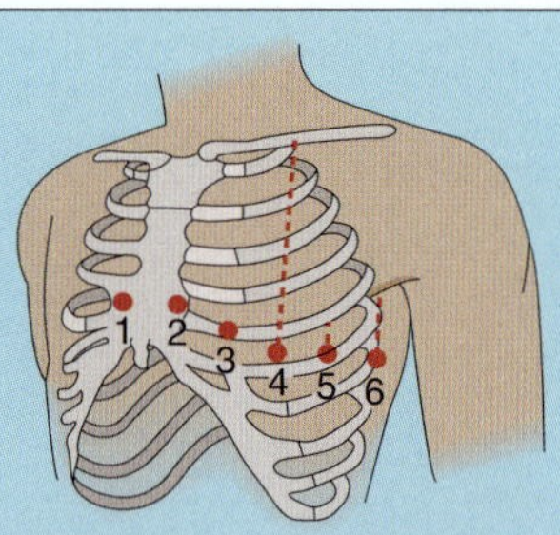

V_1 Fourth intercostal space at right margin of sternum

V_2 Fourth intercostal space at left margin of sternum

V_3 Midway between position 2 and position 4

V_4 Fifth intercostal space at junction of left midclavicular line

V_5 At horizontal level of position 4 at left anterior axillary line

V_6 At horizontal level of position 4 at left midaxillary line

FIGURE 7-10: Proper placement of electrodes for the standard routing of 12-lead and lead markings (Courtesy of Spacelabs Medical, Inc.)

Precordial leads are placed as follows (Figure 7-10):
- V_1 is on the right sternal border in the fourth intercostal space.
- V_2 is on the left sternal border in the fourth intercostal space.
- V_3 is midway between the second and fourth V leads.
- V_4 is in the fifth intercostal space measured straight down from the midclavicular notch.
- V_5 is placed between the fourth and sixth V leads in the fifth intercostal space at the anterior axillary line.
- V_6 is placed in the fifth intercostal space at the midaxillary line.

When working with a patient with an amputated limb or a cast, place the electrode at a site closest to the body. Placing electrodes in this manner will not cause inaccurate ECG tracings. Lower extremity leads may also be placed on the lower abdomen, and upper extremity leads may be placed on the upper chest just below the clavicle.

Remember that the ECG tracing is recording the electrical activity of the heart from 12 different vantage points (Figure 7-11). Each lead will look slightly different on the tracing because the deflections will vary from lead to lead. If the current is flowing toward a positive electrode, then the deflection is upward, and if it is flowing to a negative electrode, the deflection is downward.

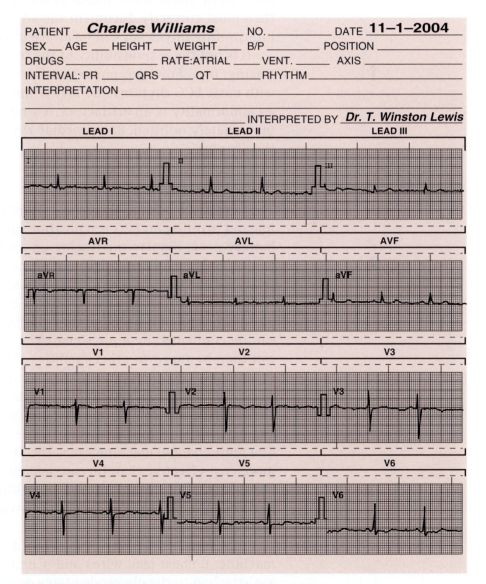

FIGURE 7-11: Mounted single-channel 12-lead ECG tracing

❶PERFORMING AN ECG

In order for a physician to use an ECG tracing as a diagnostic tool, the technician performing the ECG must be well trained. The tracing will only be as good as the technician's abilities and techniques. The interpretation, diagnosis, and treatment will be based on the accuracy of the tracings. The technician must know exactly where the electrodes are to be placed, how to prepare the patient for the procedure, how to maintain the equipment and supplies, how to recognize errors and/or artifacts that might occur, and how to correct them. There are certain situations where special techniques must be followed to ensure an accurate tracing. The technician must know under what circumstances to use these techniques, and then must correctly document the adjustments on the ECG so the interpreting physician will be aware of the situation and changes.

It is not the responsibility of the technician to interpret an ECG tracing. It is, however, important for the technician to be familiar with basic ECG rhythms and arrhythmias, in order to determine if an abnormality is an artifact, or if a nurse or physician should be immediately notified. Basic cardiac rhythms are described later in the chapter.

ECG Equipment

The new ECG machines (Figure 7-12) are capable not only of recording and printing an ECG tracing, but some models can be run by a battery pack, display the tracing on an LED screen, store tracings for later retrieval, and perform multichannel ECG functions. Some models can transmit the information via a modem to a central location for interpretation by either a computer or a physician or both. Other models have internal interpretation capabilities, which can be confirmed by a physician. The completed interpreted ECG can then be faxed to other facilities. These are quite an advancement from Einthoven's first ECG machine.

ECG machines in most facilities will either be manual, 12-lead, single-channel machines that record one lead at a time, or multichannel, 12-lead machines that record all leads simultaneously. The multichannel machine saves the facility time and paper and is more cost-effective than the single-channel machine (Figure 7-13). Today's ECG machines are also portable, and many have built-in handles for easy carrying. Machines without handles are placed on carts for transport.

On a standard 12-lead ECG, 10 lead wires are connected to the machine: 6 chest-lead wires and 4 limb-lead wires. They, in turn, are attached to the electrode plates or pads that are positioned on the patient. (Two lead wires are automatically switched internally and are used twice when performing a 12-lead ECG). The electrical impulses of the heart are detected by the electrodes, transmitted by the lead wires to the ECG machine, and then to the galvanometer. Next, they are amplified and changed into the motion of the heated stylus, and recorded on the ECG paper.

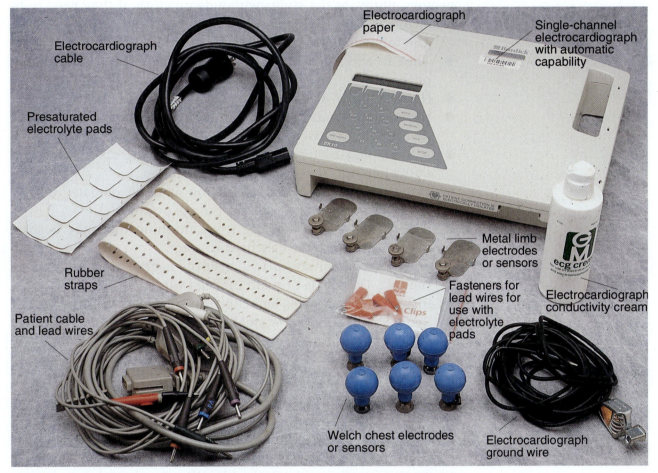

Electrocardiograph paper

Single-channel electrocardiograph with automatic capability

Electrocardiograph cable

Presaturated electrolyte pads

Metal limb electrodes or sensors

Electrocardiograph conductivity cream

Rubber straps

Fasteners for lead wires for use with electrolyte pads

Patient cable and lead wires

Welch chest electrodes or sensors

Electrocardiograph ground wire

FIGURE 7-12: Single-channel electrocardiograph and supplies needed for ECG

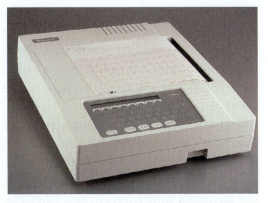

FIGURE 7-13: Multichannel ECG machine

Care of the Equipment

Most ECG machines and carts can be cleaned with a damp soft cloth and mild detergent diluted with water. It is important to ensure that the machine has been turned off and/or disconnected from its power source prior to cleaning. Do not wipe the open vents, connectors, plugs, or the stylus with a damp cloth. If they need to be cleaned, use a dry cloth.

The following are other areas of consideration:

● The cart and machine are to be wiped with a damp cloth at least once a day.
● Never write or place anything on the ECG machine.
● Never place foods or liquids on ECG carts. The machine will be damaged by spills.
● Always plug battery-powered machines into a wall electrical unit when not in use, to recharge batteries.
● Inspect electrical cords for fraying or other damage. Inspect plugs and connectors for bent prongs or pins.
● Ensure the wheels are free from anything that may become caught and make the cart hard to steer.
● Lead wires are always placed over the handle or over the top of the cart. Do not tie or bend the lead wires.
● Inspect the lead wires and clips for breaks or cracks.
● Request the services of qualified service personnel to repair ECG machines.

Patient Preparation

As with all procedures, correct identification of the patient is vital. When an ECG has been ordered for a patient, verify the patient's identification. If the patient is conscious, ask the patient to state his or her full name and check the identification bracelet. If the patient is unconscious, check the identification bracelet. In trauma situations, because the procedure is not invasive, perform the requested procedure and identify the patient later.

In order to attain an accurate ECG, the patient must be calm and relaxed. If the patient is anxious, the tracing will most likely reflect his or her anxiety. Provide privacy and a calm, relaxed environment for the patient. Explain the procedure and assure the patient that there is no pain involved and that the electrical activity is coming from within the body and not from the machine. Assure the patient that he or she will not be shocked. If performing an ECG on an inpatient, ask visitors to leave during the procedure. Pull the curtain around the patient's bed and close the door to the room. Respect the patient's modesty. Expose only the chest and the extremities as needed and cover the patient when electrodes and lead wires are in place. If the patient is cold, the tracing will be affected. Cover the patient with a warm blanket.

Patients will need to disrobe from the waist up. Provide the patient with a gown that opens in the front or a drape wrapped around the patient with the opening in the front. The patient must remove shoes and socks and all jewelry or metal items, as metal can interfere with the test.

Patient Positioning

The patient is placed in a supine position during the procedure. The legs may be slightly bent and supported by a pillow, but must not be crossed. Lying on either side, or any elevation of the chest, may alter the position of the heart within the chest cavity and render inaccurate results. If a patient is unable to lie flat, elevate the patient as minimally as possible. Document the approximate angle of elevation at which the procedure was performed. For example: HOB (the head of the bed) placed at a 45-degree angle because of SOB (shortness of breath).

Skin Preparation

It is imperative that the electrodes adhere securely to the patient's skin. Poor electrode contact with the skin is a common source of error and one that will render the tracing invalid. The skin is composed of three layers of tissue. Each layer has a different level of conductivity. The outermost layer, the **epidermis**, is composed of dead skin cells, providing very poor electrical conduction. The second layer, the **dermis**, is less resistant and is a better conductor. The dermis is composed of living cells and is the layer of skin needed to detect electrical signals for the ECG.

For optimal electrode contact, the dead skin of the epidermis and any oil, hair, or other debris must be removed. To accomplish this, the following skin preparation techniques are used:

● Shave electrode placement sites where hair will prevent optimal contact with electrode. Dry shave with a disposable razor, using quick short strokes in the direction of hair growth. Dispose of razor in appropriate sharps container. Disposable razors must be kept on the ECG cart.

● Use an alcohol wipe to remove excess oil and debris from the skin at electrode placement sites. Allow the area to air dry.

● Abrade (rough up) each electrode placement site with a 4 × 4 gauze pad to remove loose epidermal tissue.

● If a patient is **diaphoretic**, remove perspiration with a 4 × 4 gauze pad and alcohol.

EPIDERMIS
The outermost layer of skin cells.

DERMIS
The middle skin layers just under the epidermis.

DIAPHORETIC
Producing perspiration; sweating.

● Apply electrodes. Some electrodes are packaged with a conductive wet gel in the center of the electrode surrounded by an adhesive pad. The electrode tabs will leave a small residue on the patient's skin when removed. Be sure to provide the patient with tissues for cleanup. Dry electrode pads leave no residue.

● Apply pressure to the outside adhesive edges of the electrode pad, not the center of the pad, as this will disturb the conduction gel.

● Apply the electrode pads so that the tab that the lead wire is attached to points downward on the upper extremities and chest and upward on the lower extremities. These pad positions permit improved connection with the lead wires by lessening tension on the lead wires.

Mounting Single-Channel ECG Tracings

Facilities that use a singe-channel ECG machine require the ECG tracing to be mounted on an ECG mount or folder. There are several styles available (Figure 7-14). Some styles have pockets the leads slide into, and others have a self-adhesive strip that the tracing is attached to. The procedure for mounting the ECG tracing is the same for each style.

Once the technician has obtained an accurate ECG tracing, the required patient information is handwritten on the beginning of the tracing just before lead II (the rhythm strip). This is done in the event there is a delay before the technician is able to mount the tracing. The technician should then roll up the tracing, starting from the V_6 lead and ending with lead II. Do not fold the tracing.

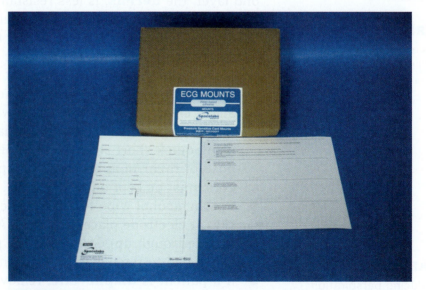

FIGURE 7-14: ECG mounts

When the ECG is ready for mounting, unroll the tracing on a clean work area. Careful handling is important as the tracing scratches easily, and folding the tracing can leave permanent marks that render the tracing unreadable. An ECG trimmer is a handy tool specifically designed to accurately trim each lead in preparation for mounting (Figure 7-15).

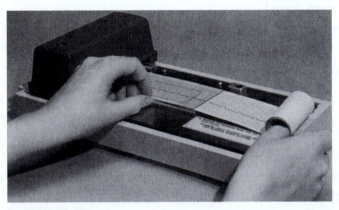

FIGURE 7-15: ECG trimmer (Courtesy of Spacelabs Medical, Inc.)

The leads should be cut so that a standardization mark is at the beginning of each lead as an identification tool (Figure 7-16). Most ECG machines at the beginning of a new lead automatically print the standardization mark. Machines that are not capable of automatically printing the standardization mark have a button that is pushed to create the mark. Some physicians prefer that a rhythm lead be mounted first. A rhythm lead is a section of lead II that can be run at the beginning of the tracing or at the end. This is mounted separately from the lead II tracing.

Once the lead has been cut, you may use scissors if the facility does not have an ECG trimmer. It is attached to the mounting card or ECG folder in the manner prescribed by the card or folder. The patient information is then written on the card or folder and given to the physician for interpretation.

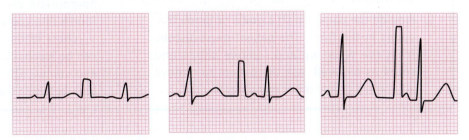

FIGURE 7-16: Standardization markings (Courtesy of Spacelabs Medical, Inc.)

Procedure 7-1

Electrocardiograph

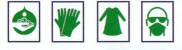

Equipment/Supplies

- Bed or exam table for patient
- ECG machine/cart with recording paper and lead wires
- Electrodes
- Razors (disposable)
- Alcohol prep pads (70% isopropyl)
- 4 × 4 gauze pads
- Gloves, goggles, and lab coat as appropriate

Method/*Rationale*

1. Assemble equipment and supplies.

   Ensures everything is available to perform the procedure.

2. Wash hands/don gloves.

   Thorough handwashing aids in controlling the spread of infection. Remember, you must comply with Standard Precautions whenever you may come in contact with body fluids or blood.

3. Identify the patient.

   Ensures the procedure is performed on the correct patient.

4. Explain the procedure.

   Helps ensure the cooperation of the patient. Remember that an anxious patient can greatly alter an ECG tracing.

5. Provide the patient with a gown or drape that opens in the front. The patient must disrobe from the waist up and remove shoes and socks as required. Ask the patient to remove all jewelry or any other metal items.

Protect the patient's privacy and modesty. Keep the patient covered as much as possible during the procedure. Provide a blanket to keep the patient warm. Metal items will interfere with the procedure and should be removed. This includes emptying pockets and removing belts if necessary.

6. Position the patient in a supine position.

   If the patient is lying on either side or if the chest is elevated it may alter the position of the heart in the chest cavity and render inaccurate test results. If the patient must be elevated for comfort, document the approximate angle of elevation on the ECG. Keep the elevation as minimal as possible.

7. Prepare the skin for electrode placement. Shave the skin as necessary. Remove excess skin oils or other debris with an alcohol prep pad and abrade the electrode area with a 4 × 4 gauze pad.

   Allows for optimal contact between the skin and the electrode.

8. Apply the electrodes in correct limb and chest lead placement.

   Place the limb leads first, positioning the leads on the upper arms and on the calves. Attach the correct color-coded lead wire to the appropriate electrode. Measure down to the fourth intercostal space on the right side for V_1 chest leads. The fourth intercostal space can be located by using the clavicle as a reference point. The first intercostal space is the area between the first and second ribs. Apply the V_1 electrode in the fourth intercostal space close to the sternum. Find the clavicle on the right side, using your right hand; place your forefinger in the space below the clavicle. This is the first intercostal space. Find the next rib with your middle finger; the space below that rib is the second intercostal space. Leaving your middle finger in place, use your next finger to locate the third intercostal space. With your little finger, locate the fourth intercostal space. Place the V_1 electrode. Place V_2 directly across from V_1 after counting down to the fourth intercostal space on the left side of the sternum. V_4 is positioned at the midclavicular line in the fifth intercostal space. V_3 is positioned halfway between V_2 and V_4 in the fifth intercostal space. V_5 and V_6 are located laterally to V_4. V_5 is in the anterior axillary line and V_6 is in the midaxillary line.

Make sure that electrodes on the chest are placed in the intercostal spaces. Placing electrodes above bone will cause artifacts on the ECG tracing. Verify correct lead placement after the leads are positioned, before recording the ECG.

9. Enter the patient information into the ECG machine as required by the facility.

If the ECG machine is not equipped with this option, all pertinent information must be handwritten onto the ECG.

10. Press the "start" or "record" button on the machine.

11. Ask the patient to lie quietly during the procedure. Correct artifacts as necessary while the tracing is being performed.

12. If you recognize a lethal arrhythmia, notify the nurse or physician immediately.

13. When the tracing is complete, quickly determine if it is an accurate tracing. If so, disconnect the patient from the machine by removing the lead wires and electrodes from the electrode site.

Providing an accurate tracing is imperative to physicians so they may correctly diagnose the patient. Provide the patient with tissue or assist the patient in cleaning the electrode site.

14. Discard electrodes and any other contaminated items in the appropriate waste receptacle.

15. Wash hands. Thank the patient.

16. Document all special information on the ECG tracing.

17. Print out ECG tracing and mount as necessary.

Artifacts

Occasionally extraneous, undesirable electrical activity is recorded from sources other than the heart on the ECG tracing. This interference is called an artifact. Its causes are varied but important for the technician to identify and correct (Figures 7-17 and 7-18).

Interference that is caused by electrical equipment is called AC interference. AC interference is a rapid vibration that produces spikes of similar amplitude that widen the baseline and make it look fuzzy and thick. In the United States the frequency of the spikes is 60 cycles per second.

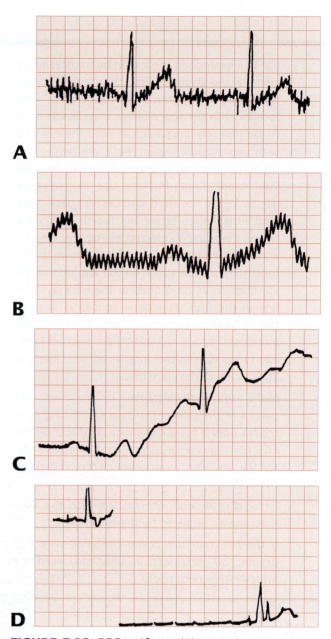

FIGURE 7-18: ECG artifacts: (A) somatic tremor; (B) alternating current (AC); (C) wandering baseline; (D) interrupted baseline. (Courtesy of Spacelabs Medical, Inc.)

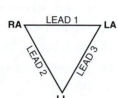

LOCATION OF SOURCE OF ARTIFACTS

Leads 1, 2, and 3 can be helpful in locating the source of interference. Refer to the triangle. Notice that each limb electrode is involved in recording two of the three leads. This means that if an artifact is observed in two leads but not in the third, the artifact is probably caused by a condition at or near the electrode that is common to the two leads. Examples: tremor on leads 1 and 3 and not on lead 2 indicates that the left arm is the probable source since it is common to leads 1 and 3. Similarly, a large amount of AC interference appearing in leads 1 and 2 and a smaller amount in lead 3, would most likely indicate that the AC source is near the right arm. If interference problems cannot be readily solved, contact your Burdick dealer or The Burdick Corporation for the name of your nearest Burdick field representative. They have equipment to help you find the interference source and can offer suggestions to eliminate or reduce the problem.

FIGURE 7-17: Sources of artifacts from leads (Courtesy of Spacelabs Medical, Inc.)

AC interference can be corrected or lessened by always positioning the ECG cart away from the patient's bed. If possible, disconnect any items plugged into the wall sockets in the patient room or exam room. This is not always possible, especially in a critical care room where the patient is on life support. Do not allow any part of the patient, especially the hands or feet, to touch any metal part of the bed.

Somatic interference is an artifact coming directly from the patient. This is patient movement of any kind during the procedure. If the patient talks, coughs, cries, and so forth during the procedure, it will affect the ECG tracing. These can all be corrected by thoroughly explaining the procedure to the patient beforehand and gaining his confident cooperation. Some somatic artifacts are more difficult to correct. Patients who have muscle tremors associated with conditions such as Parkinson's disease, hyperthyroidism, or other nervous system disorders may have a difficult time controlling their movement. In these situations, place the electrodes proximally on the limb leads. Sometimes asking the patient to lie with hands behind the buttocks will help to alleviate upper extremity tremors. The wave pattern may resemble the "F" waves of atrial flutter. Therefore, it is important for the technician to determine if there is somatic interference and to minimize or eliminate it.

The baseline of the ECG should be positioned in the middle of the paper and should be straight. Several circumstances can cause a wandering baseline. The most common is inadequate contact between the electrodes and the skin. Check to ensure a lead wire has not come loose and that all electrodes are still firmly in place. If this occurs, reprep and rerun the ECG. Another cause of a wandering baseline is an electrode pad that is too dry or too wet. Do not allow pads to dry out. This can occur if unused pads are not properly stored.

If there is a significant amount of artifact in an ECG tracing, the procedure must be repeated. The physician will be unable to accurately interpret an ECG tracing with excessive artifacts. Artifacts can often resemble any number of dysrhythmias, especially atrial and ventricular fibrillation.

Einthoven's triangle can also help to pinpoint AC interference and wandering baseline:
● If the interference is in leads I and II and not in III, check the right arm.
● If interference is in leads II and III but not in I, check the left leg.
● If interference is in leads I and III but not in II, check the left arm.
● If interference is present in the augmented leads aVR, aVL, aVF, the affected limb will also display artifact. aVR—right arm; aVL—left arm; aVF—left foot.

Box 7-4: Reminders: Artifacts

- Make sure the patient is lying quietly and arms and legs are not crossed or bent. Anxiety may cause somatic interference.
- Check for disconnected lead wires, wires not completely attached to electrode tabs, or tabs pulling away from skin.
- Place the ECG cart away from the patient's bed (if possible at a 45-degree angle to the bed). Locating the ECG cart in this way will prevent interference from other electrical equipment, especially in critical care units.

Errors in ECG recordings may also occur from reversal of lead placement. For example, if the right and left arm leads are reversed, all components of the cardiac cycle in lead I will be inverted. Another reason for cardiac cycle inversion is dextrocardia, which occurs when the heart is located in the right side of the chest cavity. Comparison of the chest leads can confirm this condition.

Special Circumstances

- Pregnant women may have a slightly abnormal ECG tracing because of the increase of blood volume during pregnancy. Place the lower extremity limb leads on the thighs. Interference from the baby may occur. Be sure to note on the ECG that the patient is pregnant and the number of weeks of pregnancy.
- If a patient has a seizure while an ECG is being performed, remain calm and stay with the patient. Do not attempt to restrain the patient. Protect the patient's head as much as possible. Call for help. Once the seizure is over, repeat the ECG and document on the ECG "s/p seizure."
- ECG electrodes are not to be placed on top of breast tissue, regardless of breast size. Document on the ECG if a patient has had a mastectomy on either or both breasts. The vector of the ECG may be altered as a result of surgery.
- Dextrocardia exists when the left ventricle, left atrium, aortic arch, and stomach of the patient are located on the right side of the thoracic cavity. When the patient has this condition, the right and left arm leads are reversed and the precordial leads are repositioned and recorded with V_1 on the left, V_2 on the right, and the other V leads progressing rightward to V_6. Document on ECG, "right side ECG."
- ECG tracings on amputees will not be affected, as limb leads can be placed on the most proximal point of the remaining limb or on the abdomen and chest.

- If a patient is in cardiac arrest or in a "code" situation, or when a patient is in SVT (supraventricular tachycardia), leave the electrodes in place if possible. A repeat ECG will probably be necessary. For repeated ECGs, the skin may be marked with a felt tip marker so that the leads may be replaced in the same positions. If the leads are not removed and the ECG is repeated, document "repeat—same lead placement." This will let the physician know that the leads were not removed.

- Document on the ECG when a deviation in lead placement is required. This may be because of surgical dressings or other equipment located at the electrode sites. For example: "V_2 and V_3 altered because of midsternal dressing." Never remove surgical dressing without a physician's order. Pay particular attention to Teguderm dressings, as they adhere tightly to the skin and can be easily overlooked. Placing an electrode on top of this type of dressing will not allow for an accurate tracing of the leads affected by that electrode. Never place an electrode over a burn or wound, as it will not provide an accurate tracing and will cause the patient discomfort and pain.

- When performing an ECG on an infant or child, use special pediatric electrodes. If unavailable or seldom used by your facility, cut standard electrodes in half lengthwise to accommodate the smaller chest. Do not allow electrode edges to touch each other.

IDENTIFYING CARDIAC RHYTHMS

Although it is not the technician's responsibility to interpret the ECG tracing, it is important that the technician be familiar with and be able to identify basic cardiac rhythms. Normal sinus rhythm is the standard electrocardial rhythm. The sinoatrial (SA) node is the pacemaker and the atria and ventricles contract at a steady continuous rate in normal sinus rhythm. The terms "arrhythmia" and "dysrhythmia" can be used interchangeably. Dysrhythmia technically is an abnormality in rhythm while arrhythmia means an absence of rhythm. However, both terms have come to mean any abnormality or disturbance of the rate, rhythm, site of origin, and/or electrical conduction of the heart. By understanding what the normal P, QRS, and T waves look like, basic abnormalities can be detected and comparisons made. When the technician recognizes an abnormal pattern, a nurse or physician must be notified immediately.

Analysis of cardiac rhythms must be consistent and thorough. Start by recognizing the normal waveforms and patterns and then associate them with what they reflect in the heart. Then look for any abnormalities and make sure that they are not artifacts.

Sinus Rhythm—Basic Arrhythmias

In normal sinus rhythm, the SA node is the site of impulse origination and forms the P wave on the ECG tracing. When the impulse travels normally through the atria and activates the ventricles, the QRS complex follows the P wave (0.10 sec). As long as the SA node continues to fire and the atria and ventricles respond, the process will continue at a set rate and rhythm. When identifying normal sinus rhythm, look for the QRS complex first, and then look for a single P wave preceding it.

Characteristics (Figure 7-19):
- 1:1 relationship between P waves and QRS complexes (one P for every QRS).
- Upright P waves in leads I, II, and III.
- Similar appearance in all wave forms.
- P-R interval is 0.12 to 0.20 seconds.
- QRS interval is 0.10 seconds or less.
- Rate is 60 to 100 beats per minute.
- Rhythm is normal.

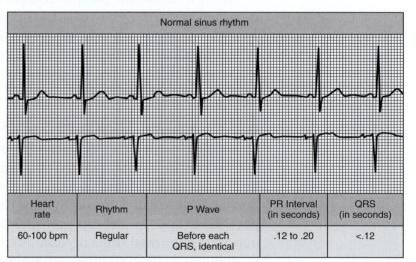

Heart rate	Rhythm	P Wave	PR Interval (in seconds)	QRS (in seconds)
60-100 bpm	Regular	Before each QRS, identical	.12 to .20	<.12

FIGURE 7-19: Normal sinus rhythm (Copyright Marquette Electronics, Marquette, Wisconsin)

Sinus Tachycardia

Impulse formation is normal, but the rate is faster. Sinus tachycardia results from increased sinus node discharge at a rate of >100 beats per minute. Sinus tachycardia can be the result of exercise, fever, hypovolemia, dehydration, pain, anxiety, anger, or cardiac failure.

Characteristics (Figure 7-20):
- P waves upright and normal.
- P-R interval is 0.12 to 0.20 seconds and constant.
- QRS complex is 0.10 seconds or less.
- Rate >100 beats per minute.
- Rhythm is normal.

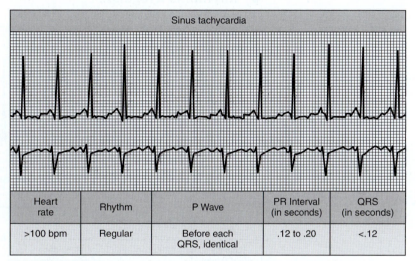

Heart rate	Rhythm	P Wave	PR Interval (in seconds)	QRS (in seconds)
>100 bpm	Regular	Before each QRS, identical	.12 to .20	<.12

FIGURE 7-20: Sinus tachycardia (Copyright Marquette Electronics, Marquette, Wisconsin)

Sinus Bradycardia

Impulse formation is normal and originates in the SA node, but the rate is slower. The heart rate is <60 beats per minute. If the heart rate becomes too slow, cardiac output will be decreased. Bradycardia may occur from certain drug effects (digoxin, propranolol, quinidine) or during vomiting, suctioning of the trachea, a Valsalva maneuver, right coronary artery disease, or intrinsic SA node disease.

Characteristics:
- P waves upright and normal.
- P-R interval is 0.12 to 0.20 seconds and constant.
- QRS complex is 0.10 seconds or less.
- Rate <60 beats per minute.
- Rhythm is regular.

Sinus Arrhythmia

Sinus arrhythmia is characterized by a "regular irregularity," a gradual slowing and then a gradual increase in rate. Impulses originate in the SA node, but speed up when the patient inhales and slow down when the patient exhales. This arrhythmia is very much related to the respiratory cycle and can also be caused by enhanced vagal tone.

Characteristics (Figure 7-21):

● Pacemaker site is the SA node.
● P waves are upright and normal.
● P-R interval is 0.12 to 0.20 seconds.
● QRS complex is ≤0.10 seconds.
● Rate is 60 to 100 beats per minute.
● Rhythm is irregular.

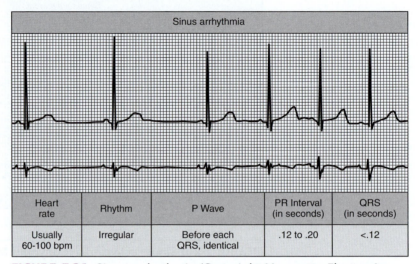

Heart rate	Rhythm	P Wave	PR Interval (in seconds)	QRS (in seconds)
Usually 60-100 bpm	Irregular	Before each QRS, identical	.12 to .20	<.12

FIGURE 7-21: Sinus arrhythmia (Copyright Marquette Electronics, Marquette, Wisconsin)

Sinus Arrest/Sinus Pause—Possible Lethal Basic Arrhythmia

Sinus arrest results from the firing failure of the SA node. Sinus pause occurs when the impulse is prevented from leaving the SA node. There is no pattern of occurrence and sinus rhythm, bradycardia, or arrhythmia precedes the pause or arrest. There is essentially no atrial activity. In sinus pause there may be long periods on the ECG tracing where there are no beats. In sinus arrest, a complete P, QRS, T cycle is missing. This results in a decrease in cardiac output. Sinus arrest can occur when there is a prolonged failure of the SA node for more than 3 seconds. If these episodes are transient (not lasting, of brief duration) they are of little significance. If the episodes become repetitive or prolonged, the condition becomes more serious because of the decrease in cardiac output, which can cause dizziness, syncope, fatigue, or angina (pain around the heart). In some cases, a secondary pacemaker may take over. Possible causes of sinus arrest or pause are SA node ischemia (lack of blood supply), right coronary artery disease, digitalis toxicity, excessive vagal tone, or degenerative fibrotic disease.

Characteristics (Figure 7-22):

● P waves are upright and normal.
● P-R interval is 0.12 to 0.20 seconds.
● QRS complex is 0.10 seconds or less. There is a sudden drop of more than one PQRST complex.
● Rate: Underlying rate is 60 to 100 beats per minute.
● Rhythm is regular except for the pause or arrest event. It is important to measure the duration of the event. Measure the distance from the last QRS to the next QRS. It is critical for the physician to know the exact duration of the event. Also document the patient's signs and symptoms during the event.

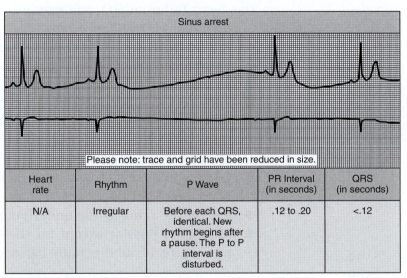

Please note: trace and grid have been reduced in size.

Heart rate	Rhythm	P Wave	PR Interval (in seconds)	QRS (in seconds)
N/A	Irregular	Before each QRS, identical. New rhythm begins after a pause. The P to P interval is disturbed.	.12 to .20	<.12

FIGURE 7-22: Sinus pause/sinus arrest (Copyright Marquette Electronics, Marquette, Wisconsin)

Atrial Arrhythmias

Atrial arrhythmias are caused by abnormal electrical activity coming from the atria. They include premature atrial contractions (PACs), tachycardias, atrial flutter, and atrial fibrillation, and are often caused by physiologic changes, myocardial infarctions, catecholamine surge, and/or atrial stretch secondary to cardiac failure.

Common characteristics of atrial arrhythmias:

● P waves often differ in size and amplitude from sinus P waves.
● P-R intervals may be shortened, prolonged, or normal.
● QRS duration is usually normal.
● PACs may or may not conduct to the ventricles.

Premature Atrial Contractions—Advanced Arrhythmia

PACs result from ectopic (displaced) foci originating within the atria. PACs are typically isolated events. PACs create P waves that appear earlier than usual in the cardiac cycle. They produce an early abnormal P wave because the impulse does not originate in the SA node. However, the AV node recognizes the impulse as if it had originated in the SA node and depolarizes the atria in a manner similar to a normal impulse. PACs can result from use of alcohol, caffeine, or nicotine, low serum potassium levels, digitalis toxicity, electrolyte imbalance, emotional stress, hypoxia, or heart or lung disease. Frequent PACs may indicate heart disease or congestive heart failure (CHF), and may provoke an atrial tachycardia.

Characteristics (Figure 7-23):

● P waves are premature and differ from sinus P waves. They may be notched, slurred, inverted, wide, or diphasic (having two phases), and are often obscured in the T wave or QRS complex.

● P-R interval: A conducted PAC usually causes a P-R interval that varies from sinus-induced P-R intervals and is typically shorter. However, P-R intervals may also be longer, depending on the site of ectopic focus.

● QRS complex is 0.10 seconds or less, or may be absent in a non-conducted PAC.

● Rate is the same as the underlying rhythm.

● Rhythm is regular except for the PAC. If every other PQRST is premature, atrial bigeminy has occurred.

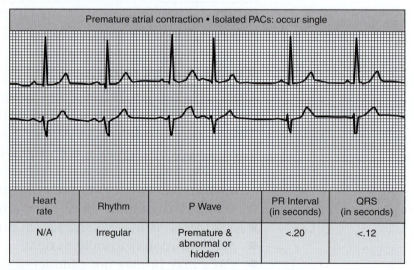

Heart rate	Rhythm	P Wave	PR Interval (in seconds)	QRS (in seconds)
N/A	Irregular	Premature & abnormal or hidden	<.20	<.12

FIGURE 7-23: Premature atrial complex (PAC) (Copyright Marquette Electronics, Marquette, Wisconsin)

Atrial Tachycardia/Supraventricular Tachycardia— Advanced Arrhythmia

Atrial tachycardia or supraventricular tachycardia (SVT) occurs with the sudden onset of rapid atrial depolarization overriding the SA node at a rate of 130 to 250 beats per minute. In SVT, the AV node tends to defer conduction, and the faster the rate of discharge from the atrial ectopic focus, the greater the AV delay. Atrial tachycardia decreases cardiac output because of the fast heart rate and the increased oxygen demand by the myocardium. It may also cause angina, hypotension, or CHF. Atrial tachycardia may deteriorate into atrial flutter or fibrillation and ventricular tachycardia, or fibrillation. Digitalis toxicity, heart disease, stress, smoking, overexertion, and caffeine may cause atrial tachycardia. It sometimes accompanies Wolff-Parkinson-White (WPW) syndrome, which manifests as supraventricular tachycardia.

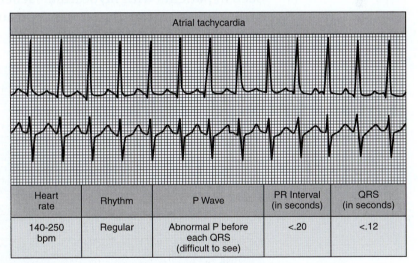

Atrial tachycardia

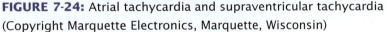

Heart rate	Rhythm	P Wave	PR Interval (in seconds)	QRS (in seconds)
140-250 bpm	Regular	Abnormal P before each QRS (difficult to see)	<.20	<.12

FIGURE 7-24: Atrial tachycardia and supraventricular tachycardia (Copyright Marquette Electronics, Marquette, Wisconsin)

Characteristics (Figure 7-24):
● Pacemaker site: Atrial ectopic focus.
● P waves cannot be clearly delineated because of the rapid rate. P wave forms may be seen with the QRS complex or may be seen distorting the end of the QRS.
● P-R interval: May not be possible to differentiate the P wave from the T wave. Look for prolonged P-R interval just before the tachycardia.
● QRS complex will be 0.10 seconds or less; greater than 0.10 seconds if related to a bundle branch block.

● Rate: 150 to 180+ beats per minute; with SVT the rate can reach 250+.
● Rhythm is regular.
● The clues to look for in atrial tachycardia and SVT are the sudden onset and rapid, regular rhythm.

Atrial Flutter—Advanced Arrhythmia

In atrial flutter, an ectopic focus generates impulses faster than the SA node and takes over the function of cardiac pacemaker. P waves will look identical because the ectopic focal point is the same for each beat. The P waves resemble a sawtooth pattern or picket fence. Therapeutic delay at the AV node may prevent many of the atrial impulses from conducting through to the ventricles. The ventricular response can be regular or irregular.

Atrial flutter is not considered to be a normal variant and is seen in patients with myocardial ischemia; it may cause re-entrant tachycardias. Atrial flutter can be caused by atrial stretch from acute illness and heart disease.

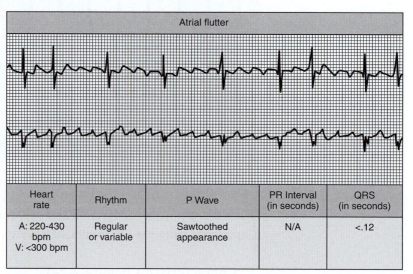

Heart rate	Rhythm	P Wave	PR Interval (in seconds)	QRS (in seconds)
A: 220-430 bpm V: <300 bpm	Regular or variable	Sawtoothed appearance	N/A	<.12

FIGURE 7-25: Atrial flutter (Copyright Marquette Electronics, Marquette, Wisconsin)

Characteristics (Figure 7-25):
● Pacemaker site is atrial ectopic focus.
● Atrial flutter waves at 250 to 300 beats per minute.
● P wave or flutter waves, sometimes referred to as "sawtooth" or "picket fence." P waves can be plotted out more easily on the negative component.

- P-R interval is constant, but will vary with irregular ventricular response. The flutter wave immediately preceding the QRS is not necessarily the wave front directly responsible for the QRS.
- QRS complex is 0.10 seconds or less. However, there may be distortion from atrial flutter waves.
- Rate varies.
- Rhythm can be regular or irregular.
- T wave may be distorted at the baseline of the flutter waves.

Atrial Fibrillation—Possible Lethal Basic Arrhythmia

The true origin of atrial fibrillation is unknown, but it occurs when ectopic foci in the atria discharge impulses at a very rapid rate and override the SA node. Although rapidly firing, only a small portion of the atrial myocardium is depolarized. Because there are multiple foci, there are no P waves. The chaotic firing produces an ECG deflection known as the "F" wave. These waves vary in size and shape and are irregular in rhythm. Possible causes of atrial fibrillation are atherosclerotic heart disease, atrial dilation, caffeine, cocaine, congestive heart failure, digitalis toxicity, alcohol, hyperthyroidism, age, hypertension, long-term chronic lung disease, chronic renal and hepatic disease, and rheumatic heart disease.

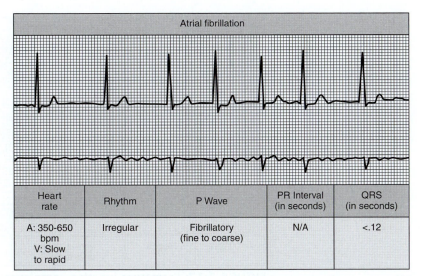

Heart rate	Rhythm	P Wave	PR Interval (in seconds)	QRS (in seconds)
A: 350-650 bpm V: Slow to rapid	Irregular	Fibrillatory (fine to coarse)	N/A	<.12

FIGURE 7-26: Atrial fibrillation (Copyright Marquette Electronics, Marquette, Wisconsin)

Characteristics (Figure 7-26):
- Pacemaker site is atrial tissue.
- P waves: none, chaotic baseline.
- P-R interval: not applicable.

- QRS complex is 0.10 seconds or less unless there is rate-related or pre-existing bundle branch block.
- Atrial rate is irregular at 350 to 750 beats per minute.
- Ventricular rate is irregular and varies with the degree of AV block.

Junctional Rhythms—Advanced Arrhythmia

Junctional beats originate from the AV junction, in the bundle of His, and can be escape (late), ectopic, or premature. The trademark of the junctional rhythm is the negative P wave. The most common junctional rhythm is the premature junctional complexes (PJCs). The PJC allows for retrograde depolarization, causing the inverted P waves. Premature junctional complexes may predispose the heart to more serious dysrhythmias. Possible causes of PJCs are caffeine, tobacco, alcohol, digitalis, ischemic heart disease, hypoxia, and rheumatic fever.

Characteristics (Figure 7-27):

- P waves may or may not be present, and are a negative waveform.
- P-R interval is approximately 0.12 seconds.
- QRS complex is 0.10 seconds or less.
- Rate: Sinus rate calculated as the underlying rate.
- Rhythm is the underlying sinus rhythm.

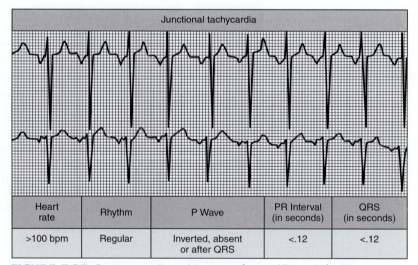

Heart rate	Rhythm	P Wave	PR Interval (in seconds)	QRS (in seconds)
>100 bpm	Regular	Inverted, absent or after QRS	<.12	<.12

FIGURE 7-27: Premature junction complexes (Copyright Marquette Electronics, Marquette, Wisconsin)

Ventricular Rhythms

The ectopic focus of ventricular rhythms occurs either in the bundle branches, Purkinje fibers, or ventricular muscle. The ventricular impulse rhythm is initiated before the impulse from the underlying rhythm starts.

Premature Ventricular Contractions (PVCs)

PVCs usually result from an ectopic focus arising from an irritable ventricular focus. PVCs are usually hypoxia-induced and replace a normally expected QRS. PVCs may be unifocal or multifocal in origin. Shape and polarity alone do not guarantee that differentiation. More correct terms are uniform and multiform in appearance.

PVCs may be coupled or may occur in various patterns:
● Bigeminy: every other beat.
● Trigeminy: every third beat.
● Quadrigeminy: every fourth beat.
● R-on-T PVC may cause ventricular tachycardia or fibrillation if it falls on the vulnerable portion of the T wave.
● Interpolated: sandwiched between two normally occurring QRS complexes. The interpolated PVC does not take the place of a normally occurring QRS.
● Frequent, multiformed.
● Couplets or runs of VT three or more in succession.

Possible causes of PVCs are acid-base abnormalities, digitalis, electrolyte abnormalities, hypertension, hypovolemia, hypoxia, myocardial ischemia, inadequate perfusion, and stress.

PVCs often indicate ventricular irritability in the patient with ischemia. Patients often sense "skipped beats."

Characteristics (Figure 7-28):
● Pacemaker site—underlying rhythm.
● P waves—underlying rhythm.
● P-R interval—underlying rhythm.
● QRS complex—underlying rhythm.
● QRS of the PVC is different.
● QRS/T wave polarity is opposite.
● Sinus P wave usually plots through.
● QRS duration is usually greater than 0.10 seconds.

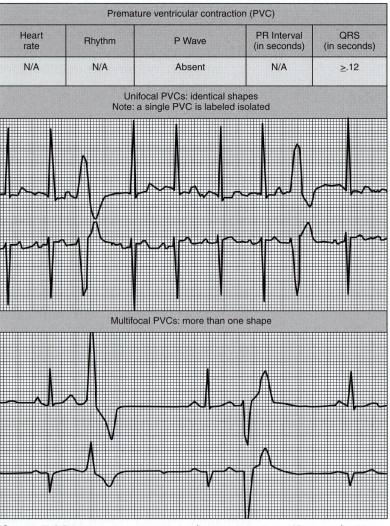

Premature ventricular contraction (PVC)				
Heart rate	Rhythm	P Wave	PR Interval (in seconds)	QRS (in seconds)
N/A	N/A	Absent	N/A	≥.12

Figure 7-28A: Premature ventricular contractions (Copyright Marquette Electronics, Marquette, Wisconsin)

Ventricular Tachycardia—Possible Lethal Basic Arrhythmia

Ventricular tachycardia (V-tach) is defined as three or more ventricular complexes in succession, with ventricular ectopic focus at a rate in excess of 100 beats per minute overriding the underlying rhythm. In association with myocardial infarction, V-tach may represent a life-threatening situation. Possible causes of V-tach are the same as for PVCs. Altered automaticity after depolarization is another probable cause.

Sustained V-tach results in low cardiac output. The faster the rhythm, the less perfusion. It is critical to confirm the presence or absence of pulses, as the patient may be perfusing, poorly perfusing, or dead. Sustained V-tach may deteriorate to ventricular fibrillation or asystole.

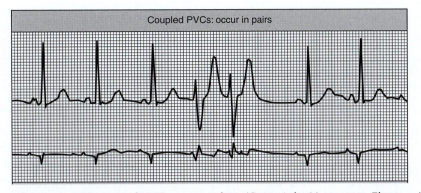

Figure 7-28B: Paired PVCs or couplets (Copyright Marquette Electronics, Marquette, Wisconsin)

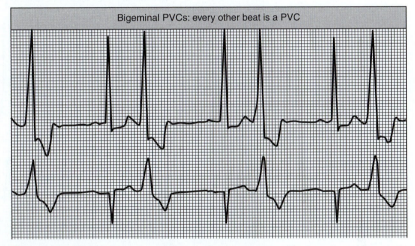

Figure 7-28C: Bigeminy (Copyright Marquette Electronics, Marquette, Wisconsin)

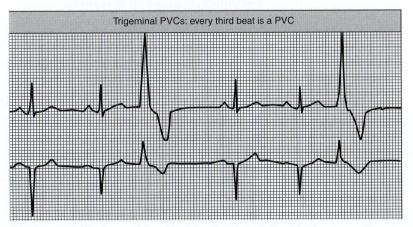

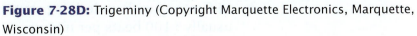

Figure 7-28D: Trigeminy (Copyright Marquette Electronics, Marquette, Wisconsin)

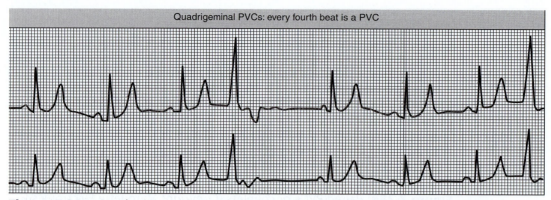

Figure 7-28E: Quadrigeminy (Copyright Marquette Electronics, Marquette, Wisconsin)

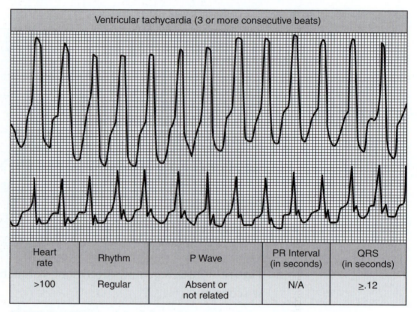

Heart rate	Rhythm	P Wave	PR Interval (in seconds)	QRS (in seconds)
>100	Regular	Absent or not related	N/A	≥.12

FIGURE 7-29: Ventricular tachycardia (Copyright Marquette Electronics, Marquette, Wisconsin)

Characteristics of V-tach (Figure 7-29):
● Pacemaker as with underlying rhythm.
● P waves as with underlying rhythm.
● P-R interval as with underlying rhythm.
● QRS complex as with underlying rhythm.
● The QRS of the PVC is different.
● QRS/T wave polarity is opposite.
● Sinus P wave usually plots through.
● Rate-sustained V-tach is 100 to 250 beats per minute.
● Rhythm is regular.
● QRS rate as with underlying rhythm. The episodes of V-tach are usually >100 beats per minute.

Characteristics of sustained V-tach:
- Pacemaker site: ventricular focus.
- P waves: not always visible; depends on the rate of V-tach.
- P-R interval is not applicable.
- QRS complex >0.10 with QRS/T opposite polarity.
- Rate is >100 beats per minute.
- Rhythm is regular.

Ventricular Fibrillation—Possible Lethal Basic Arrhythmia

Ventricular fibrillation (V-fib) exists when the ventricular rhythm is chaotic, resulting from multiple areas within the ventricle exhibiting varying degrees of depolarization and repolarization. Typically there is no ventricular depolarization or contraction. The patient may display agonal breathing or jerking movements of the extremities, but there is no pulse and no cardiac output. Rapid identification and defibrillation are critical in treating the patient in V-fib. Notify the nurse or physician immediately upon recognition of this arrhythmia. The longer the delay in intervention, the less success in conversion to a higher order of rhythm. Possible causes of V-fib are advance coronary artery disease, R-on-T, frequent paired or multiformed PVCs in the setting of acute myocardial infarction, drug abuse, traumatic event, or electrical injuries.

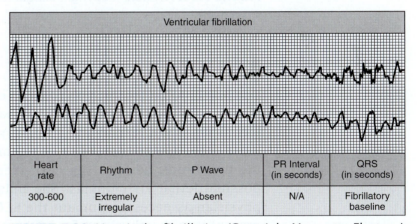

Heart rate	Rhythm	P Wave	PR Interval (in seconds)	QRS (in seconds)
300-600	Extremely irregular	Absent	N/A	Fibrillatory baseline

FIGURE 7-30: Ventricular fibrillation (Copyright Marquette Electronics, Marquette, Wisconsin)

Characteristics (Figure 7-30):
- Pacemaker site: numerous ectopic foci in ventricle
- P waves: none.
- P-R interval: none.
- QRS complex: none.
- Rate nondiscernible.
- Rhythm not discernible.

Other Malignant Arrhythmias

Agonal—Possible Lethal Basic Arrhythmia

An agonal rhythm consists of very irregular and widely spaced complexes originating from several different ventricular pacemakers. Agonal rhythm has a very poor prognosis.

Asystole—Possible Lethal Basic Arrhythmia

Asystole implies the absence of all cardiac activity (Figure 7-31). There is no ventricular depolarization and no contraction of the heart. However, the atria may continue to beat on their own for a short time.

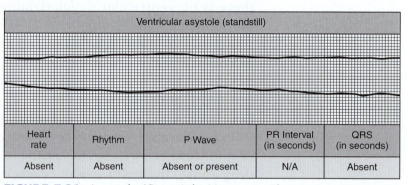

		Ventricular asystole (standstill)		
Heart rate	Rhythm	P Wave	PR Interval (in seconds)	QRS (in seconds)
Absent	Absent	Absent or present	N/A	Absent

FIGURE 7-31: Asystole (Copyright Marquette Electronics, Marquette, Wisconsin)

● SUMMARY

The phlebotomy technician's role has expanded to include the performance of electrocardiography in many health care settings. The technician is not responsible for interpretation of ECG results, but must know how to care for the equipment, prepare the patient for the procedure, perform the ECG, identify artifacts, and identify possible lethal arrhythmias. She must also notify the nurse or physician as necessary, mount the ECG tracing as applicable, and present it to the physician for interpretation.

The technician must remember that an ECG tracing is only as good as the technician who performs it. Be meticulous with details and provide the physician with an accurate, interpretable electrocardiograph.

COMPETENCY CHECK-OFF SHEET
Electrocardiography Competency Check

Given all the equipment and supplies, the student will be required to perform, within 15 minutes, an electrocardiography on a classroom volunteer. A "0" in more than two areas or an overall percent less than 80 will require the procedure to be repeated for competency.

Points to Be Awarded:	5 pts	2.5 pts	1 pt	0 pts	total pts
1. Assemble and prepare equipment and supplies					
2. Wash hands/don PPE					
3. Identify patient					
4. Explain the procedure					
5. Position patient					
6. Prepare the skin for electrode placement					
7. Apply limb leads					
8. Apply precordial leads					
9. Enter patient information into ECG as appropriate					
10. Run tracing with lead II rhythm strip					
11. Correct for artifacts as appropriate					
12. Disconnect the patient					
13. Respect the patient's privacy					
14. Discard electrodes/contaminated items					
15. Wash hands/thank the patient					
16. Document patient information					
17. Mount ECG as appropriate					

Total points possible: _____ Total points earned: _____

Start time: _____ End time: _____

Instructor signature: _____ Date: _____

Student signature: _____ Date: _____

● STUDY AND REVIEW EXERCISES

Defining Key Terms

Write the definition for each of the following key terms.

1) apex _____

2) arrhythmia _____

3) artifact _____

4) atria _____

5) atrioventricular node _____

6) bipolar _____

7) bundle of His _____

8) cardiac cycle _____

9) complexes _____

10) coronary circulation _____

11) dermis _____

12) depolarization _____

13) diaphoretic _____

14) electrocardiogram _____

15) electrodes _____

16) endocardium _____

17) epicardium _____

18) epidermis _____

19) galvanometer _____

20) intervals _____

21) ischemia _____

22) mediastinum _____

23) myocardium _____

24) P wave _____

25) polarized _____

26) P-R interval _____

27) precordial leads _____

28) pulmonary circulation _____

29) Purkinje fibers _____

30) QRS complex _____

31) QT interval _____

32) repolarization _____

33) segments _____

34) septum _____

35) sinoatrial node _____

36) somatic interference _____

37) ST segment _____

38) systemic circulation _____

39) T wave _____

40) U wave _____

41) unipolar_____

42) vector _____

43) ventricles _____

44) waves _____

Reviewing Key Points

1) List the components of the electrical conduction system of the heart and the sequence of impulse origination.

2) Differentiate between unipolar, bipolar, and precordial leads.

3) Describe Einthoven's triangle and how it measures the electrical polarity of the heart.

4) Distinguish between systemic, pulmonary, and coronary circulation.

5) Describe the effects of proper patient positioning during an ECG.

Sentence Completion

1) _____ was awarded the Nobel Prize for his invention of the electrocardiograph machine in 1903.

2) The two lower, pumping chambers of the heart are called _____.

3) The middle layer of cardiac muscle is called the _____.

4) Four unique qualities of the myocardial cells are _____, excitability, conductivity, and contractility.

5) The _____ is the site of original electrical impulse formation and is known as the heart's natural pacemaker.

6) The ECG machine is composed of a _____, a heated stylus, lead wires, electrodes, and recording paper.

7) Each small square of ECG graph paper is _____ × _____.

8) The _____ is the first initial upward deflection of the cardiac cycle and represents the depolarization of the atria.

9) The _____ represents depolarization of the ventricles.

10) Leads I, II, and III are standard limb leads and are considered to be _____ leads with one positive electrode and one negative electrode.

Multiple Choice

1) In an ECG tracing aVR, aVL, and aVF leads are considered to be _____ leads.
   A. unipolar
   B. bipolar
   C. precordial
   D. arbitrary

2) _____ or chest leads demonstrate electrical activity of the heart by viewing the impulses that transverse the heart from anterior to posterior.
   A. Unipolar
   B. Bipolar
   C. Precordial
   D. Arbitrary

3) The chest lead _____ is placed on the right sternal border in the fourth intercostal space.
   A. V_1
   B. V_3
   C. V_4
   D. V_5

4) On a standard 12-lead ECG, 10 lead wires are connected to the machine: _____ chest-lead wires and _____ limb-lead wires.
   A. 8, 2
   B. 7, 3
   C. 6, 4
   D. 5, 5

5) When performing an ECG on a patient, it is possible that the patient may feel a slight shock from the electrodes. You should assure the patient that the discomfort will only be slight.
   A. True
   B. False

6) When preparing the patient for an ECG, the patient should be placed in a _____ position.
   A. Trendelenburg
   B. prone
   C. dorsal recumbent
   D. supine

7) _____ is an artifact that is caused directly by the patient. The patient may have been talking, sneezing, or moving during the procedure.
   A. Somatic
   B. AC
   C. DC
   D. Wandering baseline

8) A(n) _____ is most commonly caused by inadequate electrode contact with the patient's skin.
   A. somatic interference
   B. AC interference
   C. DC interference
   D. wandering baseline

9) If interference is located in leads I and II and not in lead III, you should check the _____ to locate the source of the interference.
   A. right leg
   B. right arm
   C. left leg
   D. left arm

10) If the patient has a condition called _____ the right and left arm leads are reversed and the precordial leads are repositioned and recorded with V_1 on the left and the remaining V leads on the right.
   A. Wolff-Parkinson-White Syndrome
   B. bradycardia
   C. premature ventricular contraction
   D. dextrocardia

Critical Thinking

1) You have been asked to perform an ECG on Mr. Greenbaum, an 82-year-old patient in Room 712. While running the ECG you notice that the rhythm is abnormal, as in the strip below. What is the arrhythmia? What action, if any, must be taken?

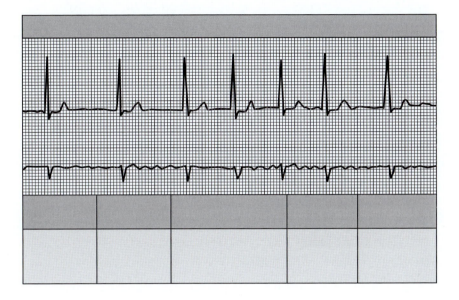

2) While performing an ECG on Gennie Larkin, A 34-year-old patient, you see the following arrhythmia. Identify the arrhythmia. Describe what action, if any, must be taken.

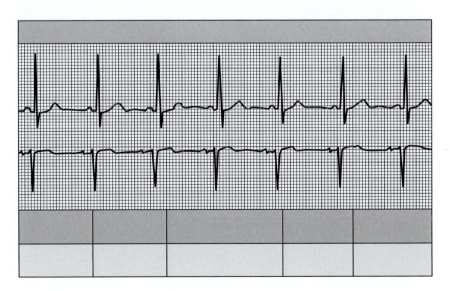

Blood Collection Equipment and Supplies

KEY TERMS

bevel (**BEV**-el)
butterfly infusion set
centrifuge (**SEN**-tri-fuj)
hemolysis (he-**MOL**-ih-sis)
lancet (**LAN**-set)
microcollection container
needle gauge
palpation (pal-**PAY**-shun)
personal protective
 equipment (PPE)
sharps container
syncopal (**SIN**-ko-pal)
tourniquet (**TOOR**-ni-ket)

OBJECTIVES

Upon completion of this chapter the student should be able to:

- Define and correctly spell each of the key terms.
- Identify, list, and describe the equipment and supplies necessary for general blood collection.
- Identify and describe the equipment and supplies specific to capillary punctures.
- Identify and describe the equipment and supplies needed for a venipuncture blood collection, using the syringe, butterfly, and evacuated tube methods.
- Identify and describe the equipment and supplies used for arterial blood gas collection.
- Describe the varieties of needles used for phlebotomy.
- Identify the color-coded Vacutainer™ tubes and the additives associated with each.

OUTLINE

- General Blood Collection Equipment and Supplies
- Capillary Puncture Equipment and Supplies
- Venipuncture Equipment and Supplies
- Arterial Blood Gas Equipment and Supplies

GENERAL BLOOD COLLECTION EQUIPMENT AND SUPPLIES

The primary responsibility of the phlebotomist is to collect blood specimens safely, accurately, and in the most cost-effective manner. In order to perform these tasks efficiently, the phlebotomist must have the correct "tools of the trade."

In today's market there is a wide array of blood collection equipment and supplies. It is important for the phlebotomist to keep informed about new technology and equipment. The safety of the patient and the phlebotomist should be the main objective when selecting the correct tools.

Gloves

The Occupational Safety and Health Administration (OSHA) has mandated that gloves be worn by health care providers during every invasive procedure. Gloves are considered a part of **personal protective equipment (PPE)** and act as a barrier precaution. Gloves are made of materials such as latex, vinyl, and nitrile. Latex gloves are the most commonly used. They come in a variety of sizes and are available with talcum powder inside for ease in putting on and removing. If the phlebotomist is allergic to talcum powder, low-powder and powder-free gloves are available. Some talcum powder will interfere with test results. Talcum powder made with calcium products, for example, is not recommended for phlebotomists because the calcium in the talcum powder may increase the patient's calcium values. If the phlebotomist or the patient is allergic to latex, vinyl or nitrile gloves may be used. Some phlebotomists prefer nitrile gloves because they are more durable, harder to tear, and are more comfortable to wear. Nitrile gloves, however, are more expensive. The phlebotomist may wear a pair of cotton or vinyl gloves under the latex gloves to prevent an allergic reaction. If the patient is allergic to talcum powder or latex, the same precautions are taken. Latex tourniquets and bandages are also not used if the patient is allergic to latex.

Nonsterile gloves come prepackaged in dispenser boxes of 100 per box. Sterile, individually packaged pairs of gloves are also available. Nonsterile gloves may be worn for routine blood collections.

Goggles

Safety goggles protect the phlebotomist from possible aerosol exposure or splashing blood into the eyes. Safety goggles are a PPE item and, although not mandated for routine blood collection,

PERSONAL PROTECTIVE EQUIPMENT (PPE)

Disposable gloves, lab coats or aprons, and/or protective face gear, such as masks and goggles with side shields, required by OSHA to be worn when handling body fluids.

their use is highly recommended. They should be readily available to every phlebotomist who wishes to use them.

Antiseptics

Alcohol pads or alcohol wipes, containing a 70% isopropyl alcohol solution, are used prior to the puncture to disinfect the patient's skin at the site of needle insertion. Alcohol pads are individually packaged and are supplied 200 to a box. Alcohol pads are used for most routine blood collections. However, when performing a puncture for collecting blood cultures or when blood is drawn for testing blood alcohol levels, povidone-iodine (Betadine®) swab sticks are used to disinfect the skin.

Gauze Pads

Gauze pads are made of loosely woven cotton fabric and come in a variety of sizes. The phlebotomist most commonly uses a gauze pad that is a 2 inch by 2 inch square and is simply referred to as a "2 × 2". Gauze pads are supplied in sterile and nonsterile sleeves of 100 to 200 pads. Sterile 2 × 2s are not to be placed on any contaminated surface prior to placing directly over the puncture site upon completion of the draw.

Bandages

After the collection of a blood specimen, a slight pressure bandage dressing is applied. The most common dressing is a sterile 2 × 2 folded in quarters placed directly over the puncture site and secured in place with a prepackaged adhesive bandage or a piece of tape. If the patient is allergic to adhesive, nonallergenic tape, such as Transpore™, is used. Some patients will decline a bandage of any type. When patients refuse a bandage the phlebotomist makes sure that the puncture site has completely stopped bleeding by applying manual pressure over the site before releasing the patient.

Box 8-1: Did You Know?

Instruct patients to remove the bandage 5 to 10 minutes after the draw. Patients should also be instructed not to carry a purse or anything heavy with the punctured arm for at least 1 hour after the venipuncture or to lift weights in a gym for 4 to 6 hours.

Bandages should not be used on children under the age of 2, because of danger of aspiration and suffocation by a loose bandage.

Needle Disposal Equipment

To aid in prevention of contaminated needle sticks, the phlebotomist always uses specially designed puncture-proof containers, commonly referred to as "**sharps containers**" (Figure 8-1). These units come in a wide variety of shapes and sizes. Some containers are designed to fit into phlebotomy drawing trays.

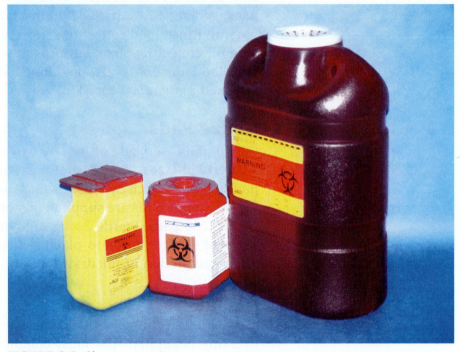

FIGURE 8-1: Sharps containers

After collection of the blood specimen, the safety shield needle guard is "clicked" into place, covering the end of the needle. The entire unit is then disposed of in the sharps container. Other items, including syringes, butterfly infusion sets, and lancets are also disposed of in the larger puncture-proof containers as whole units. Sharps containers are available from most medical supply companies.

Box 8-2: OSHA ALERT

Never re-cap needles. Never bend, cut, or unscrew a needle from the tube adapter or syringe prior to disposal.

CAPILLARY PUNCTURE EQUIPMENT AND SUPPLIES

Lancets

Lancets are small, sterile, single-use instruments used to puncture the capillaries of the skin.

LANCET

A sterile, disposable, sharp-pointed instrument used to pierce the skin to obtain droplets of blood used for testing.

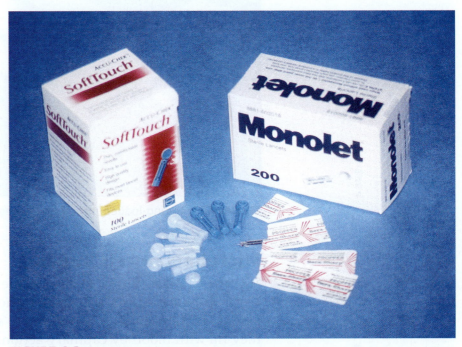

FIGURE 8-2: Lancets

Lancets are primarily used on infants, children, and the elderly, or when microcollection techniques are required. Lancets are available in a variety of point lengths. Point length is especially important when performing capillary punctures on infants. The point length for capillary punctures on infants, particularly newborn infants, should not exceed 2.4 mm. A puncture deeper than this could penetrate the calcaneous bone, which could cause complications such as sepsis and osteomyelitis. For premature infants, lancet length is even shorter. The phlebotomist must use a special premie-length lancet on these babies.

Spring-Loaded Puncture Devices

A variety of spring-loaded puncture devices is available (Figure 8-3). The advantage of using a spring-loaded puncture device is the consistency of the depth of the puncture. These devices are very useful to patients who need to perform routine blood-glucose tests at home.

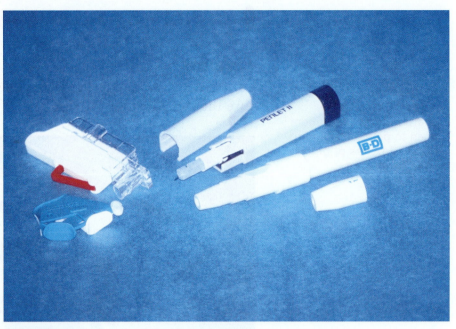

FIGURE 8-3: Spring-loaded puncture devices

Microhematocrit Tubes

Microhematocrit tubes are disposable glass pipettes, resembling small drinking straws designed to hold 50 to 75 microliters of blood. They are commonly referred to as "capillary tubes," because they fill with blood by capillary action. Microhematocrit tubes are available with and without anticoagulants and are color-coded for easy identification. Ammonium-heparin-coated tubes have a red band at one end; plain tubes have a blue band. These tubes are routinely used to collect samples from capillary punctures and are spun down in a specifically designed microhematocrit **centrifuge** to determine the patient's hematocrit values.

Clay Sealer Trays

A clay sealer tray is a small plastic tray filled with clay (Figure 8-4). It is used to plug the open end of microhematocrit tubes and to hold filled tubes until the specimens are ready to be centrifuged. The tray has small numbered holes in which the microhematocrit tube is placed once the end has been filled with clay.

CENTRIFUGE

A machine used for the process of separating substances of different densities, such as plasma and RBCs in the blood. The centrifuge spins substances at high speeds.

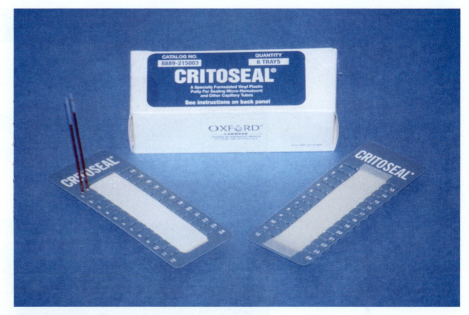

FIGURE 8-4: Clay sealer trays

Microcollection Systems

In recent years, with the development of **microcollection containers**, the process of collecting capillary puncture samples has been greatly simplified. Microcollection devices are typically plastic disposable tubes with color-coded tops that match the evacuated tube color-coded system, and contain the same anticoagulants. The tube cap accommodates its own blood collector, which is shaped like a small scoop. Microcollection tubes provide for easy measuring, storing, color-coding, and centrifugation of the capillary specimen.

VENIPUNCTURE EQUIPMENT AND SUPPLIES

There are three commonly used methods of venipuncture collection, each requiring its own specific equipment.

Syringe

In past years syringe draws were the norm. Today syringe draws are generally the exception. There are particular circumstances, however, when the phlebotomist will want to perform a venipuncture by means of a syringe draw. A syringe should be used when drawing blood from fragile veins, whereby the pressure behind the vacuum in evacuated tubes could cause a patient's vein to collapse.

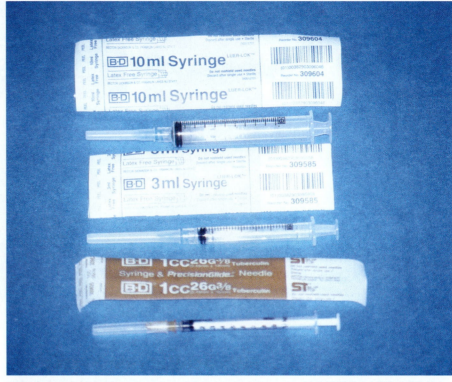

FIGURE 8-5: Syringes

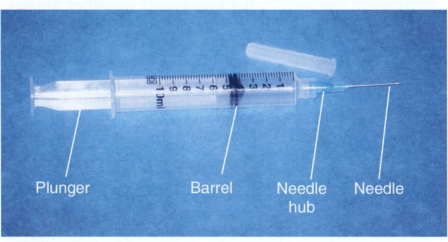

Plunger   Barrel   Needle hub   Needle

FIGURE 8-6: Parts of a syringe

BUTTERFLY INFUSION SET

A ½- to ¾-inch stainless steel needle connected to a 5- to 12-inch length of tubing. It is called a butterfly because of its wing-shaped plastic extensions, which are used for gripping the needle.

A syringe is a plastic disposable tube consisting of a barrel and a plunger (Figures 8-5 and 8-6). The plunger is situated within the barrel and, when pulled back, slowly fills the barrel with blood. Syringes come in a variety of sizes: 3 cc, 5 cc, 10 cc, 20 cc, and 60 cc. The 10 cc syringe is most commonly used for routine venipuncture. A syringe may be used with either a **butterfly infusion set** or a hypodermic needle.

Once the specimen is collected in the syringe, the blood must be transferred into the appropriate evacuated tube for transport and testing. Transferring blood from a syringe to an evacuated tube poses a greater risk to the phlebotomist for accidental contaminated needle sticks than collection from an evacuated tube.

Butterfly Collection Device

The butterfly infusion set consists of a needle, which is attached to tubing, and a connector, which attaches to the syringe (Figure 8-7). Butterfly infusion sets are also available with connectors that make them adaptable for the evacuated tube system.

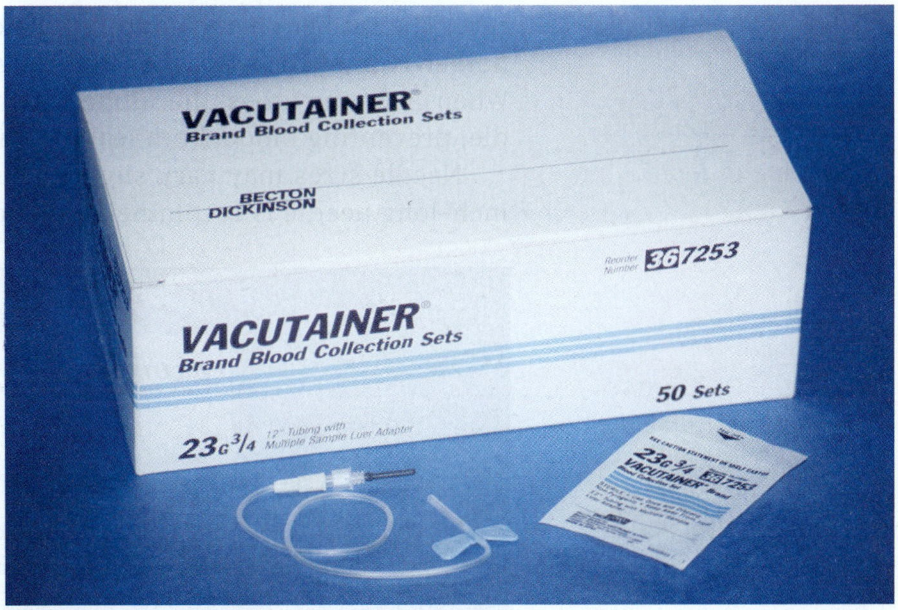

FIGURE 8-7: Butterfly infusion set

This method of venipuncture offers several advantages. Because the butterfly needle is a smaller **needle gauge** (23 gauge is standard—anything smaller will cause the red blood cells to lyse), it is generally less painful. Using a butterfly infusion set is less likely to collapse the patient's vein, because of the smaller needle gauge and length of attached tubing, which dissipates the strength of the vacuum when using the evacuated tube system. This system is the best choice when a patient's veins are small, as is often the case with children and the elderly. The drawbacks to this method include: 1) The risk of **hemolysis** because of the small gauge of needle; 2) it is difficult to collect large quantities of blood using this method; 3) it takes longer to fill the syringe or evacuated tubes when using butterfly infusion sets.

NEEDLE GAUGE

A standard for measuring the diameter of the lumen of a needle.

HEMOLYSIS

The destruction of the membrane of red blood cells and the liberation of hemoglobin, which diffuses into the surrounding fluid.

Needles

Two basic types of needles are used when performing venipuncture: multisample needles and single-sample or hypodermic needles.

Multisample Needles

Multisample needles are most commonly used with the evacuated tube system (Figure 8-8). The needle has two sharp ends; one end is **beveled** and is used to penetrate the patient's skin. The other end is covered with a rubber sheath and is generally shorter; it is used to penetrate the evacuated tube. The shorter end of the needle is screwed into the tube holder. Multisample needles allow the collection of more than one tube of blood, with only one skin puncture. The rubber sheath covering the end of the needle in the tube holder is pushed back when the tube is pushed onto the needle. When changing tubes, the rubber sheath once again covers the needle, preventing blood from leaking (Figures 8-9 and 8-10).

Needle sizes may vary slightly, but a 20 to 21 gauge, 1 to $1\frac{1}{2}$ inch–long needle is recommended and most commonly used.

BEVEL

The point of a needle that has been cut on a slant for ease of entry.

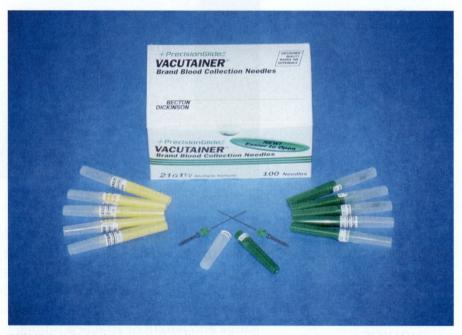

FIGURE 8-8: Multisample needles

> **Box 8-3: OSHA ALERT**
>
> In an effort to reduce the risk of contaminated needle sticks to the health care worker, OSHA has mandated the following:
>
> Where engineering controls will reduce employee exposure either by removing, eliminating, or isolating the hazard, they **must** be used. Significant improvements in technology are most evident in the growing market of safer medical devices that minimize, control, or prevent exposure incidents. Ideally, the most effective way of removing the hazard of a contaminated needle is to eliminate the needle completely by converting to needleless systems. When this is not possible, removal of the hazard as soon as possible after contamination is required. This is best accomplished by using a sharp with engineered sharps injury protection, which shields the sharp from exposure as soon as it is withdrawn from the patient. No one medical device is appropriate in all circumstances of use. Employers must implement the safer medical devices that are appropriate, commercially available, and effective.
>
> Medical supply manufacturers have produced some innovative new products to accommodate these new regulations. These include needles with safety shields that click into place after removal of the needle from the vein, needles that are self-blunting, in which the standard tube holders can still be used, to tube holders with automatic needle release.

Hypodermic Needles

Hypodermic needles are typically single-sample needles, used when performing syringe draws. The gauge and length of needle options are the same as multisample needles.

Tube Holder/Adapter

The tube holder, often referred to as the tube adapter, is a plastic tube slightly larger than the evacuated tube. It is designed to hold the needle at one end and allow insertion of the evacuated tube onto the needle at the other (Figure 8-11). Tube holders are disposable, and should remain attached to the needle and placed in the sharps container upon completion of the procedure.

Tube holders are available in a variety of sizes to accommodate both adult and pediatric evacuated tubes. Tube holders that retract the needle into the barrel to reduce the risk of accidental needle sticks are also available.

Saf-T-Clik Shielded Blood Needle Adapter

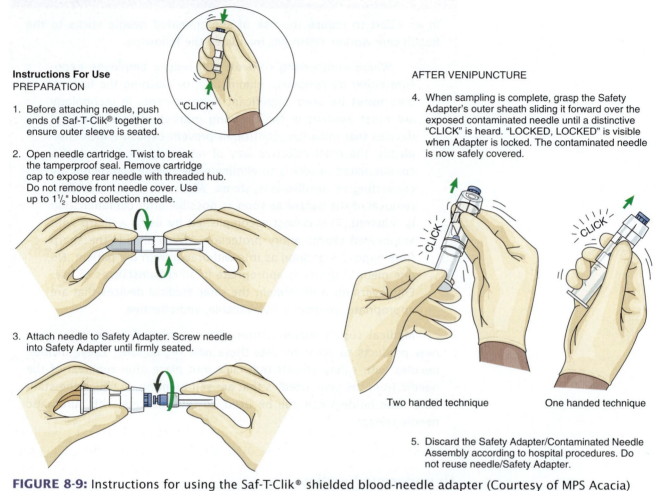

Instructions For Use
PREPARATION

1. Before attaching needle, push ends of Saf-T-Clik® together to ensure outer sleeve is seated.

2. Open needle cartridge. Twist to break the tamperproof seal. Remove cartridge cap to expose rear needle with threaded hub. Do not remove front needle cover. Use up to 1½" blood collection needle.

3. Attach needle to Safety Adapter. Screw needle into Safety Adapter until firmly seated.

AFTER VENIPUNCTURE

4. When sampling is complete, grasp the Safety Adapter's outer sheath sliding it forward over the exposed contaminated needle until a distinctive "CLICK" is heard. "LOCKED, LOCKED" is visible when Adapter is locked. The contaminated needle is now safely covered.

Two handed technique   One handed technique

5. Discard the Safety Adapter/Contaminated Needle Assembly according to hospital procedures. Do not reuse needle/Safety Adapter.

FIGURE 8-9: Instructions for using the Saf-T-Clik® shielded blood-needle adapter (Courtesy of MPS Acacia)

FIGURE 8-10: The Saf-T-Clik® adapter locked after use (Courtesy of MPS Acacia).

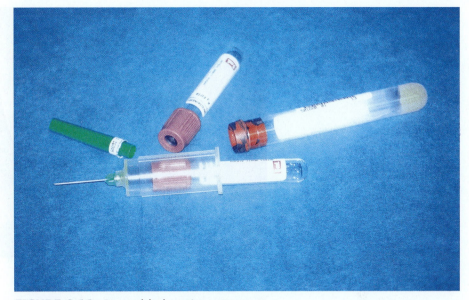

FIGURE 8-11: Assembled venipuncture set

Tourniquets

Tourniquets are designed to temporarily stop the flow of venous blood in the arm. When applied prior to venipuncture, the tourniquet will cause the veins to distend, providing better visualization and **palpation** of the vein.

Tourniquets are available in a variety of styles, but are most commonly a length of rubber tubing called a Penrose Drain (Figure 8-12). The tubing is 18 to 20 inches in length and $\frac{1}{2}$ to 1 inch wide. Other styles include rubber straps, Velcro tourniquets, and blood pressure cuffs. Blood pressure cuffs, however, are not recommended for routine use, as they can cause tissue damage and discomfort to the patient.

Tourniquets should not be left in place for longer than 1 to 2 minutes as blood may become more concentrated when constricted. This is called hemoconcentration and adversely affects test results. Prolonged use of a tourniquet will also cause the patient discomfort and may cause tissue damage.

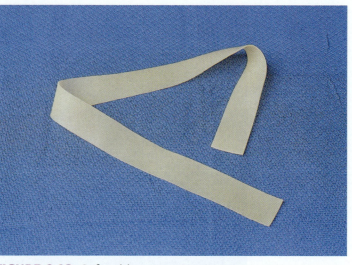

FIGURE 8-12: Soft rubber tourniquet

Evacuated Tubes

These vacuum tubes are made of either glass or plastic and are available in a range of sizes from 2 to 15 mL. Considerations for tube size are: amount of blood required for a test, stability of the patient's veins, and amount of vacuum in the tube. Larger tubes contain stronger vacuum, and smaller tubes, less vacuum. Patients with fragile veins, such as children or the elderly, require a smaller tube with less vacuum. Using the wrong size tube can collapse a fragile vein.

Evacuated tubes fill immediately with blood because of the precisely premeasured amount of vacuum. However, the vacuum in a tube will be lost if the cap is removed prior to the draw, the tube is dropped, the tube has been pushed too far into the needle holder prior to insertion of the needle, or the needle is pulled slightly out of the vein during the draw. Manufacturers place an expiration date on each tube and guarantee that the vacuum is accurate until the expiration date.

Evacuated tubes have a color-coded cap system used to identify which additive, if any, has been added to the tube. It is important that the phlebotomist learn to identify the additive that is associated with each color cap. The lab will discard specimens that are drawn into the wrong tube, necessitating blood to be redrawn from the patient.

Color-coded evacuated tubes must be drawn in the correct order; this is called the "Order of Draw." Table 8-1 describes each color-capped tube, the additive it contains, the type of specimen being drawn, and what test(s) will be performed. They are listed in the correct evacuated tube order of draw.

Table 8-1: Evacuated Tube System Listed in Order of Draw Sequence

Color	Additive	Specimen Type	Tests Performed	Special Requirements	Minimum Volume per Tube
Yellow sterile tubes or bottles	Acid-citrate-dextrose (ACD) or Sodium polyanetholesul-fonate (SPS)	Whole blood preservation of red blood cells or sodium	Immunodeficiency panels or for collection of blood cultures	Tube inversion must occur for proper mixing	Full draw required
Red	None	Serum	Serology–routine chemistries–blood banking–therapeutic drug levels	Must not be inverted	Not affected
Light Blue	Sodium citrate	Plasma	Coagulations studies–prothrombin time (PT)–activated partial thromboplastin time	Tube inversion must occur for proper mixing	Full draw required
Green	Lithium heparin Ammonium heparin Sodium heparin	Plasma	Chemistry determinations and cytogenics	Tube inversion must occur for proper mixing	No less than ¾ of a tube. Full draw preferred
Lavender	Ethylenediamine-tetra-acetate EDTA	Whole blood	Hematology Complete Blood Count (CBC)	Tube inversion must occur for proper mixing	No less than ¾ of a tube. Full tube preferred
Gray	Potassium oxalate/ sodium fluoride Sodium fluoride Lithium iodoacetate Lithium iodoacetate/ lithium heparin	Plasma	Glucose determinations	Tube inversion must occur for proper mixing	No less than ¾ of a tube. Full tube preferred
Royal Blue	EDTA (Na$_2$) Sodium heparin None	Plasma or serum	Trace element and nutrient studies and toxicology profiles	None	For tubes with anticoagulants a full draw is preferred but should be no less than 50%
Brown	Na heparin	Plasma	Lead determinations	Tube inversion must occur for proper mixing	No less than ¾ of a tube. Full draw preferred

(continues)

Table 8-1: Evacuated Tube System Listed in Order of Draw Sequence *(continued)*

Color	Additive	Specimen Type	Tests Performed	Special Requirements	Minimum Volume per Tube
Red-Gray Yellow-Black Red-Green Green-Black	The mottled cap colors indicate the tube has a gel barrier. The tube may or may not contain an anticoagulant	Serum	Tests requiring blood serum; not recommended for blood banking or drug levels	Clot activator and polymer gel	Not affected
Black	3.8% buffered sodium citrate	Whole blood	Hematology–Westergren Sedimentation Rate	Tube inversion must occur for proper mixing	No less than ¾ of a tube. Full draw preferred
Green-Gray	Lithium heparin and polymer gel	Plasma	Chemistry polymer gel separates plasma from cells when properly centrifuged	Tube inversion must occur for proper mixing	No less than ¾ of a tube. Full draw preferred

The order of draw is discussed in further detail in Chapter 10.

Blood-Drawing Trays

Phlebotomists can easily carry their equipment between stations and hospital rooms if they use blood-drawing trays (Figure 8-13). The trays should be made of a sturdy material with a handle and divided storage areas to keep equipment organized. Trays must be large enough to allow the phlebotomist to carry an adequate supply of equipment.

A variety of commercially designed trays are manufactured specifically for this purpose. Other commonly used utility trays, although not specifically designed as blood-drawing trays, are available at the local hardware store and will work just as efficiently. The tray should always be kept clean and restocked frequently.

Table 8-2 describes the most commonly found items in a well-stocked blood drawing tray.

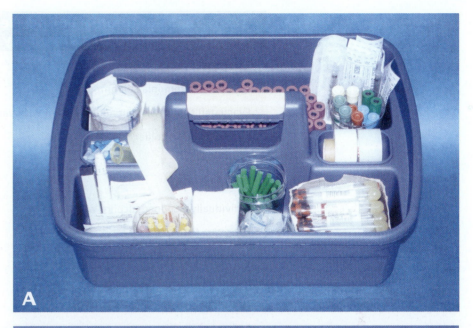

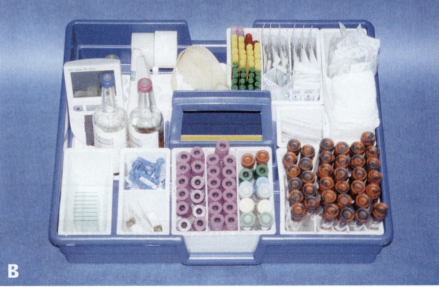

FIGURE 8-13: Phlebotomy trays: (A) utility tray; (B) manufactured phlebotomy tray

Table 8-2: Commonly Found Items in a Well-Stocked Blood-Drawing Tray
10 cc syringes
Blood culture bottle (aerobic/anaerobic)
Butterfly infusion sets

(continues)

Table 8-2: Commonly Found Items in a Well-Stocked Blood-Drawing Tray *(continued)*

Clay sealant trays

Disposable ammonia salt ampules

Evacuated tubes (without additives and with various additives)

Evacuated tube holder/adapter

Glass slides

Gloves

Individually wrapped alcohol wipes

Lancets—Autolets®

Microcollection containers

Microhematocrit tubes

Multidraw needles 21 gauge, 1 to $1\frac{1}{2}$ inch

Pediatric collection equipment (as needed)

Povidine-iodine swabs

Self-adhesive bandages

Sharps container

Sterile 2×2 gauze squares

Syringe needles 21 to 23 gauge, 1 to $1\frac{1}{2}$ inch

Tape—paper/cloth/nonallergenic—various widths

Tourniquets

Box 8-4: Critical Thinking

You have just come on shift and a STAT order for a CBC, chemistry panel, and blood cultures on Mrs. Thompson in room 213 is thrust into your hand. The technician just finishing his shift tells you on his way out the door that this lab request is already past due and the physician has called twice to check on its status. You say no problem; you will take care of it immediately. When you arrive at room 213 you first identify that the patient is indeed Mrs. Maureen Thompson. You then begin accumulating the equipment necessary from your blood-drawing tray for the ordered tests. However, because you did not have time to check and restock the tray before you left the lab, you had not noticed that you are completely out of Lavender top tubes. What would you do, knowing that the physician is waiting for the results, which are already very late?

Blood-Drawing Chair

Blood-drawing chairs are used in most outpatient labs. There are numerous models of blood-drawing chairs available. All have several features in common. All are equipped with a comfortable seat for the patient, with an arm support (Figure 8-14). The blood-drawing chair also has a restraint system to secure the patient in the chair should they have a **syncopal** episode. Most chairs have a storage area attached to keep supplies. Chairs are equipped with either a built-in blood-drawing tray or a surface area to set the tray.

SYNCOPAL

A transient loss of consciousness resulting from an inadequate flow of blood to the brain, relating to or marked by syncope.

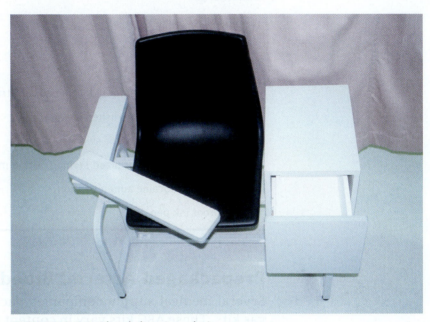

FIGURE 8-14: Blood-drawing chair

A bed or rest area should also be available for a patient to lie down, as it is not uncommon for a patient to feel dizzy or faint during a blood draw. Sometimes a patient will advise the phlebotomist if he or she is prone to this reaction. As a courtesy, the phlebotomist should ask the patient about prior adverse reactions during phlebotomy.

● ARTERIAL BLOOD GAS EQUIPMENT AND SUPPLIES

Arterial blood gases provide the physician with vital information about the respiratory status and acid-base balance of a patient. Arterial blood is used for blood gases because its composition is the same throughout the body, whereas venous blood has various compositions relative to the metabolic activities in surrounding tissues.

General Supplies

The equipment and supplies needed to perform a successful arterial puncture are listed in Table 8-3. Note that several items are used in a venipuncture as well.

Table 8-3: Equipment and Supplies for Arterial Puncture
Adhesive bandage
Alcohol pad
Gauze 2 × 2 squares
Lidocaine ½ to 1% to numb site
Needle 20 to 22 gauge, for ABG collection
Needle 25 to 26 gauge, for Lidocaine administration
Plastic bag or cup with crushed ice and water
Povidone-iodine (Betadine®) swabs
Syringe—prefilled heparinized syringe, 1 to 5 mL (specific to ABG collections)
Syringe, for Lidocaine administration
Waterproof ink pen

Prepackaged Arterial Blood Gas Kits

Several medical supply companies package special arterial blood gas kits. These ABG kits vary in content from manufacturer to manufacturer. The most standard ABG kit contains the following items:

- 1 cc syringe
- 25 g × ⅝ inch preattached needle
- 23 g × 1 inch packaged needle
- Vented tip cap
- Needle stopper
- 2 gauze pads
- Povidone-iodine prep
- Alcohol prep
- Patient identification label
- Adhesive bandage
- Zip-lock ice bag

SUMMARY

One of the most important tasks of the phlebotomist is to safely and accurately collect blood specimens in the most cost-effective manner. Learning the proper tools of the trade and when to use them are the first steps in accomplishing this task. With experience, the phlebotomist will choose the right equipment for each individual patient's specific needs.

STUDY AND REVIEW EXERCISES

Defining Key Terms

Write the definition for each of the following key terms.

1) personal protective equipment _____

_____

2) lancet _____

3) centrifuge _____

4) microcollection container _____

5) needle gauge _____

6) hemolysis _____

7) bevel _____

8) tourniquet _____

9) palpation _____

10) sharps container _____

11) syncopal _____

12) butterfly infusion set _____

Reviewing Key Points

The following is a list of equipment and supplies required for blood collection.

Categorize the list by placing in the blank a (**G**) if the item is used for all types of blood collections, a (**V**) if it is specific to venipuncture, a (**C**) if the item is specific for capillary puncture, or an (**A**) if the item is specific for arterial puncture. It is possible to have more than one letter per blank.

_____ 1) 2 × 2 gauze

_____ 2) 23 gauge needle

_____ 3) Adhesive bandage

_____ 4) Alcohol prep

_____ 5) Blood-drawing tray

_____ 6) Butterfly infusion set

_____ 7) Evacuate tube holder

_____ 8) Evacuated tube

_____ 9) Gloves

_____ 10) Ice

_____ 11) Lancet

_____ 12) Lavender top tube

_____ 13) Lidocaine $\frac{1}{2}$ to 1%

_____ 14) Microcollection containers

_____ 15) Microhematocrit tube

_____ 16) Patient identification label

_____ 17) Povidone-iodine prep

_____ 18) Sharps container

_____ 19) Syringe

_____ 20) Tourniquet

_____ 21) Zip-lock bag

Sentence Completion

1) The primary responsibility of the phlebotomist is to _____.

2) OSHA encourages every phlebotomist to wear goggles, but they mandate every phlebotomist wears _____.

3) Alcohol preps should contain a _____ solution to be effective.

4) Alcohol preps should not be used for draws when testing for _____.

5) The phlebotomist should instruct the patient to remove any adhesive bandage _____ to _____ minutes after the draw.

6) Needles, lancets, blood capillary tubes, and glass slides are all examples of _____ and should be disposed of properly.

7) The recommended point length of a lancet particularly for use on a newborn infant is _____.

8) _____ are disposable glass pipettes, resembling a small drinking straw.

9) Microhematocrit tubes must be _____ in order to determine the patient's hematocrit values.

10) The three commonly used methods of venipuncture are _____, _____, and _____.

11) A _____ is a plastic disposable tube consisting of a barrel and plunger.

12) A _____ set consists of a needle, which is attached to tubing and a connector, which attaches to a syringe.

13) The standard needle gauge for venipuncture is _____. Anything smaller will cause the red blood cells to _____.

14) A _____ is most commonly used with the evacuated tube system, because it has two sharp ends, one beveled and the other covered with a rubber sheath.

15) A _____ is used to temporarily stop the flow of venous blood in the arm.

16) _____ are not recommended for routine venipunctures as a method of stopping blood flow. They can cause tissue damage and discomfort to the patient.

17) A tourniquet should not be left in place for any longer than _____.

18) Evacuated tubes fill immediately with blood because of the precisely premeasured amount of _____.

19) Color-coded evacuated tubes must be drawn in the correct order, called the _____.

20) Arterial blood gasses provide the physician with vital information about the _____ and _____ of the patient.

Multiple Choice

1) A _____ top evacuated tube would be drawn for glucose determinations.
   A. brown
   B. blue
   C. gray
   D. lavender

2) A _____ top evacuated tube must not be inverted.
   A. red
   B. lavender
   C. yellow
   D. black

3) Lithium heparin and polymer gel are the additives in a(n) _____ top evacuated tube.
   A. red-gray
   B. orange-blue
   C. yellow-black
   D. green-gray

4) A _____ top evacuated tube would be drawn if the physician ordered a complete blood count.
   A. yellow
   B. green
   C. red
   D. lavender

5) Sodium citrate is the additive in the _____ top evacuated tube.
   A. royal blue
   B. light blue
   C. light gray
   D. green-black

6) Chemistry determinations and cytogenics are tests performed from the blood in a _____ top evacuated tube.
   A. yellow
   B. green
   C. royal blue
   D. red

7) A _____ top evacuated tube contains 3.8% buffered sodium citrate.
   A. black
   B. yellow
   C. red
   D. lavender

8) Toxicology profiles may be performed on blood from a _____ top evacuated tube.
   A. yellow
   B. red
   C. royal blue
   D. green

9) A red-gray top evacuated tube is/is not affected by the volume of blood collected in the tube.
   A. is
   B. is not

10) A _____ top evacuated tube would be drawn for collection of blood cultures.
   A. red
   B. light blue
   C. brown
   D. yellow

Critical Thinking

A patient is allergic to latex. What considerations should be taken during a venipuncture?

Collection by Capillary Puncture

CHAPTER

9

KEY TERMS

calcaneous (**kal-KA**-nee-us)
differential (**dif**-er-**EN**-shal)
inpatient
interstitial fluid
   (**in**-ter-**STISH**-al)
osteochondritis
   (**os**-tee-o-**kon**-**DRY**-tis)
osteomyelitis
   (**os**-tee-o-**my**-el-**EYE**-tis)
perpendicular
   (**per**-pen-**DIK**-yoo-lar)
superficial (**soo**-per-**FISH**-al)

OBJECTIVES

Upon completion of this chapter the student should be able to:

- Define and correctly spell each of the key terms.
- Identify and describe the equipment and supplies necessary to perform a capillary puncture.
- Properly identify the patient and explain the procedure.
- Describe the proper procedure for selecting a capillary site and the precautions associated with site selection.
- Identify the circumstances under which a capillary puncture is inappropriate.
- Describe the circumstances under which a capillary puncture is preferred.
- Identify the composition of capillary blood, describing the components that vary from venous blood.
- Describe the proper procedure for collecting a blood specimen when performing a capillary puncture on adults, infants, and children.
- Describe techniques used to obtain a free-flowing, well-performed capillary puncture.
- Describe the steps taken to ensure that the patient is properly cared for after completion of the puncture.
- List the appropriate "Order of Draw" for collecting capillary puncture specimens.
- Describe the procedure for filling microcollection containers from a capillary puncture.
- Describe the procedure for preparing a blood smear.

❶ INTRODUCTION

Capillary puncture, also referred to as a "skin puncture," "micro-capillary stick," or "fingerstick," is the procedure by which the skin is punctured with a lancet. This procedure is used to obtain a blood specimen when only a small amount of blood is needed to perform testing.

Capillary blood is a mixture of arterial blood from the arterioles and venous blood from the venules. It contains more arterial blood than venous blood because of the pressure behind the arteries. Therefore, it more closely resembles the composition of arterial blood rather than venous blood. This is important to the phlebotomist because the reference values for certain tests are affected. Glucose levels are higher in capillary blood specimens, while potassium, calcium, and total proteins are lower.

INTERSTITIAL FLUID
Fluid between the tissues, surrounding a cell.

Tissue fluid called **interstitial fluid** is located between the tissues of the skin and is released into the blood during the process of a capillary puncture. Interstitial fluid will contaminate the blood sample, so the first drop of blood must always be wiped away with a sterile 2 × 2 gauze square. Blood specimens that have been contaminated by interstitial fluid will not produce accurate test results, because the specimen will be diluted.

The following are circumstances under which it is more appropriate to perform a capillary puncture rather than a venipuncture:

- When only a small amount of blood is required to perform a test
- When collecting specimens on children and infants
- When a substantial vein cannot be located
- When a patient is not cooperative or is overly apprehensive about having a venipuncture
- When the client has severe burns or scar tissue over venipuncture sites

SUPERFICIAL
Pertaining to or situated near the surface.

- When the patient has very fragile or **superficial** veins

PHLEBOTOMIST PREPARATION—ASSEMBLING AND PREPARING EQUIPMENT

Prior to performing any specimen collection it is imperative that you assemble all the required equipment and supplies. As discussed in Chapter 8, the following items must be available prior to capillary puncture:

- 2 × 2 gauze pads
- Adhesive bandages
- Alcohol prep pads
- Clay sealer tray
- Glass slides
- Gloves
- Lancets
- Microcollection containers
- Microhematocrit tubes
- Spring-loaded puncture device (as appropriate)

CLIENT/PATIENT IDENTIFICATION AND PREPARATION

Once the equipment and supplies have been assembled the next step is to identify the client/patient. First, introduce yourself:

"Hi, my name is Sandra Brown and I am the phlebotomist who will be drawing your blood today. Your name is?" Ask the client/patient to state his or her full name. The phlebotomist should not ask, "Are you Mrs. Wilson?" A patient on medication may not be able to respond appropriately. If the client/patient is an **inpatient** at the hospital, verify the information on the patient's identification bracelet against the laboratory orders and the information supplied by the patient. If an identification bracelet is not present, the patient's nurse or physician must be asked to confirm the patient's identification. The nurse's or physician's name is then documented on the requisition form. If the client/patient is an outpatient, verify the patient's name and date of birth using the client/patient's driver's license or some other picture identification card.

The phlebotomist may be required to perform a procedure on a patient who is unable to verbally communicate (i.e., unconscious, in shock, or with a mental or physical disability). Often these patients will come into the emergency room. In these situations, a

INPATIENT
A patient who is hospitalized overnight.

temporary identification number will be assigned by the hospital, and a temporary identification bracelet issued. The temporary identification number will later be cross-referenced with a permanent identification number when the patient's identify is confirmed.

The next step is to wash your hands and put on gloves. Then you must select the appropriate capillary site.

◖ SITE IDENTIFICATION

Capillary punctures may be performed on fingertips, heels, toes, or earlobes. Earlobes, however, are not recommended as a site of choice, but may be used in extreme cases, such as severe burn victims.

Fingertips

Fingertips are the recommended sites for adults and older children. All fingertips may be used, with the exception of the fifth digit. The tissue on the fifth digit is much thinner and is generally more painful when punctured. The third and fourth digits are more commonly used. The second digit has thicker tissue and is harder to puncture. Although it can be used, it should not be the first choice. The fingertip should be punctured in the area illustrated in Figure 9-1 to obtain the best sample.

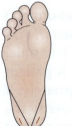 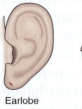 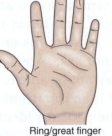 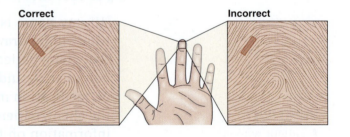

Infant's heel   Earlobe   Ring/great finger

FIGURE 9-1: Capillary blood collection sites

The site on either side of the pad of the finger allows a more generous blood flow than the tip and sides of the fingers. The risk of puncturing bone in these areas is another reason for only using the finger pad.

PERPENDICULAR

Being at right angles to the plane of the horizon.

The puncture should be made **perpendicular** to the fingerprint, causing a drop to form. Punctures made horizontal to the fingerprint cause blood to run down the finger instead of forming a drop.

Patient's requiring frequent finger sticks, such as diabetic patients, should be reminded to rotate their sites because repeated punctures at the same site can cause tissue damage.

Areas that are swollen, scarred, cyanotic, or cold are to be avoided. Blood obtained from these sites may have inaccurate test results, such as elevated hemoglobins or cell-count values.

Heel and Toes

Toes can be used instead of fingers when fingers are either not available or not usable. The site location on the toes is comparable to site locations on the fingertips.

The heel is the recommended site when performing capillary punctures on infants less than 1 year old. Care should be taken when performing the puncture, so that an area is not used that is directly over bone. Puncturing the bone may not only be painful, but can cause **osteomyelitis** and/or **osteochondritis**. Additional punctures at the same site can spread the infection.

The **calcaneous** bone of an infant's heel can be a little as 2.4 mm below the skin surface. The National Committee for Clinical Laboratory Standards (NCCLS) guidelines state which areas may be punctured and how deep the puncture may be. According to the guidelines recommended by NCCLS in document H4-A3, to avoid puncturing the bone, heel punctures should only be performed on the side of the infant's heel pad (see Figure 9-2), medial to an imaginary line extending from the middle of the great toe to the heel, or lateral to an imaginary line drawn from between the fourth and fifth toes to the heel. In addition, the depth of the puncture should not exceed 2.4 mm in depth.

Tenderfoot® makes infant and premie spring-loaded lancets that puncture precisely at the depth NCCLS recommends.

● PERFORMING THE PUNCTURE
Finger Stick
See Procedure 9-1.

Heel Stick
When performing a heel stick on an infant (Figure 9-2), extra precaution must be taken. The area in which the puncture is made and the depth of the puncture are extremely important. There are several things to remember when performing a heel stick. When performed in the hospital nursery, isolation techniques are required.

OSTEOMYELITIS

Inflammation of the bone (especially the bone marrow) caused by a pathogenic organism.

OSTEOCHONDRITIS

Inflammation of the bone and cartilage.

CALCANEOUS

The heel bone.

Procedure 9-1

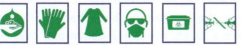

Finger Stick

Equipment/Supplies

- Lancet (Figure 9-3)
- Latex gloves
- Alcohol prep pads
- 2 × 2 gauze pads
- Microcollection container
- Required point-of-care testing equipment
- Biohazardous waste container
- Bandage
- Pen

Method/*Rationale*

1. Assemble equipment and supplies.

   Ensures everything is available to perform the procedure.

2. Wash hands/put on gloves.

   Thorough handwashing aids in controlling the spread of infection. Remember that you must comply with Standard Precautions whenever you may come in contact with body fluids or blood.

3. Identify the patient.

   Ensures the procedure is performed on the correct patient.

4. Explain the procedure to the patient.

   Helps ensure you will have the cooperation of the patient.

5. Position the patient seated or lying down with the palmar side of the hand facing up. Support the arm.

   The patient must be placed in a comfortable position with the arm secure and supported.

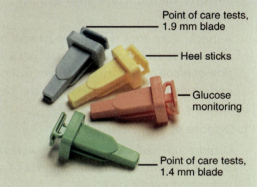
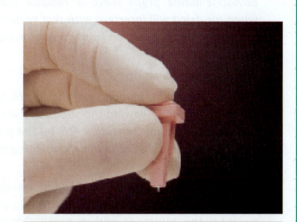

FIGURE 9-3: Microtainer® brand lancets—varying depths (Courtesy of Becton-Dickinson Vacutainer Systems)

6. Select the puncture site.

   Correct selection of the site will ensure an adequate blood flow, without risking injury to the patient.

7. Warm the site as needed.

   Blood flow can be greatly increased when the site is warm. Warming can be accomplished by massaging the finger, wrapping the finger in a warm moist towel no hotter than 108° F (hotter temperatures will burn the skin), or running the hand under warm water.

(continues)

P r o c e d u r e   9 - 1   *(continued)*

8. Clean the site.

   Use a 70% isopropyl alcohol prep pad. Do not use povidone-iodine for capillary punctures. Povidone-iodine preps leave a residue that when air-dried will interfere with test results. Clean in a circular motion from point of puncture out.

9. Allow the site to air dry.

   Air drying prevents hemolysis of the specimen from the alcohol. Allowing the site to dry also lessens the stinging sensation felt by the patient. Alcohol residue may interfere with glucose test results.

10. Grasp the patient's finger firmly but gently between your thumb and index finger and perform the puncture with a quick, "dart-like" motion.

    A quick, deep stick is no more painful than a slow superficial stick, but you will get a better flow of blood and spare the patient from a second puncture when you stick quickly and deeply only once.

11. Dispose of the lancet.

    Dispose immediately in the biohazardous sharps container to prevent the risk of a contaminated needle stick.

12. While applying gentle pressure to the patient's finger, wipe away the first drop of blood with sterile 2 × 2 gauze pad.

    Remember that the first drop of blood contains interstitial fluid that can dilute the sample.

13. Continue to apply a firm, even pressureproximal to the puncture site.

    This will ensure a steady blood flow. If necessary, massage or "milk" the patient's finger to increase blood flow. Note, however, that this should be kept to a minimum, as excessive massaging can cause interstitial fluid to dilute the specimen.

14. Collect the blood samples in the appropriate microcollection containers.

15. Once the specimens have been collected, place a clean, dry 2 × 2 gauze pad over the puncture site.

    Ask the patient to apply direct pressure to stop any further bleeding.

16. Place a bandage over the puncture site of an adult or older child.

    Never use a bandage on a child under the age of two, as the child may choke on it if it becomes loose.

17. Mix any collection containers that contain an additive.

    This ensures that anticoagulants will be thoroughly mixed with the blood to prevent coagulation.

18. Dispose of contaminated material in the appropriate biohazardous waste container and remove all equipment from the area.

    Disposing of contaminated material immediately reduces the risk of spreading infections.

19. Label the specimens with the appropriate information.

    Labeling the specimens before leaving the area ensures that the correct specimen will be tested for the correct patient.

20. Remove gloves and dispose of in the appropriate biohazardous waste container.

21. Wash your hands.

    Washing your hands reduces the risk of infection.

22. Transport the specimens to the lab for testing, or put on a new pair of gloves and perform point-of-care testing.

Procedure 9-2

Heel Stick—Infant

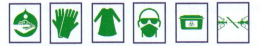

Equipment/Supplies

- Lancet—*must be less than 2.4 mm in length*
- Latex gloves
- Alcohol prep pads
- 2 × 2 gauze pads
- Microcollection container
- Required point-of-care testing equipment
- Biohazardous waste container
- Bandage
- Pen

Method/*Rationale*

1. Assemble equipment and supplies.

   Ensures everything is available to perform the procedure.

2. Wash hands/put on gloves.

   Thorough handwashing aids in controlling the spread of infection. Remember that you must comply with Standard Precautions whenever you may come in contact with body fluids or blood.

3. Identify the patient.

   Ensures the procedure is performed on the correct patient. Have the infant's or small child's parent or guardian provide identification.

4. Explain the procedure.

   Helps ensure you will have the cooperation of the patient. Because your patient is an infant, explain the procedure to the parent or guardian.

5. Position the patient lying down in a supine position, or lying across the parent's or guardian's lap. It is also possible to position the infant securely in a parent's or guardian's arms, leaving the foot exposed. The "burp" position on an adult's shoulder is also very effective; the infant's foot is in a down position, thereby allowing gravity to help with the flow of blood.

   The patient must be placed in a comfortable position but securely supported.

6. Select the puncture site.

   Correct selection of the site will ensure an adequate blood flow, without risking injury to the patient.

7. Warm the site as needed.

   Blood flow can be greatly increased when the site is warm. Warming the heel can be accomplished by massage, wrapping the heel in a warm moist towel, no hotter than 108°F (hotter temperatures will burn the skin). Commercially prepared heel warmers may also be used.

8. Grasp the patient's heel firmly but gently (see Figure 9-2). Hold the heel with your thumb below the puncture site and your index finger above the site in the curve of the arch of the infant or young child's foot; your remaining fingers and palm of your hand will cradle the patient's foot.

9. Clean the site.

   Use a 70% isopropyl alcohol prep pad. Do not use povidone-iodine for capillary punctures. Povidone-iodine leaves a residue that when air-dried will interfere with test results. Clean in a circular motion from point of puncture out.

(continues)

Procedure 9-2 *(continued)*

10. Allow the site to air dry.

    Air drying prevents hemolysis of the specimen from the alcohol. Allowing the site to dry also lessens the stinging sensation felt by the patient. Alcohol residue may interfere with glucose test results.

11. Perform the puncture.

    A quick, deep stick is no more painful than a slow, superficial stick, but you will get a better flow of blood and spare the patient a second puncture when you stick quickly and deeply only once.

12. Dispose of the lancet.

    Dispose immediately in the biohazardous sharps container to prevent the risk of a contaminated needle stick.

13. Apply a firm, even pressure proximal to the puncture site. Wipe away the first drop of blood.

    This will ensure a steady blood flow. If necessary, massage or "milk" the patient's heel to increase blood flow. Note, however, that this should be kept to a minimum as excessive massaging can cause interstitial fluid to dilute the specimen.

14. Collect the blood samples in the appropriate microcollection containers or filter paper test cards.

15. Once the specimens have been collected place a clean, dry gauze pad over the puncture site.

    Apply direct pressure until all bleeding has stopped. Never use a bandage on a child under the age of 2, as the child may choke on it if it becomes loose.

16. Mix any collection containers that contain an additive.

    This ensures that anticoagulants will be thoroughly mixed with the blood to prevent coagulation.

17. Dispose of contaminated material in the appropriate biohazardous waste container and remove all equipment from the area.

    Disposing of contaminated material immediately reduces the risk of spreading infections.

18. Label the specimens with the appropriate information.

    Labeling the specimens before leaving the area ensures that the correct specimen will be tested for the correct patient.

19. Remove gloves and dispose of in the appropriate biohazardous waste container.

20. Wash your hands.

    Washing your hands reduces the risk of infection.

21. Transport the specimens to the lab for testing, or perform point-of-care testing as appropriate.

Never take the blood-drawing tray into the nursery with you. The nursery has its own equipment and supplies. Hands must be washed thoroughly for a minimum of 3 minutes. Don a gown and mask as required. Follow all hospital protocols for working with infants. Never puncture areas that are bruised or have been previously punctured. Ensure that the infant's heel is warmed adequately prior to the puncture. If it is not, use a commercially prepared heel warmer.

PROCESSING THE SPECIMEN

Order of Draw

It is important to collect specimens in the correct order. To minimize the risk of platelets clumping in the collection device, smear slides first, then collect any hematology samples, then collect all other samples. Use the order of draw listed in Chapter 8 for microcollection containers with anticoagulants.

Microcollection Containers

There are a wide variety of microcollection containers available for use by today's phlebotomist. The proper collection container must be selected according to the type of test requested. Most microcollection containers are made of plastic, with built-in scoops in their lids. Microcollection containers may also contain the same additives as evacuated tubes, and are color-coded in the same manner (i.e., lavender top collection containers contain EDTA in both the evacuated tube and the microcollection tube). Some laboratories prefer to use a specific type of container. It is important to become familiar with the different varieties used by the laboratory.

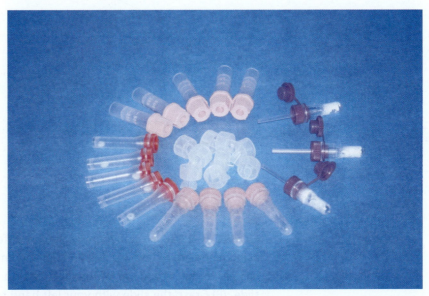

FIGURE 9-4: Microcollection containers

Blood Smears

The phlebotomist performs blood smears so the medical laboratory technician (MLT) or physician can interpret the results by using a microscope. A blood smear is a drop of blood that is placed on one end of a glass slide and then spread in a thin, even smear using another glass slide (Figure 9-5). Most laboratories prefer blood smears to be made from fresh capillary blood. Whole blood from a lavender top tube may also be used, but fresh capillary blood provides a better slide.

As it is the responsibility of the phlebotomist to smear the slide at the time of the puncture, it is imperative that he or she knows the criteria for a readable slide and how to perform the procedure.

The blood smear is performed immediately after wiping away the first drop of blood of a capillary puncture. It is the first specimen obtained according to the capillary order of draw.

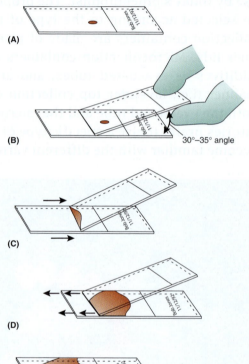

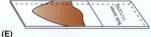

FIGURE 9-5: Making a blood smear for a differential white blood cell count using a spreader slide: (A) Position labeled end to right if you are right-handed, or left if you are left-handed. Place a small drop of blood on the slide. (B) Grasp the slide with your left hand to steady it. (C) Pull the spreader slide back into the drop of blood. Let the blood spread along the back side of the spreader slide. (D) Quickly, without jerking, push the spreader slide to the left. (E) Allow the blood smear to air-dry before it is stained.

Making a good blood smear is an art that takes practice to perfect. Blood smears that are improperly done will have an uneven distribution of cells, which will give inaccurate test results.

Procedure 9-3

Making a Blood Smear

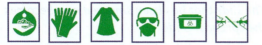

Equipment/Supplies

- Latex gloves
- Two glass slides
- Fresh capillary blood or EDTA venous blood
- Pipette or DIFF-SAFE®
- 2 × 2 gauze pads
- Biohazardous waste
- Sharps container
- Pen

Method/*Rationale*

1. Assemble equipment and supplies.

   Ensures everything is available to perform the procedure.

2. Wash hands/put on gloves.

   Thorough handwashing aids in controlling the spread of infection. Remember that you must comply with Standard Precautions whenever you may come in contact with body fluids or blood.

3. Select two glass slides.

   Slides must be clean and free from chips or cracks.

4. Place on each slide one medium-sized drop of blood (1 to 2 mm).

   This is approximately ¹/₂ inch, centered from the end of the slide.

5. Use one of the slides as the first spreader slide.

6. Place it in front of the drop of blood. Hold the spreader slide in your dominant hand at a 45˚ angle.

7. Slowly back the spreader slide into the drop of blood.

   Allow the drop of blood to spread all the way across the slide. This ensures that the smear will be wide enough.

8. Lower the angle of the spreader slide to a 30˚ angle and quickly push the slide along the length of the stationary glass slide.

   This movement is like that of striking a match or pretending the spreader slide is like an airplane taking off the runway.

9. Evaluate the smear.

   The smear should be at least 1/2 of the slide's length; 3/4 of the slide's length is preferable. The blood starts out thicker at the end closest to the original drop of blood and gradually thins as it gets closer to the other end.

   The smear should have a feathered edge at the thin end of the smear, and when held to the light, a rainbow should be seen. The feathered edge is only one cell thick and is the most important area of the slide. It is the location where the **differential** *is read (Figure 9-6).*

   DIFFERENTIAL

   The number and type of cells; determined by microscopic examination of a thin layer of blood on a glass slide.

   The smear should be free from any holes, lines, or jagged edges, and must be centered on the slide.

(continues)

Procedure 9-3 *(continued)*

Applying too much pressure can cause the smear to have ridges of blood in the feathered end or little strings of blood past the feathered edge. These strings of blood may be caused by using an unclean or chipped spreader slide.

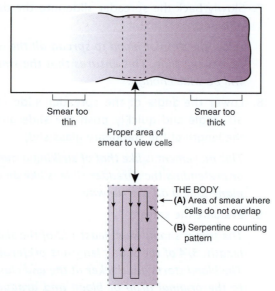

Smear too thin

Smear too thick

Proper area of smear to view cells

THE BODY

(A) Area of smear where cells do not overlap

(B) Serpentine counting pattern

FIGURE 9-6: Proper area of slide to be viewed for differential count: (A) Close-up of proper body; (B) counting pattern.

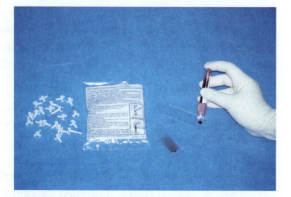

FIGURE 9-7: DIFF-SAFE®

10. Once the smear has been made on the first slide, repeat the procedure on the second slide.

    The slide that has been smeared now becomes the spreader slide.

11. When both slides have been made they are left to air dry, standing on end with the drop of blood end down.

    If you are using frosted slides you may write the patient's name in pencil on the frosted end of the slide. Otherwise, attach a paper label to the blood end of the slide. Do not use ink as it will be washed off during the staining process.

12. Transport the slide to the laboratory.

    The slide will be stained and interpreted in the laboratory.

Box 9-1: Blood Smears and DIFF-SAFE®

Blood smears may be made using anticoagulated venous blood. A specimen drawn in a lavender top evacuated tube can be used. Make sure the specimen has been thoroughly mixed with the EDTA.

There are several methods for dispensing a drop of blood from an evacuated tube onto the glass slide. Using a pipette or capillary tube are two methods. Both require removing the cap from the evacuated tube. Another method is using the DIFF-SAFE® (Figure 9-7). The DIFF-SAFE® allows a slide to be prepared from an EDTA tube without removing the stopper. The DIFF-SAFE® is pushed through the stopper of the EDTA tube and then pressed against the slide to deliver a uniform drop of blood.

● SUMMARY

Capillary puncture is an excellent method for collecting blood specimens when only small amounts of blood are required. With practice, this procedure can be accomplished with minimal discomfort to the patient and can provide accurate test results to the physician.

COMPETENCY CHECK-OFF SHEETS
Capillary Finger Stick Competency Check

Given all the equipment and supplies, the student will be required to perform, within 5 minutes, a capillary finger stick on a classmate/patient. A "0" in more than two areas or an overall score of less than 80% will require the procedure to be repeated for competency.

Points to Be Awarded:	5 pts	2.5 pts	1 pt	0 pts	total pts
1 Assemble and prepare equipment and supplies					
2 Identify the patient					
3 Explain the procedure					
4 Select the puncture site					
5 Warm the site as needed					
6 Gloving					
7 Position patient (palmar side of hand up)					
8 Clean site with alcohol					
9 Air dry site					
10 Grasp patient's finger					
11 Perform the puncture					
12 Dispose of lancet					
13 Squeeze patient's finger					
14 Wipe first drop of blood					
15 Collect sample in appropriate microcollection containers					
16 Apply direct pressure					
17 Bandage puncture site					
18 Mix any collection containers w/additives					
19 Dispose of any contaminated materials					
20 Label specimens					
21 Remove gloves					

Chapter 9 Collection by Capillary Puncture ● **369**

Points to Be Awarded:	5 pts	2.5 pts	1 pt	0 pts	total pts
22 Wash hands					
23 Transport specimen to lab or perform point-of-care testing					

Total Points Possible: _____   Total Points Earned: _____

Start Time: _____   End Time: _____

Instructor Signature: _____   Date: _____

Student Signature: _____   Date: _____

STUDY AND REVIEW EXERCISES

Defining Key Terms

Write the definition for each of the following key terms.

1) calcaneous _____

2) differential _____

3) inpatient _____

4) interstitial fluid _____

5) osteochondritis _____

6) osteomyelitis _____

7) perpendicular _____

8) superficial _____

Reviewing Key Points

1) Describe the composition of capillary blood.

2) Identify the circumstances when a capillary puncture is appropriate.

3) List the appropriate "Order of Draw" for specimens collected by capillary puncture.

4) Describe the procedure for preparing a blood smear.

5) Describe two precautions associated with capillary puncture site selection.

Sentence Completion

1) Capillary punctures can also be referred to as _____, _____, or _____.

2) Capillary blood more closely resembles _____ blood in composition.

3) _____ levels are higher in capillary blood specimens.

4) _____ is located between the tissues of the skin and is released into the blood during the process of a capillary puncture.

5) When performing a finger stick, all fingertips may be used with the exception of the _____ digit.

6) A capillary puncture of the finger should be made _____ to the fingerprint.

7) The _____ is the recommended site when performing capillary punctures on infants less than 1 year old.

8) The calcaneous bone of an infant's heel is approximately _____ below the skin's surface.

9) _____ sets the guidelines that state which areas can be punctured and how deep to puncture when performing a capillary stick.

10) Whole blood from a _____ top evacuated tube may also be used when preparing a blood smear.

Multiple Choice

1) Of the following supplies, which item is *NOT* required to perform a capillary puncture?
   A. Gloves
   B. Tourniquet
   C. Lancet
   D. Microcollection container

2) When performing a capillary puncture, the phlebotomist runs the risk of puncturing bone in which one of the following locations?
   A. Heel
   B. Second digit
   C. Fifth digit
   D. It is possible to puncture bone in all the above

3) Punctures made _____ to the fingerprint cause blood to run down the finger instead of forming a well-rounded drop of blood.
   A. distal
   B. perpendicular
   C. horizontal
   D. medial

4) Puncturing a bone is not only painful but can cause which one of the following disorders?
   A. Diabetes
   B. Osteomalacia
   C. Melanoma
   D. Osteochondritis

5) In the following list, which activity would be done first when performing a finger stick?
   A. Explain the procedure to the patient.
   B. Dispose of the lancet.
   C. Identify the patient.
   D. Assemble and prepare equipment and supplies.

6) When performing a capillary puncture, position the patient seated or lying down with the _____ side of the hand facing up.
   A. dorsal
   B. palmar
   C. ventral
   D. plantar

7) It is imperative to wipe away the first drop of blood immediately following the capillary puncture because:
   A. It is contaminated with alcohol and interstitial fluid.
   B. The patient may see it and faint.
   C. You will not be able to see the puncture site to collect the specimens.
   D. It is not necessary to wipe away the first drop of blood.

8) "Milking" the patient's finger causes severe tissue damage and should never be performed.
   A. True
   B. False

9) When performing a capillary puncture, the blood will flow more freely if the area to be punctured is slightly cold to the touch.
   A. True
   B. False

10) When making blood smears, which one of the following statements is correct?
   A. The smear should be less than 1/2 the length of the slide.
   B. Once the slide has been made you should blow on it to dry it quickly.
   C. The feathered edge is the most important area of the slide.
   D. Only mark on the slide with black ink.

Critical Thinking

1) You have a STAT order for a white blood count via a heel stick on an infant in the nursery. The infant's mother is holding the baby when you arrive. Explain the procedure to the new mom.

Collection by Routine Venipuncture

CHAPTER 10

KEY TERMS

aliquot (**AL**-ih-kwot)
antecubital (**an**-tee-**KU**-bi-tal)
bevel (**BEV**-el)
hemoconcentration
 (**he**-mo-**kon**-sen-**TRAY**-shun)
hemolysis (he-**MOL**-ih-sis)
occluded (**o**-**KLUDE**-ed)
palpate (**PAL**-payt)
periphery (**per**-**IF**-eh-ree)
reflux (**RE**-fluks)
sclerosed (skle-**ROZT**)
thrombosed (**THROM**-bosd)
venipuncture
 (**VEN**-ih-**punk**-chur)

● OBJECTIVES

Upon completion of this chapter the student should be able to:

- Define and correctly spell each of the key terms.
- List the supplies and equipment required to perform a venipuncture.
- Identify the essential information on a laboratory requisition slip.
- Describe the patient identification process, the information that must be verified, and how to handle discrepancies.
- Describe how to prepare patients for testing.
- Identify the location of antecubital, hand, and wrist veins.
- Describe the procedure for applying a tourniquet, including the time constraints.
- Describe each step of the venipuncture procedure.
- Describe the variance in collection using the evacuated tube method, the syringe method, and the butterfly infusion set.
- List the information that is required when labeling tubes.
- Describe the situations that would lead to a "short draw" or failure to obtain a specimen, and the techniques to overcome or correct each.
- List the necessary precautions involved in performing a venipuncture if the patient has an intravenous infusion, is an outpatient, or has a hematoma over the venipuncture site.
- Describe the procedure for handling routine specimens.

(continues)

- Describe the processing of specimens that require special handling, such as: specimens requiring protection from light, specimens that must be chilled, specimens that must be kept warm, and timed specimens.
- Describe the procedure for centrifuging blood specimens.
- Describe the procedure for separating plasma and serum into aliquot tubes.
- List reasons why specimens are rejected.
- Describe the process of prioritizing patients.

OUTLINE

- Introduction
- Phlebotomist Preparation—Assembling and Preparing Equipment
- Client/Patient Identification and Preparation
- Sequence of Venipuncture Procedure
- Specimen Identification and Tube Labeling
- Failure to Obtain Blood and Other Considerations
- Other Considerations Regarding Routine Venipuncture
- Specimen Integrity—Quality Assurance
- Processing a Blood Specimen
- Specimen Rejection
- Prioritizing Patients

INTRODUCTION

VENIPUNCTURE

Puncture of a vein for any purpose.

Routine **venipuncture** is the main method used to obtain a blood sample for diagnostic testing. Chapter 8 discussed the equipment required to perform the three methods of venipuncture collection: evacuated tube collection, syringe collection, and butterfly infusion set collection. This chapter addresses the techniques and procedures used for obtaining blood samples by each of these methods.

It is important that the phlebotomist learn the correct venipuncture techniques, using each of these methods. Most patients have only a limited number of accessible veins, and maintaining the integrity of these veins is always the primary goal. The phlebotomist must learn to assess the patient's veins accurately and must use the appropriate method of collection to prevent damage to existing collection sites. Vein assessment becomes even more important when drawing blood from a hospitalized patient. Inpatients may have repeated venipunctures for diagnostic testing to monitor therapeutic drug levels, or to assess the progression of their condition.

Every phlebotomist will establish a routine for performing a venipuncture. There are a variety of accepted techniques and routines. This text focuses on the most widely accepted and most commonly used methods, thereby establishing a basic standardized guideline (Box 10-1) that can be adapted to fit individual facility requirements and protocols.

Box 10-1: Guidelines for Venipuncture Routine

- Collect equipment
- Review laboratory requisition form
- Identify patient
- Wash hands
- Don gloves
- Explain procedure to patient
- Assemble equipment
- Apply tourniquet
- Select site
- Clean site
- Air dry
- Insert needle
- Collect specimen
- Release tourniquet
- Apply direct pressure to site
- Mix tubes
- Apply dressing
- Instruct patient on site care
- Thank patient
- Label tubes
- Remove gloves
- Wash hands
- Transport specimen to laboratory

PHLEBOTOMIST PREPARATION— ASSEMBLING AND PREPARING EQUIPMENT

As presented in Chapter 8, the following equipment is assembled prior to blood collection by venipuncture:

- Personal protective equipment (PPE)
- Antiseptic: 70% isopropyl alcohol pads or povidone-iodine pads
- 2 × 2 gauze pads
- Bandages
- Sharps container

- Biohazardous waste container
- Tourniquet
- Evacuated tubes
  —Evacuated Tube Method
  - Tube adapter/holder
  - Evacuated tube multidraw needles, 20 to 21 gauge, 1 to 1½ inches
  —Syringe Method
  - Syringe—3 cc, 5 cc, or 10 cc
  - Needle—single-sample, 20 to 21 gauge, 1 to 1½ inches
  —Butterfly Method
  - Syringe—10 cc or pediatric evacuated tube equipment
  - Butterfly infusion set

The next step is to review the laboratory requisition form. Make sure all information is complete, as was discussed in Chapter 5. Verify the date and time of the collection, as well as all specific requirements, such as diet restrictions or priority of testing. Determine the identity of the ordered tests and make sure the required supplies and equipment are assembled prior to the draw.

● CLIENT/PATIENT IDENTIFICATION AND PREPARATION

Patient identification is critical. Follow the same procedure outlined in Chapter 9. Introduce yourself first and then ask the client or patient to state his or her full name. For inpatients, verify the information on the patient's identification bracelet against the laboratory orders and the information supplied by the patient. At this time also verify that the patient has followed required diet restrictions, for example, nothing by mouth (NPO) after midnight, or fasting for 12 hours.

The next step is to perform proper handwashing and don a pair of gloves.

The phlebotomist now assembles the equipment (Figure 10-1). Secure the needle on the tube adapter or assemble syringe or butterfly infusion set, open the antiseptic, set out the required tubes in the correct order of draw, open the bandage, and set out a small stack (5 to 6) of 2 × 2 gauze pads.

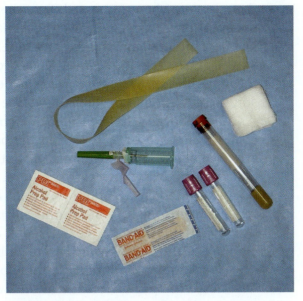

FIGURE 10-1: Routine venipuncture equipment

Patients are generally nervous about having their blood drawn. The phlebotomist should reassure and calm the patient. Explain to the patient each step of the procedure prior to beginning it. Patients may be afraid that it will be painful. Tell the patient to expect some discomfort, but that it will be over quickly. Never tell a patient "It won't hurt," especially when the patient is a child. If it does hurt, and the patient has been told that it won't hurt, the patient will lose trust in the medical profession and in you in particular. Rewarding children when the procedure is over is a great incentive to be "good" during the draw. Stickers, cartoon character bandages, or badges work well. Although children may prefer it, giving candy is generally discouraged.

Position the patient in either a sitting or lying down position prior to the blood draw. Never draw a patient's blood while the patient is standing. If the patient is sitting, ensure the patient can sit with the feet comfortably on the ground. Do not use a chair with rollers or allow a patient to sit in a chair that keeps the feet from comfortably reaching the ground. Place a box or book under the feet if necessary.

Gain the patient's cooperation by being honest and efficient. Talk to your patient throughout the entire procedure. Focusing on conversation takes the patient's mind off the needle. Or if you feel it might help keep the patient involved, you may ask the patient to take an active role in the procedure by holding gauze pads or by handing you the evacuated tubes. Backup gauze and tubes should be accessible if the patient cannot follow through with handing them to you when requested. Do not surprise the patient with the needle stick. Always tell the patient that you are ready to insert the needle. State it in a matter-of-fact tone: "Mrs. Carter, now you'll feel a little stick," and move on with the collection. Once the needle is through the skin and has passed the nerve endings, there is no reason the patient should feel any further discomfort.

Most laboratories have special blood-drawing, or "phlebotomy," chairs. When seated in the chair, the patient's arm is placed on the attached armrest and extended in a straight line from shoulder to wrist in a slightly downward position. Hospital inpatients are generally situated in a supine position, as are outpatients who feel faint or have a history of fainting during blood draws. As with the seated patient, the arm is extended in a straight line and is in a position with the hand lower than the elbow. Pillows or rolled towels are used to help accommodate this position as necessary.

There are special considerations when drawing blood from an inpatient in a hospital bed. The bed rails are lowered on the side of the bed where the phlebotomist will be working. The phlebotomist must be careful to avoid catching IV lines, catheter bags, or other tubing or equipment when lowering the bed rails. The rails are raised when the draw is complete, for the safety of the patient. As a member of the professional health care team, the phlebotomist will be held liable for any injury to the patient that occurs because of carelessness in not raising the bed rails. It is because of this liability that some hospital protocols state *never* to lower the bed rails to perform a venipuncture. The phlebotomist must also learn how to collect the blood specimen without lowering the bed rails when there is a risk of the patient falling from the bed.

While having blood drawn, patients must not be permitted to eat, drink, or have anything in their mouths, such as candy thermometers or lozenges. The patient could reflexively bite down or choke on anything in his or her mouth at the time of the draw.

● SEQUENCE OF VENIPUNCTURE PROCEDURE

Site Identification

ANTECUBITAL

In front of the elbow; at the end of the elbow.

Most frequently, venipuncture is performed in the **antecubital** area of the arm where the median cubital, cephalic, and basilic veins are located close to the surface (Figure 10-2). Examine this area first, being sure to check both arms. Patients who have had their blood drawn in the past will often tell you where their "best vein" is located. If you examine their "best vein" and you are not comfortable with it, do not hesitate to check for other veins before drawing. The most prominent veins are generally in the arm of the patient's dominant hand.

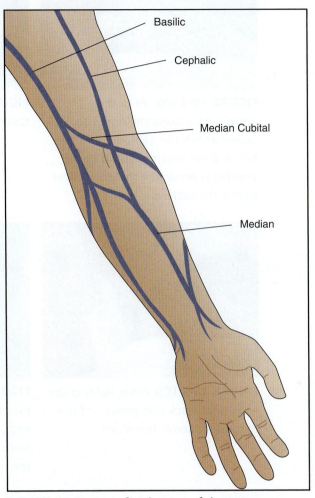

FIGURE 10-2: Superficial veins of the arm

Application of Tourniquet

● Select the appropriate tourniquet, as presented in Chapter 8.
● Inspect the patient's arms for the most likely vein.
● Wrap the tourniquet around the patient's arm approximately 3 to 4 inches above the venipuncture site. A method for gauging this distance is to place your hand, with your index finger on the site, and measure up four fingers.
● Bring both ends of the tourniquet around to the front of the patient's arm. (See Figure 10-3.)

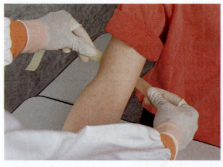

FIGURE 10-3 (A): Wrap the tourniquet around the arm 3 to 4 inches above the venipuncture site. Keeping the tourniquet flat to the skin helps minimize the discomfort felt by the patient.

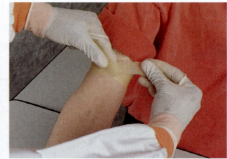

FIGURE 10-3 (B): Stretch the tourniquet tight and cross the ends.

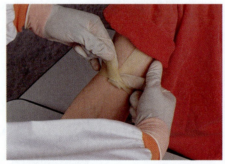

FIGURE 10-3 (C): While holding the ends tight, tuck one portion of the tourniquet under the other.

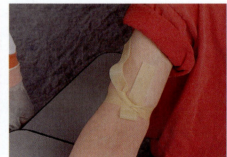

FIGURE 10-3 (D): Check that the tourniquet will not come loose. The ends of the tourniquet should be pointed upward and not hang into the intended venipuncture site.

● Pull the left end of the tourniquet taut, and hold steady.
● Pull the right end tighter as you pull across the front of the patient's arm, crossing the right end over the top of the left end and grasping both sides of the tourniquet with the thumb and forefinger of one hand.
● Pull the right loose end slightly down and create a loop.
● Tuck the loop up under the area of the tourniquet that has been crossed.
● The loose ends should be running up the patient's arm and away from the venipuncture site. The tourniquet will cause the veins to bulge, which will make them appear more prominent.
● To release the tourniquet, gently tug on the right free end.

When applying a tourniquet to a patient with fragile skin that tears or bruises easily, apply the tourniquet on top of the patient's shirt or blouse, as this will reduce the friction applied directly to the skin. You may also wrap gauze around the area prior to application of the tourniquet.

Box 10-2: Do's and Don'ts of Tourniquets

Improper application or use of tourniquets during a venipuncture can cause hemoconcentration of the specimen. The sample will render inaccurate test results and the specimen will be rejected. The sample will need to be recollected.

● Do place the tourniquet 3 to 4 inches above the venipuncture site.
● Do remove the tourniquet within 1 minute of application.
● Do remove the tourniquet prior to withdrawing the needle from the patient.
● Do *not* apply the tourniquet over an open sore or burn.
● Do *not* apply a tourniquet to an arm on the same side as a recent mastectomy.
● Do *not* apply the tourniquet so tightly that all circulation is compromised.

HEMOCONCENTRA-TION

A relative increase in the number of red blood cells resulting from a decrease in the volume of plasma.

PALPATE

To examine by touch; to feel.

SCLEROSED

Hardened; having sclerosis.

Asking your patient to make a fist will also help make the vein more prominent. Do not, however, request the patient to vigorously open and close the fist, as this can contribute to **hemoconcentration**, which causes some test results to be inaccurate.

Do not rely on visually locating a vein. Frequently patients have veins you cannot see. Using the tip of the index finger to **palpate** the vein is the most accurate method of locating a vein. Gently "bounce" your index finger across the antecubital area. Veins will bounce back; arteries will pulsate. Do not rub your finger across the patient's arm. Veins cannot bounce back if you are rubbing. If you are having difficulty locating a vein, close your eyes and feel. Closing your eyes increases your sense of touch. Train yourself to locate veins while wearing gloves because this will save you time in the long run. For example, if the phlebotomist places the tourniquet, palpates the vein, and then puts on gloves the tourniquet will be in place too long, causing hemoconcentration. Palpating veins allows you to identify the direction of the vein, how deep beneath the surface of the skin the vein is located, and the size of the vein. Select a vein that feels large and well anchored, and one that will not "roll" off to one side when pushed by the needle. Try not to select a vein that feels hard or cord-like, as these veins may be **sclerosed** and are more difficult to penetrate with the needle. A

THROMBOSED

Denoting a vessel containing a thrombus.

thrombosed vein also feels hard and should not be used as a venipuncture site. Veins that are located beneath scar tissue, burns, tattoos, or moles should not be used; select another site. IV drug users often have scar tissue surrounding their veins. If this is the case, ask patient for the location of their "best" vein.

Once a vein is selected, keep a mental picture of its location. Reference the location to an existing landmark such as a mole or freckle. This technique makes it easier to return to the location after disinfecting the area.

Box 10-3: Tips for Marking Venipuncture Site

There are several methods for temporarily marking the location of a vein. With practice, keeping a mental picture of the vein location will become easier. However, even an experienced phlebotomist will occasionally have difficulty locating a vein and will need to "mark" the vein once it has been located. One of the ways to accomplish this is to take the end of a pen with the ink cartridge retracted and gently push in over the site, leaving a small round indentation over the area the needle will be inserted.

Another method that works well is to leave your index finger over the vein with the distal joint line of the finger directly lined up with where the needle will be inserted. Move the finger just slightly above the insertion site, to allow for cleansing of the area.

Yet another method is to locate the vein, then keep your index finger over the site, clean the area, and with your free hand position the corner of a clean alcohol prep pad in direct line with the vein and remove the finger. Keep the prep pad far enough away from the site so it will not interfere with the draw.

If an antecubital site is not suitable on either arm, check the wrists and backs of each hand for a vein. If a suitable site cannot be located, warm the arm or hand by wrapping a warm, moist towel (42° C) around the site, leave in place for 3 to 5 minutes, reapply tourniquet, and then try to locate a vein again. Warming the area increases the blood flow to make the veins more prominent.

When no other site can be located, ankle veins may be used, but only with written permission from the patient's physician. As lower extremity circulation may be compromised, especially in bedridden patients, inaccurate test results frequently occur. Drawing blood specimens from a patient's ankle also increases the risk of blood clots and additional impaired circulation. Some facilities do not permit ankle draws at all because of liability issues.

There may be occasions when the phlebotomist cannot locate an acceptable vein. When this is the case, you must follow institutional protocols which may include asking another phlebotomist, a nurse, or physician to perform the draw.

Cleansing the Venipuncture Site

Venipuncture sites must be cleansed thoroughly prior to insertion of the needle. Remember that skin tissue can never totally be sterilized, so it must be cleansed as thoroughly as possible. When cleaning the venipuncture site there are two options. The first option, and the most frequently used, is cleansing with alcohol wipes. The second option, povidone-iodine, is used for blood cultures, when a patient is allergic to alcohol, or for collection of specimens for blood-alcohol level testing. The following guidelines apply to both alcohol and povidone-iodine cleansing procedures.

- Remove the alcohol prep or povidone-iodine prep from its package.
- Cleanse the venipuncture site in a circular motion from the center to the **periphery**. Use sufficient pressure to remove surface debris and dirt. If the site is especially dirty, repeat the procedure with a new alcohol prep or povidone-iodine swab until the site appears clean.
- Allow the area to air dry for 30 to 60 seconds. Do not wipe the cleansed area with a gauze pad, because this will introduce new microorganisms to the site. Do not fan or blow on the site to dry it faster. Blowing and fanning introduce airborne contaminants. Evaporation helps to destroy the microbes. In addition, not allowing the site to dry thoroughly causes the patient to feel a burning sensation when the needle is inserted and may hemolyze the specimen.
- Do not touch the site once it has been cleansed. If it is necessary to repalpate the vein, the site must be recleansed.
- Being very careful not to touch the cleansed site, reapply the tourniquet. Once the venipuncture technique has been mastered, you should be able to apply the tourniquet, locate the vein, clean the vein, and draw the specimen without removing the tourniquet and reapplying it. *Remember:* A tourniquet must not be left in place for longer than 1 minute.

Performing the Puncture

Evacuated Tube Draw

Place the first evacuated tube in the tube adapter. Do not push it onto the needle. Remove the needle cover. Examine the needle for

PERIPHERY

The outer part or surface of a body; the part away from the center.

defects such as chips or burrs. Needles that are defective must be replaced. Once the needle cover has been removed, the needle cannot touch any surface prior to insertion into the patient's vein. If the needle touches any surface it is considered contaminated and must be replaced.

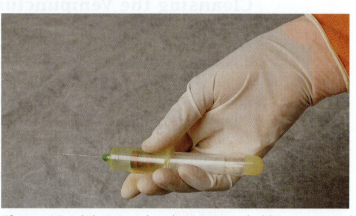

Figure 10-4 (A): Proper hand position to hold an evacuated tube system

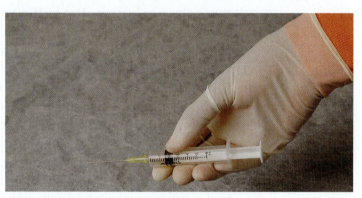

Figure 10-4 (B): Proper hand position to hold a syringe

Hold the blood-drawing equipment in your dominant hand (Figure 10-4). Rest the blood-drawing equipment on your *fingertips*, with your index and middle finger holding the tube adapter, and your ring and little finger holding the evacuated tube. Press up gently on the evacuated tube so the tube is firmly against the top of the inside of the tube adapter. Your thumb will be resting on the top of the tube adapter. Using this method gives you a more secure hold when inserting the needle. Do not push the tube onto the needle.

Some phlebotomists prefer not to put the evacuated tube into the adapter until after the needle has been inserted into the vein. Either method is acceptable.

With your nondominant hand, grasp the patient's arm approximately 1 to 2 inches below the venipuncture site. Pull the skin taut

BEVEL

The point of a needle that has been cut on a slant for ease of entry.

with your thumb. This procedure secures the vein and helps to keep it from rolling. Pulling the skin taut also eases the insertion of the needle into the patient's skin. Using the two-finger technique—thumb and index finger—to pull the skin taut is not recommended. It increases the risk of an accidental needle stick if the patient should suddenly jerk or pull his arm back. The needle may bounce into the phlebotomist's finger.

Insert the needle, holding it at a 15 to 30-degree angle. Adjust the angle according to the angle of the patient's vein. Deeper veins will need a greater angle. Position the needle to follow the line of the patient's vein. It is recommended that the **bevel** of the needle be facing up upon insertion. Insert the needle, penetrating the skin and then the vein in one quick, smooth motion. A slight "give" and less resistance are felt when the needle enters the vein. As soon as you sense the needle is in the vein, stop advancing the needle and anchor the tube adapter. The needle is generally inserted so that the entire bevel is in the vein.

Some phlebotomists like to switch hands at this point, anchoring the tube adapter with their nondominant hand. If the phlebotomist chooses to use this method, the fingers of the nondominant hand are gently slid underneath the tube adapter with the thumb on top. The needle in the patient's arm must not move as the dominant hand releases the tube. This method allows the phlebotomist to have more control while pushing the evacuated tubes onto the needle. Phlebotomists who are left-handed generally do not switch hands and continue to hold the tube adapter steady while changing tubes with their nondominant hand.

Whichever method is used, it is most important to hold the blood-drawing equipment steady. Moving the needle not only causes the patient discomfort but can cause damage to underlying tissues and nerves.

Once the needle is successfully inserted into the vein, push the evacuated tube onto the needle. Securely anchor the blood-drawing equipment before doing so. Grasp the flanges of the tube adapter with the index and middle finger. While gently pulling with these fingers, push the evacuated tube onto the needle with your thumb. This push/pull counteraction will help prevent the needle from moving. Blood will begin to fill the tube immediately if the needle is in the vein.

Keep the needle steady in the patient's arm. Do not push or pull down on the needle while it is in the vein, as this will cause pain. Keep the patient's arm and the tube in a downward position, with the tube filling from the bottom up. This positioning will prevent

REFLUX

A return or backward flow.

reflux. It will also prevent the carryover of additives from tube to tube because of blood left on the needle as tubes are changed.

Because of the amount of vacuum pressure, evacuated tubes will fill approximately two-thirds of the way full. They will not fill completely to the top of the tube. The vacuum inside the tube will exhaust at approximately the two-thirds point and blood flow will stop. If the vacuum seems to have exhausted before the blood is at this point, the tube may be defective or out-of-date. Another tube of blood will be needed if this occurs. The ratio of blood to additive is critical and will be incorrect if the tube is not filled appropriately. Test results will be inaccurate.

If you are drawing only one tube of blood, loosen the tourniquet as soon as blood begins to fill the tube. Blood will continue to fill the tube without the tourniquet. If you are drawing more than one tube of blood, wait to remove the tourniquet until the last tube is filled. Keep in mind, however, that the tourniquet must not be kept on for more than 2 minutes. Three to four tubes can generally be filled in less than 1 minute. If drawing on an elderly patient or a patient with fragile veins, keep the tourniquet in place until just prior to removing the needle. Removing the tourniquet earlier on these patients may cause the vein to collapse and the blood flow to stop.

Using the reverse motion of inserting the tube onto the needle, to remove or change tubes, pull and twist gently on the end of the evacuated tube while bracing the thumb on the flange of the tube adapter. Again, this push/pull counteraction prevents needle movement.

If the tube contains an additive, after removing the tube from the needle and tube adapter, gently invert the tube 5 to 8 times before setting it down. Different additives and manufacturers may require more or less mixing. Never shake the tube vigorously to mix the additive and blood, as this will cause the blood to hemolyze. Inadequate mixing of the blood and additive can lead to clot formation. Tubes without additives do not require mixing.

When the last tube has filled, remove it from the needle and the tube adapter prior to removing the needle from the patient's arm. If the last tube is not removed from the needle prior to its withdrawal from the vein, the needle will leak blood, causing unnecessary contamination.

As the needle is removed from the vein, a clean 2×2 gauze pad is simultaneously placed directly over the site and the needle's safety guard is "clicked" into place covering the contaminated needle (Figure 10-5). *Do not* press down on the gauze pad until the needle is safely removed from the patient's arm.

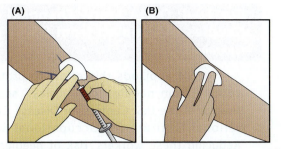

(A)   **(B)**

FIGURE 10-5: (A) Apply sterile pad before withdrawing needle. (B) Have patient apply pressure to the site until clot forms.

Apply direct pressure to the site with the gauze pad for 3 to 5 minutes. The patient, if able, may hold this pressure for you while you finish the collection procedures. Inadequate or insufficient pressure will cause leakage into the surrounding tissues and will cause a hematoma. *Do not* allow the patient to bend his or her arm. Bending the arm keeps the vein open and allows blood to leak into the surrounding tissues causing a hematoma. If the patient is unable or unwilling to hold pressure, the phlebotomist must maintain pressure on the puncture site until bleeding has stopped.

Box 10-4: OSHA Alert—Disposal of Contaminated Needles (As quoted from OSHA Trade News Release)

"OSHA is clarifying its policy on the prohibition of removing contaminated needles from blood tube holders in order to reduce the dangers of needlesticks for health care workers and others who handle medical sharps."

"Removing contaminated needles and reusing blood tube holders can expose workers to multiple hazards," said OSHA Administrator John Henshaw. "We want to make it very clear that this practice is prohibited in order to protect workers from being exposed to contaminated needles."

OSHA explained in a letter of interpretation that the blood-borne pathogens standard requires blood tube holders with needles attached to be immediately discarded into a sharps container after the device's safety feature is activated.

In the revised blood-borne pathogens compliance directive, the agency outlines its contaminated needle policy and explains that removing a needle from a used blood-drawing/phlebotomy device is rarely, if ever, required by a medical procedure. Because these devices involve the use of a double-ended needle, removing the needle exposes employees to additional risk, as does the increased manipulation of a contaminated device.

(continues)

Box 10-4: OSHA Alert—Disposal of Contaminated Needles (As quoted from OSHA Trade News Release) *(continued)*

"NIOSH applauds this effort to protect the nation's health care workers from needlestick injuries," said Kathleen M. Rest, Acting Director of the U.S. Centers for Disease Control and Prevention's (CDC) National Institute for Occupational Safety and Health (NIOSH). "Reducing these workers' risk of needlesticks decreases their risk of infection from hepatitis C, HIV, and other blood-borne pathogens."

The blood-borne pathogens standard also prohibits contaminated needles and other contaminated sharps from being bent, recapped, or removed, unless the employer demonstrates that no alternative is feasible or that such action is required by a specific medical or dental procedure.

Disposing of the needle immediately after withdrawing from the patient's vein is critical and is a habit to be remembered and adopted from the beginning (Figure 10-6). With the new OSHA policy, needles should never be removed from a Vacutainer™ holder or a syringe. The entire unit should be disposed of in the sharps container. *Never* cut, bend, break, or recap needles or stick a used needle into a pillow or mattress of a patient's bed. If a sharps container is not available, use the one-handed scoop method (Box 10-5) to resheath the needle until a sharps container can be located.

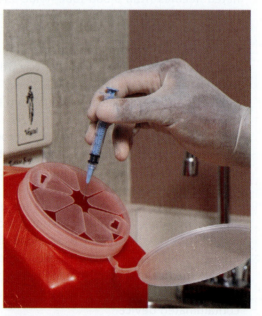

Figure 10-6: Discard entire used syringe and needle intact into biohazardous sharps container to prevent dangerous needle sticks.

Box 10-5: Recapping a Needle by the One-Handed Scoop Method

Ideally the phlebotomist has a sharps container accessible for the proper disposal of the venipuncture needle at every draw. However, the phlebotomist may find him or herself in a situation where a used venipuncture needle will need to be recapped for the safety of the patient and the phlebotomist. Knowing how to accomplish this safely reduces the risk of a contaminated needle stick.

Place the needle cover on a steady, level surface. Keeping the non-dominant hand away from the needle cover, hold the tube adapter and attached needle in the dominant hand. Scoop the needle into the needle cover. Once the needle is covered, snap the cover on tightly. With the development of safety guards the chance of ever re-capping a venipuncture needle is almost nonexistent.

Vacutainer and syringe needles are now available with an attached plastic safety sheath that can be clicked into place once the needle is withdrawn from the patient's vein, adding one more level of safety to the prevention of contaminated needle sticks. These devices should be used whenever possible as part of routine venipuncture. Refer to Chapter 8 for a description of their use.

Once the needle has been disposed of, the tubes are labeled with the following information:
● Patient's name
● Patient number or hospital ID number
● Patient's room number, if an inpatient
● Time and date of collection
● Phlebotomist's initials

Some requisition slips have preprinted numbered tracking labels that are peeled off and placed on the tubes as well. The numbers are the patient's identification numbers. Be sure to compare these tracking numbers to the patient's identification bracelet.

Never allow the patient to leave the area or facility without first properly labeling his or her tubes (Figure 10-7). Never use a pencil to label tubes. Indelible ink must be used. Never leave a patient's room before labeling tubes. Do not label tubes prior to the collection.

Some specimens for particular tests require special handling. Special handling is covered in greater detail in Chapter 12. Follow all requirements. As necessary, place the specimen in ice to keep it cool (e.g., ammonia), or place the specimen in a heat block to keep the specimen warm (e.g., cold agglutinin), or wrap the specimen in aluminum foil to protect it from light (e.g., bilirubin).

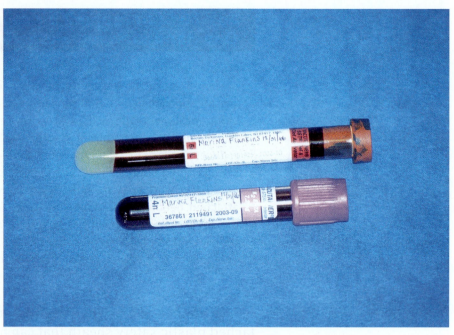

FIGURE 10-7: Tubes labeled with pertinent patient information

Check on the patient. Make sure that the bleeding has stopped. Patients who are on anticoagulant therapy or have bleeding disorders must be monitored closely for a minimum of 30 minutes. Place a slight pressure dressing over the site. Fold a 2 × 2 gauze pad into fourths, place it over the site, and secure with either tape or a self-adhesive bandage strip. If the patient is allergic to adhesive, use paper tape. Some patients have very sensitive skin and even paper tape can cause tissue damage. In this situation, use rolled gauze and wrap around the patient's arm. Apply the tape over the gauze. Instruct the patient to leave the bandage on for at least 15 minutes, at which time it may be removed. Instruct patients not to carry or lift any heavy objects with the arm the venipuncture occurred on for approximately 1 hour. Doing so may cause the vein to start bleeding again and may cause a hematoma. Tell patients who have been fasting that it is okay to eat now. Thank patients for their cooperation.

Now is the time to dispose of all contaminated items in the biohazardous waste container. Do not leave any supplies or equipment in the patient's room. Thank the patient. Remove gloves (see Procedure 4-1 in Chapter 4) and dispose in the appropriate biohazardous waste container. Wash hands.

Promptly transport the specimen to the laboratory for processing. Enter the specimen information into the computer system or logbook. Each facility has its own method for logging invasive procedures. Regardless of the facility's protocol, the venipuncture must be documented. Collections not documented have not legally been done. Refer to Chapter 5 for the correct method of logging invasive procedures.

Syringe Draw

The pressure exerted by the evacuated tube method may be too great for some patients' veins, such as children and the elderly (pediatric venipuncture will be presented in Chapter 12). The syringe draw and butterfly draw method of obtaining blood specimens are excellent alternatives to the evacuated tube method of collection. Using the syringe method, the phlebotomist can control the amount of pressure by pulling the plunger of the syringe back slowly (Figure 10-8).

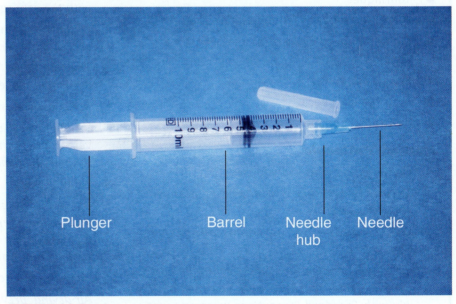

Plunger   Barrel   Needle   Needle
                            hub

FIGURE 10-8: 10 cc syringe

When drawing blood by the syringe method, patient identification, patient preparation, and site selection are the same as in the evacuated tube procedure. Prepare the syringe and needle by removing them from their sterile wrappers. To comply with OSHA regulations, only needle-locking syringes (e.g., Luer-lock syringes) are to be used. Pull the plunger of the syringe back to ensure it moves freely in the barrel. Replace the plunger to its original position. Attach the needle to the syringe. (*Note:* Syringes may come supplied with needles preattached.) Make sure that the needle is securely locked into place. Do not uncap the needle at this time. Apply the tourniquet, cleanse the site, remove the needle cap, inspect

Procedure 10-1

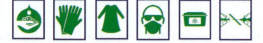

Evacuated Tube System of Venipuncture

Equipment/Supplies

- Personal protective equipment (gloves, gown, face mask/shield)
- Alcohol prep or povidone-iodine prep
- 2 × 2 gauze pads
- Tube adapter/holder
- Tourniquet
- Evacuated tubes as required for ordered tests
- Multidraw needle, 20 to 21 gauge, 1 to 1½ inches
- Sharps container
- Indelible ink pen
- Adhesive bandage/tape

Method/Rationale

1. Gather equipment and supplies.

   Ensures everything is available to perform the procedure.

2. Wash hands/don personal protective equipment.

   Thorough handwashing aids in controlling the spread of infection. Remember, you must comply with Standard Precautions whenever you may come in contact with body fluids or blood.

3. Identify the patient.

   Ensures the procedure is performed on the correct patient.

4. Assemble equipment.

   Attach the needle to the tube adapter, open the antiseptic, set out the required tubes in the correct order of draw, open the adhesive bandage, and set out a small stack of gauze pads. Assembling your equipment prior to applying the tourniquet diminishes the amount of time the patient has the tourniquet on his or her arm.

5. Explain the procedure.

   Helps ensure you will have the cooperation of the patient.

6. Position the patient seated or lying down with the arm at an angle and the palmar side of the hand facing up. Support the arm.

   The patient must be in a comfortable position with the arm securely supported.

7. Apply the tourniquet approximately 2 inches above the bend of the arm.

   The tourniquet will cause the veins to bulge, which will make them more prominent.

8. Select a venipuncture site.

   Visibly inspect both arms for the most likely vein. Start in the antecubital area and move to the hands and wrists as appropriate.

9. Clean the site.

   Use a 70% isopropyl alcohol prep or a povidone-iodine prep depending on the requested test. Clean in a circular motion from point of insertion outward.

10. Allow the site to air dry.

    Air-drying prevents hemolysis of the specimen from the alcohol. Allowing the site to dry also lessens the stinging sensation felt by the patient. The evaporation and drying process helps to destroy microbes.

11. Place the evacuated tube in the holder and uncap the needle.

    Inspect the needle for defects such as chips or burrs. Discard and replace defective needles.

12. Hold the blood-drawing equipment in your dominant hand.

    Rest the blood-drawing equipment on your fingertips with your index and middle finger hold-

ing the tube adapter and your ring and little finger holding the evacuated tube. Without allowing the adapter needle to penetrate the tube, press up gently on the evacuated tube so that the tube is firmly against the top of the inside of the tube adapter, and your thumb is resting on the top of the tube adapter.

13. Pull the patient's skin taut.

    Grasp 1 to 2 inches below and slightly to the side of the venipuncture site. This will secure the vein and help to keep it from rolling. This also helps to ease insertion of the needle.

14. Insert the needle.

    Bevel up. Use a 15 to 30-degree angle—adjust the angle in accordance with patient's vein. Position the needle to follow the line of the vein. Insert the needle in one quick smooth motion. As soon as you sense the needle is in the vein, stop advancing (generally just past the bevel) and push the tube onto the needle.

15. Allow the tubes to fill.

    Evacuated tubes fill because of the vacuum inside the tube. The tube will stop filling when the vacuum is exhausted, typically two-thirds of the way full.

16. Remove the tourniquet.

    If drawing only one tube, remove the tourniquet as soon as blood begins to fill the tube. If drawing more than one tube, remove the tourniquet when the last tube is filling.

17. Withdraw the needle.

    Prior to withdrawing the needle, pull the last tube from the adapter. Have a 2 × 2 gauze pad ready to place directly on the venipuncture site immediately following withdrawal of the needle. Pull the needle out at the same angle it was inserted. Click safety guard into place covering the end of the contaminated needle.

18. Apply direct pressure over the site.

    You may ask the patient to apply the direct pressure to stop any further bleeding. Do not allow the patient to bend his or her arm.

19. Mix the tubes.

    Gently invert the tubes 8 to 10 times to mix the additive with the collected blood. Red top tubes must not be mixed, as the blood must clot prior to centrifugation and serum separation.

20. Dispose of the needle and tube holder.

    Place the entire unit into the sharps container. Do not remove the needle from the tube holder.

21. Label the tubes.

    Be sure to use indelible ink. Write the patient's name, patient ID number, room number (if inpatient), time and date of collection, and your initials. Apply the hospital-preprinted labels and tracking numbers as appropriate.

22. Check on your patient.

    Make sure that the bleeding has stopped. Remember that patients on anticoagulation therapy or outpatients on daily aspirin therapy will take longer to stop bleeding and must be monitored closely for a minimum of 30 minutes.

23. Apply a bandage to the site.

    Fold a 2 × 2 gauze pad in fourths and apply an adhesive bandage or tape over the 2 × 2 to create a slight pressure bandage. Instruct your patient to remove the bandage in 15 minutes.

24. Instruct the patient on proper wound care.

    Tell the patient to not carry or lift heavy objects with the drawn-on arm for approximately 1 hour. Tell patients who have been fasting that it is okay to eat now.

(continues)

Procedure 10-1 *(continued)*

25. Thank your patient.

    Common courtesy to the patient promotes healthy client/patient relationships.

26. Dispose of any contaminated items in the biohazardous waste container.

    All items that are contaminated with blood must be disposed of in an approved biohazardous waste container. All other waste may be disposed of in a regular waste receptacle.

27. Transport the specimen to the laboratory.

    This must be done as promptly as possible.

28. Document the procedure according to the facility's protocol.

    All venipunctures must be documented, either manually in a logbook or on a computer.

for defects, and enter the vein with the bevel up in the same manner as you would if using the evacuated tube method. When the needle is in the vein, blood appears in the hub of the needle. This is called flash. You may remove the tourniquet at this point.

Secure the syringe in the same manner as with the evacuated tube system, by resting the supporting hand on the patient's arm. Slowly pull back on the plunger of the syringe until the barrel is filled with blood. When an adequate amount of blood has been collected, remove the needle in the same manner as with the evacuated tube method. Click the needle's safety shield into place and dispose of the entire unit in the appropriate sharps container.

If one syringe is not enough blood for the tests requested, it is possible to "pull" more than one syringe, *although this procedure is not recommended.* Place a short stack of gauze pads under the inserted syringe at the point it attaches to the needle. Holding the needle securely in the vein, unscrew the syringe off the needle and quickly attach a second syringe. It is helpful to have another person assist with this procedure by filling evacuated tubes with the collected blood while you draw the second syringe. Remember, blood left sitting in the first syringe will clot and render some test results inaccurate. Once the appropriate amount of blood has been collected, remove the needle from the vein and continue with the procedure in the same manner as with the evacuated tube method.

Box 10-6: Transferring Blood from a Syringe to an Evacuated Tube

When the syringe method of venipuncture is used the specimen must be transferred to an evacuated glass tube so that the specimen is mixed with the appropriate anticoagulant. To perform this task, select the tubes required for the requested tests.

(Remember that the correct order of tube filling from a syringe draw is slightly different from that of an evacuated tube draw. The syringe order is: **S**terile specimens, **L**ight blue stopper, **L**avender stopper, **G**reen stopper, **G**ray stopper, **R**ed stopper or red/gray stopper.)

Place the tubes in the correct order in a tube rack or slots in the collection tray. Insert the needle on the syringe into the first tube and allow the tube to fill using the vacuum draw of the tube. *Do not* push the blood into the tube as this will lyse the cells and cause inaccurate test results.

To further minimize the chance of hemolysis, slant the needle toward the side of the tube so that the blood runs down the side of the tube.

Never hold tubes in your hand while filling from a syringe.

If a tube is not to be filled completely, pull back on the plunger to stop the flow of blood at the appropriate point.

Dispose of the syringe and needle as one unit in the sharps container.

Butterfly Infusion Set Draw

If the phlebotomist is drawing blood from a patient who has small, fragile veins, such as an elderly patient, an infant, or a small child, or from an adult patient who has small antecubital, wrist, or hand veins, a winged-infusion set (butterfly infusion set) should be selected for the blood draw.

The butterfly infusion set may be used with either a syringe or the evacuated tube system. Butterfly infusion kits come prepackaged with a syringe attached, or with a multiple-sample Luer adapter that is attached directly to the evacuated tube adapter. The butterfly needle is typically 23 gauge and ⅝ inches in length. This size is ideal for accommodating small, fragile veins. It is recommended that pediatric-sized 2 mL evacuated tubes be used with pediatric-sized tube adapters. The force of the vacuum in the 5 mL evacuated tube is too great for fragile veins and will cause them to collapse. In addition, the use of 5 mL tubes with a 23 gauge needle may cause **hemolysis** (Box 10-7) of the specimen.

HEMOLYSIS

The destruction of the membrane of red blood cells and the liberation of hemoglobin, which diffuses into the surrounding fluid.

Box 10-7: What Causes Hemolysis?

- Using a needle with a bore too small for venipuncture.
- Using too large of an evacuated tube with a butterfly infusion set.
- Mixing additive tubes too vigorously.
- Rough-handling of the specimen after collection.
- Pulling back the plunger of a syringe too quickly.
- Drawing blood from a vein with a hematoma.
- Forcing blood from a syringe into an evacuated tube.
- Improper attachment of a needle on a syringe (causes frothing of the blood).
- Not allowing the alcohol to dry completely prior to collection (alcohol residue will cause hemolysis).

The procedure for using a butterfly infusion set is the same as for the syringe method, with a few exceptions. When assembling the equipment, the tubing attached to the needle is coiled. Uncoil the tubing and stretch it slightly to help prevent it from recoiling during the draw. Attach the butterfly infusion set to the syringe or evacuated tube system. If using the evacuated tube method, rest the first tube in the adapter.

If drawing from an antecubital vein, the draw continues from this point in the same manner as with an evacuated tube draw. When drawing blood from a hand or wrist vein the following adjustments are made:

- Apply the tourniquet above the wrist.
- Ask the patient to make a fist or bend the fingers. It is helpful for the patient to grasp a ball, or if a ball is not available, the patient can grasp an unopened package of 2 × 2 gauze pads.
- The hand must be well-supported. Use rolled towels or an armrest.
- Select the vein and cleanse the site. For hand draws, use your thumb to pull the skin taut over the top of the patient's knuckles. For wrist draws, pull the skin taut with your thumb just below the venipuncture site.
- Hold the tube adapter/syringe and tubing in your dominant hand or lay it next to the patient's hand. With the bevel up, grasp the "wings" and fold them together with your thumb and index finger.

- Align the needle with the vein. Using a 10 to 15-degree angle, enter the vein with a quick but steady motion. Entering the tissue slowly when using a butterfly needle will only push the vein off to the side. Once the vein has been entered you will see a "flash" of blood in the tubing. When this occurs you can pull the plunger back to fill a syringe or push the evacuated tube onto the needle in the tube adapter.
- Because venipunctures done with a butterfly infusion set are most commonly performed on difficult veins, the tourniquet may be left in place until the draw is complete as long as the draw is accomplished within the 2-minute window.
- Keep the tube adapter and tube lower than the patient's arm, pointing downward so that the tube fills from the bottom up.
- When the last tube is filled, release the tube from the needle, place gauze over the venipuncture site, remove the needle, and apply pressure in the same way as with a routine evacuated tube venipuncture.
- Dispose of the butterfly infusion set by releasing the needle and tubing from the tube adapter, placing the needle, attached tubing, and tube adapter into the sharps container. If a syringe has been attached, the blood must be transferred to an appropriate evacuated tube prior to disposal. Remove the butterfly infusion set and dispose of it in the sharps container. Replace with a sterile needle and follow procedure from this point as described previously for a syringe draw.

SPECIMEN IDENTIFICATION AND TUBE LABELING

Every facility has its own specific requirements for labeling tubes. These requirements are outlined in their Policies and Procedures Manual. General guidelines for labeling tubes require that indelible ink be used when writing on prefixed tube labels. The following information must be included:

- Patient's full name
- Patient number or hospital identification number
- Patient's room number, if an inpatient
- Time and date of collection
- Phlebotomist's initials

Specimens must be labeled immediately following collection. Tubes are not to be prelabeled. A tube might not be used after a draw because of an insufficient amount of blood, or a tube not required for testing might inadvertently have been drawn. A prelabeled tube may be accidentally picked up and sent to the lab for testing. The patient may be charged for a lab test not required or inaccurate test results. If the tube has been prelabeled with a phlebotomist's initials and another phlebotomist finishes the collection, the label is inaccurate. Removing an already attached label is difficult; a new patient's label must be placed over the old label. This could cause the unused tube to be wastefully discarded.

Many hospitals generate preprinted labels for each patient upon admission (Figure 10-9). In this situation the preprinted label may simply be attached upon completion of the draw. Be sure to match the preprinted labels to the patient's identification bracelet.

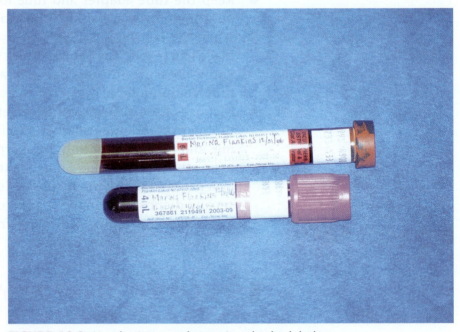

FIGURE 10-9: Handwritten and preprinted tube labels

FAILURE TO OBTAIN BLOOD AND OTHER CONSIDERATIONS

There are several situations leading to an incomplete or "short" draw, or to a complete failure to obtain a blood specimen. Knowing what these situations are and how to avoid or correct them is instrumental in becoming an accomplished professional phlebotomist.

An incomplete, partial, or "short" draw refers to an evacuated tube or syringe that does not contain the required amount of blood to perform the requested tests. One or more of the following can cause an incomplete draw:

- Collapsed vein
- Damaged or occluded veins
- Obesity
- Incorrect needle and/or tube position
- Removal of tube before correct amount of blood has been collected

Collapsed Vein

A patient's vein can collapse because of the pressure caused by the vacuum of an evacuated tube, or because the plunger of a syringe is pulled back too quickly or forcefully. Once the vein has collapsed, do not probe for it with the needle. Tightening the tourniquet by grasping the ends with one hand and twisting is a possible remedy for collapsed veins. Although it is often difficult and is not recommended, on occasion it will work to "pump" the vein back up. Applying pressure to the vein several inches above the needle is another remedy. Wait a few seconds to remove the attached evacuated tube and insert a smaller one or pull back more slowly on the syringe plunger. If the blood flow does not return, withdraw the needle and attempt a second venipuncture at another site.

Damaged or Occluded Veins

Sclerosed or **occluded** veins are often the result of inflammation and disease or occur in patients who have had repeated punctures to veins. Sclerosed or occluded veins will feel hard when palpated and will not allow blood to properly flow through them. They should be avoided for venipuncture.

Obesity

OCCLUDED

Closed or obstructed or joined together.

Patients who are obese commonly have antecubital veins that are difficult to either see or palpate. Probing excessively for these veins is not recommended, as probing can cause damage to the tissues and may rupture red blood cells. Excessive probing may also increase the concentration of intracellular fluid and release tissue clotting factors, which will cause inaccurate test results. Inspect the patient's wrists and hands for veins that can be seen or palpated. If this is not successful, attempt to locate the cephalic vein in the antecubital space by rotating the patient's arm so that the hand is prone. In this position, the weight of the arm tissue pulls downward with gravity, often allowing the cephalic vein to become visible or palatable. With experience, a "blind stick" may be performed, although this is not encouraged. A "blind stick" requires approximation of the anatomic location of the vein. Typically the phlebotomist will return to the antecubital area to do a "blind stick" as the antecubital veins tend to be in the same location from patient to patient. Hand and wrist veins vary. Increase the angle of needle insertion on obese patients as appropriate, as their veins tend to be located deeper than those of nonobese patients.

Incorrect Needle and/or Tube Position

The first item to check if the tube is not filling with blood is whether or not the tube has been properly seated onto the needle. If not, reseat the tube. Another possibility is that the tube has lost its vacuum. Tubes lose their vacuum over time. Inspection of tube expiration dates must be done prior to the draw. If you suspect that the tube has lost its vacuum, insert another tube into the tube adapter and push onto the needle.

A third possibility for the inability to obtain blood is incorrect positioning of the needle (Figure 10-10). This may be caused by one of the following:

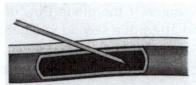

Correct — blood flows freely into the needle

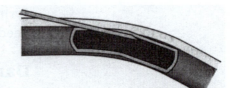

Incorrect — bevel against the upper wall impedes flow

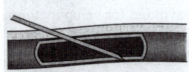

Incorrect — bevel against the lower wall impedes flow

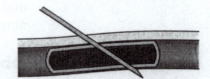

Incorrect — needle is inserted too far

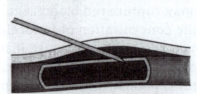

Incorrect — needle partially inserted, causing hematoma

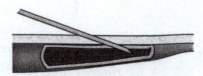

Incorrect — a collapsed vein

FIGURE 10-10: Incorrect needle positions

● Needle not inserted deeply enough: If the needle has not been inserted deeply enough into the vein, blood may fill the tube very slowly. If the needle has not been inserted deeply enough into the tissue to reach the vein, the tube will not fill with blood at all. Push the needle further into the tissue or vein. Correct blood flow should be established. By positioning the needle only partially in the vein (bevel is half in and half out of the vein), blood will seep into the surrounding tissue, causing a hematoma. If this occurs, immediately remove the tourniquet, withdraw the needle, and apply pressure.

● Needle inserted too deeply: The needle may have been inserted through the vein. This may occur if the tube adapter is not held securely while pushing the tube onto the needle or if the needle has been pushed in too far on initial insertion. Slowly withdrawing the needle should establish blood flow if this has occurred. Blood will seep into the tissues and cause a hematoma if this is not corrected immediately.

● Needle bevel against the wall of the vein: If the needle, once inserted, is held against the wall of the vein, blood flow will be impaired. Relax the needle angle slightly. If blood flow returns, maintain this position throughout the draw. Rotating the needle slightly may determine if this is the cause of low or no blood flow.

● Needle is alongside the vein: Veins are often tough to penetrate. If the vein has not been securely anchored, the vein may "roll" off to the side when force is exerted against its wall by the needle, causing the needle to lie alongside the vein. Occasionally the needle is inserted just next to the vein. In either of these situations, remove the evacuated tube from the needle so as not to lose the vacuum, slightly withdraw the needle until the bevel is just below the skin surface, reanchor the vein, and redirect the needle into the vein. Replace the tube on to the needle.

● Unable to determine position of needle: If you are unable to tell exactly where the needle is located in relation to the vein, it is acceptable to "feel" for the vein with the needle still in the patient's arm. To locate the vein, remove the tube from the needle so that the vacuum is not lost, and withdraw the needle until the bevel is just below the surface of the skin. With a gloved finger, feel for the vein above the site of insertion. Do not feel for the vein directly over the point of insertion or too close to the needle, as it is painful to the patient. Once the vein has been relocated, redirect the needle into the vein and proceed with the venipuncture. If the vein cannot be located, release the tourniquet and withdraw the needle. Apply direct pressure over the site. Then select another site.

It is recommended and accepted practice that the phlebotomist not "stick" a patient more than twice. If a third attempt is necessary, it is to be performed by another phlebotomist. Other considerations of concern to the phlebotomist when performing venipuncture include:

1. The number of times a day blood may be drawn from a patient. Although the maximum number may vary from facility to facility, the average is typically three times a day. Physicians, nurses, and health care workers should coordinate their efforts to minimize the number of venipunctures per day.

2. The total volume of blood per day that may be drawn on a patient. This is especially important when the patient is an infant or child, although each facility has its own guidelines. The amount of blood drawn is based on the patient's weight. For example a 21 lb child should only have 10 mL of blood drawn per day.

3. The type of information the phlebotomist may share with the patient regarding the tests being performed. It is acceptable for the phlebotomist to share basic information with the patient, such as the name of the test that has been ordered. However, the phlebotomist should not speculate but should emphasize that the patient's physician has ordered the tests and should encourage the patient to address further questions to the physician.

4. The procedure to follow if a patient refuses to have his or her blood drawn. All competent patients have the right to refuse treatment. The phlebotomist has the responsibility to make every effort, using his or her best judgment, to persuade the patient to agree to the blood draw. However, take care to not harass the patient. By underscoring the value of accurate laboratory results in determining the patient's diagnosis, treatment, and prognosis, the phlebotomist may convince a reluctant patient to agree and consent to the procedure. If the patient continues to refuse, the phlebotomist must remain professional and respect the patient's right to refuse. Note the refusal in the patient's chart and explain to the patient that the physician will be notified.

OTHER CONSIDERATIONS REGARDING ROUTINE VENIPUNCTURE

● Do not insert a needle above an intravenous infusion (IV). It is important to check the institution's protocols regarding IVs. However, a typical protocol states that if an IV is running in both arms and there is no other alternative except for the IV site, the phlebotomist may draw blood at least 2 inches below the IV site once permission has been given by the patient's physician. Ask the nurse to turn off the IV for a minimum of 2 minutes prior to the draw. Apply the tourniquet below the IV site. Use a vein other than the one the IV is attached to. Discard the first 5 mL of blood, and then draw the sample to be used for testing.

● Outpatients should remain sitting for 15 minutes before attempting a venipuncture for certain procedures. Sitting allows the body to recover from stress and/or exercise prior to collection of the specimen. Stress and exercise can increase the test values for lactate dehydrogenase (LDH), AST (aspartate aminotransferase), platelet count, and creatine kinase (CK) levels.

● If the venipuncture site begins to swell during the venipuncture process, immediately release the tourniquet and remove the needle. Apply firm, direct pressure, using several gauze pads on the site for 8 to 10 minutes. Elevate the patient's arm while continuing to apply pressure. An ice pack may be applied to the area as well (never place an ice pack directly on the patient's skin; place on a towel or other protective material first). Monitor the patient for signs of shock, fainting, or vomiting.

SPECIMEN INTEGRITY—QUALITY ASSURANCE

Proper handling of the specimen begins the moment the blood is drawn into the evacuated tube or syringe, and continues throughout the collection process. It includes transporting the specimen to the laboratory and its processing there. Improper handling of the specimen compromises its integrity and renders the specimen useless for testing. Every specimen must be handled with the utmost concern for the blood-borne pathogen safety guidelines which protect the phlebotomist and others from accidental exposure to potentially infectious substances. The integrity of the specimen is dependent on the phlebotomist's following these general guidelines:

1. Handling routine specimens
   - Immediately after the blood draw, additive tubes must be gently inverted 8 to 10 times. Vigorous mixing of the tubes causes hemolysis and inaccurate test results. Inadequate mixing causes the blood to form clots, which may also cause inaccurate test results, especially on hematology tests. Nonadditive tubes are not to be mixed, as the blood must be allowed to clot.
   - Blood specimens should be transported carefully to prevent tube breakage. Tubes should be transported stopper-up, which helps prevent hemolysis and aids in clot formation. Specimens being transported through pneumatic tube systems, or being transported offsite, are placed in a zipper-locked plastic bag to contain spills and then placed in a rigid plastic transport container. Specimens that are being sent via mail must be specifically packaged. Transport mailer kits contain rigid plastic containers with a cutout foam insert for tube placement. The lid is then screwed on and the container is placed in a leakproof bag supplied by the mail service. Medical specimens transported by the U.S. Post Office or private carrier such as Federal Express or UPS must be labeled with biohazardous labels affixed to the outside of all bags. Be sure to follow all current regulations.

2. Specimens requiring special handling
   - Specimens requiring protection from light—Several tests are affected by the presence of light, which can cause falsely low values. Bilirubin is the most common of these tests. Vitamin B$_{12}$, carotene, and red blood cell folate are also affected. To protect a specimen from light, wrap it in aluminum foil. Specifically designed amber-colored microcollection containers are available for collection of bilirubin specimens from infants.
   - Specimens required to be chilled—Specimens that require chilling after collection are those for blood gases, ammonia, lactic acid, renin, prothrombin time, partial thromboplastin time, and glucagon tests. Chilling a specimen after collection slows down the metabolic processes which would continue after the draw. Without chilling, test results would be inaccurate. Chilling a specimen can be accomplished by making a "slurrey" out of crushed ice and water in a disposable cup and placing the specimen in the cup directly after collection and throughout transporting the specimen to the lab. The specimen can then be refrigerated as required.

● Specimens required to be kept warm—Some specimens need to be kept at or near body temperature (37° C), such as cold agglutinins, cryoglobulin, and cryofibrinogen. Warming can be accomplished by transporting the specimen in a commercially manufactured, 37° C heat block.

Some tests, such as the activated clotting time, require that the tube used for testing be kept warm prior to drawing the blood for the test. For manual activated clotting times, the tube must be kept warm during as well as before the procedure.

● All specimens must be transported to the lab in a timely manner. However, some tests require specific timing. Routine specimens should arrive at the laboratory within 45 minutes of collection and are to be centrifuged within 1 hour. NCCLS sets the maximum time limit for separating serum and plasma from the cells at 2 hours from time of collection. Potassium and cortisol specimens must reach the laboratory within a 45-minute window.

Specimens are often sent to the laboratory from another off-site facility, such as a doctor's office. These specimens will not reach the laboratory within the time limit requirements. These off-site specimens must be allowed to clot, be centrifuged, and the serum or plasma separated and transferred into a separate serum tube for transport.

If specimens have been drawn in serum separator tubes (SSTs) or plasma separator tubes (PSTs) they only need to clot and be centrifuged. Once centrifuged, the separator gel will prevent glycolysis for up to 24 hours.

● Exceptions to the above guidelines—Lavender top tubes (EDTA) drawn for hematology studies are never centrifuged. EDTA specimens are stable for 24 hours. However, blood smears made from EDTA tubes must be completed within 1 hour of collection to preserve the integrity of the specimen. Specimens drawn for glucose determination in tubes containing sodium fluoride, a glycolytic inhibitor, are stable for 24 hours at room temperature and for up to 48 hours when refrigerated.

PROCESSING A BLOOD SPECIMEN

Most laboratories are equipped with a specific area where specimens are processed, called Central Processing. Once a specimen is received it is logged in, prioritized, and prepared for testing. Specimens that require centrifuging are spun down, and the serum or

ALIQUOT

A portion of the specimen used for testing.

plasma is pipetted off and transferred into **aliquot** tubes. Specimens are matched to the correct aliquot tubes and laboratory requisition form. Specimens are then sent to the appropriate area of the laboratory for further testing. For example, hematology studies are sent to hematology, and blood-banking specimens are sent to blood banking.

Once a blood specimen has fully clotted, it may be centrifuged. A centrifuge is a machine that spins the blood at high revolutions per minute (rpm's). The spinning creates a force that causes the formed elements (red blood cells, white blood cells, and platelets) to separate from the serum or plasma. The formed elements are heavier than the serum or plasma and travel to the bottom of the tube. The tubes must remain stoppered during this procedure to prevent blood from splashing out of the tube, the specimen from evaporating, the pH of the specimen from changing, or from forming aerosol. If stoppers are removed to add a separator device, they must be restoppered prior to centrifugation.

The centrifuge contains stainless steel tubes placed in a circle, in which the evacuated glass tubes are placed. It is important that the machine be balanced by placing equal tubes and volumes of specimens opposite each other. An unbalanced machine will spin unevenly and cause the evacuated glass specimen tubes to break, creating aerosols. If there are not an equal number of blood-filled evacuated glass tubes available for testing, an empty evacuated glass tube is filled with water and is used in place of a blood specimen to balance the centrifuge (Figure 10-11).

OSHA requires wearing protective apparel during the processing of specimens. This includes a buttoned lab coat, gloves, and protective face gear.

Specimens requiring centrifugation are one of two categories: plasma or serum. Tests requiring plasma specimens are collected in tubes containing an anticoagulant specific for the requested test. These specimens may be centrifuged immediately. Tests requiring serum are collected in tubes that do not contain an anticoagulant and must be left to clot prior to centrifuging. If the specimen is not allowed to fully clot prior to centrifuging, the serum may clot and interfere with accurate test results. The specimen must be allowed to clot at room temperature from a minimum of 20 minutes up to 45 minutes. Specimens taken from patients on anticoagulant therapy such as Coumadin or heparin may take longer to clot. Specimens from patients with high white blood cell counts or specimens that have been chilled may also take longer to clot.

The lid of the centrifuge must be closed and latched in place during the spinning of the specimens. Always allow the centrifuge to come to a complete stop before opening the lid.

Centrifuge the specimens only once. Repeating centrifugation will cause hemolysis and inaccurate test results. As centrifugation generates heat, specimens that require chilling must be spun down in a temperature-controlled centrifuge.

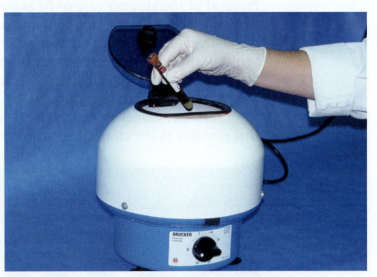

FIGURE 10-11 (A): Loading specimens in centrifuge

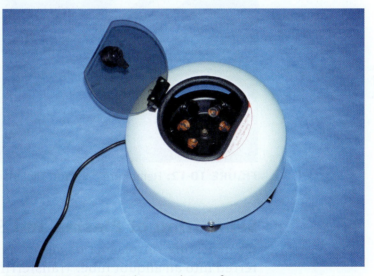

FIGURE 10-11 (B): Balance tube configuration

If an evacuated glass tube breaks during the process of centrifugation, clean up the broken glass using wet paper towels while wearing a pair of heavy-duty utility gloves. Disinfect the centrifuge, following the facility's blood spill cleaning protocols. Dispose of broken glass in the appropriate sharps container.

Stopper Removal

To perform testing on serum or plasma, the stopper of the tube may be removed. However, devices designed to allow penetration through a stopper are now available for some tests. When required removal of the stopper cannot be accomplished using a stopper removal device, or if the device is not available, it may be removed manually using a 4 × 4 gauze pad placed over the stopper. This prevents any aerosol that might be released. Pull the stopper straight up; do not "pop" it off. Becton Dickinson manufactures tubes with easy release stoppers called Hemogards™ (Figure 10-12), which are designed to protect personnel from splatters and aerosols caused by blood that remains in the stopper or around the outer rim of the tube.

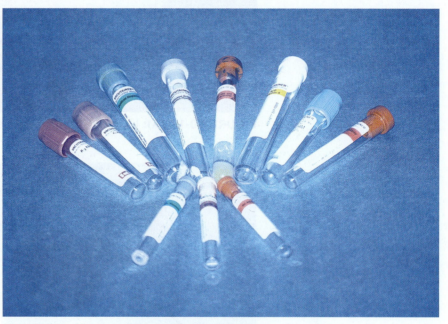

FIGURE 10-12: Hemogard™ Becton Dickinson tubes

Separation of Plasma and Serum

When testing on plasma or serum is required, it must be transferred into an aliquot tube. Transferring must be done in a manner that minimizes the risk of splashes, aerosol formation, and contact with the blood. Disposable plastic calibrated pipettes are used, rather than pouring the serum or plasma. If plasma or serum samples are to be used in other departments for testing, then measured amounts may be transferred into several aliquot tubes, labeled, and distributed.

SPECIMEN REJECTION

Each health care facility has its own requirements for specimen rejection. The requirements are located in the Policies and Procedures Manual. The following are basic specimen rejection guidelines common to most facilities:

● Discrepancies between requisition forms and labeled tubes (e.g., names and ID numbers, dates and times do not match)
● Unlabeled tubes
● Hemolyzed specimens.
● Specimens collected in wrong tube (e.g., CBC collected in red top tube)
● Expired tubes
● Insufficient specimen for the test ordered (labeled QNS—**Q**uantity **N**ot **S**ufficient)
● Specimen collected at the wrong time interval (e.g., a specimen for a fasting glucose-tolerance test collected just after the patient ate lunch)

The phlebotomist must collect new specimens as quickly as possible. If this will not correct the problem, the phlebotomist's supervisor and the patient's physician are to be notified immediately. Errors are to be acknowledged and documented immediately.

Box 10-8: Specimen Contamination

Inadvertent contamination of a specimen can occur by using the wrong antiseptic to cleanse the puncture site. For example, cleansing a site with alcohol can contaminate a blood-alcohol level test. Using povidone-iodine to clean a site can contaminate the specimen and cause erroneously high levels of potassium, uric acid, and phosphate.

Not allowing an antiseptic to completely air dry prior to collection can also contaminate specimens used for blood cultures. Traces of the antiseptic in the culture media may inhibit the growth of bacteria and cause false-negative blood cultures.

Contamination of blood cultures can occur if the site or blood culture bottles have not been properly cleaned prior to collection.

Powder from gloves can contaminate blood slides and skin puncture specimens.

PRIORITIZING PATIENTS

The phlebotomist is required to continuously make decisions regarding the order in which patients will be drawn. Priorities must be set and maintained or test results will be rendered inaccurate. Areas of consideration when making these decisions include:

● Timed specimens—When tests are ordered to be done at a particular time, the phlebotomist must collect the specimens at the time ordered. Glucose levels are the most commonly ordered timed test. They must be drawn 2 hours after meals. If the specimen is collected too early, the glucose levels in the blood will be falsely elevated. If collected too late they may register a false normal result. Other timed tests include drug therapy levels and hormone levels such as cortisol and aldosterone. The highest levels of cortisol occur at 8:00 AM whereas by 8:00 PM levels have dropped by two-thirds. Aldosterone requires a different type of timed testing. The patient must be in a recumbent position for at least 30 minutes prior to blood collection. Another example is the collection of blood for renin activity. In this case, the patient must be on a special diet for 3 days prior to collection of the specimen, and it must be documented whether the patient is in an upright or prone position when the specimen is collected.

● Fasting specimens—Fasting levels for glucose, cholesterol, and triglycerides are important in the diagnosis and monitoring of a patient's progress. Fasting means that the patient has had nothing to eat or drink except water for a specified period of time. The phlebotomist must determine if the patient has been fasting, and, if not, the patient's physician must be contacted for further instructions.

● Stat specimens—The term *stat* means immediately and indicates that a patient is critical and must be treated or responded to as a medical emergency. The phlebotomist must draw the blood quickly and efficiently and ensure that the specimen is delivered to the laboratory stat. Despite the emergency nature of the collection, the phlebotomist must not take shortcuts; the specimens must be drawn and labeled correctly. If specimens must be redrawn, this will cause the results to be delayed, thereby placing the patient at increased risk.

◖SUMMARY

Routine venipunctures are the phlebotomist's most commonly performed procedures. Through practical experience the phlebotomist will establish an individual routine that encompasses the guidelines set forth by NCCLS, OSHA, and the health care facility. The phlebotomist will perform this procedure with ease, gain the patient's cooperation and confidence, and obtain a satisfactory specimen to provide the physician and patient with accurate test results.

● COMPETENCY CHECK-OFF SHEETS
Evacuated Tube Venipuncture Competency Check

Given all the equipment and supplies, the student will be required to perform, within 5 minutes or less, an evacuated tube venipuncture on a classroom volunteer. A "0" in more than two areas or an overall score of less than 80% will require the procedure to be repeated for competency.

Points to Be Awarded:	5 pts	2.5 pts	1 pt	0 pts	total pts
1 Assemble and prepare equipment and supplies					
2 Wash hands/don PPE					
3 Identify patient					
4 Explain the procedure					
5 Position patient					
6 Apply tourniquet					
7 Select site					
8 Remove tourniquet					
9 Clean site with alcohol					
10 Air-dry site					
11 Reapply tourniquet					
12 Inspect needle					
13 Pull patient's skin taut					
14 Insert needle					
15 Fill evacuated tubes in correct order of draw					
16 Remove tourniquet					
17 Apply direct pressure					
18 Mix tubes					
19 Dispose of needle/tube adapter					
20 Label tubes					
21 Check on patient—hemostasis					
22 Apply bandage					

Points to Be Awarded:	5 pts	2.5 pts	1 pt	0 pts	total pts
23 Instruct patient in wound care					
24 Thank patient					
25 Dispose of waste					
26 Package specimen for transport					
27 Remove gloves/wash hands					
28 Document procedure in log book					

Total Points Possible: _____ Total Points Earned: _____

Start Time: _____ End Time: _____

Instructor Signature: _____ Date: _____

Student Signature: _____ Date: _____

Syringe Venipuncture Competency Check

Given all the equipment and supplies, the student will be required to perform, within 5 minutes, a syringe venipuncture on a classroom volunteer. A "0" in more than two areas or an overall score of less than 80% will require the procedure to be repeated for competency.

Points to Be Awarded:	5 pts	2.5 pts	1 pt	0 pts	total pts
1 Assemble and prepare equipment and supplies					
2 Wash hands/don PPE					
3 Identify patient					
4 Explain the procedure					
5 Position patient					
6 Apply tourniquet					
7 Select site					
8 Remove tourniquet					
9 Clean site with alcohol					
10 Air-dry site					
11 Reapply tourniquet					
12 Inspect needle/work plunger					
13 Pull patient's skin taut					
14 Insert needle					
15 Fill syringe					
16 Remove tourniquet					
17 Apply direct pressure					
18 Transfer blood to evacuated tubes in correct order of draw					
19 Mix tubes					
20 Dispose of needle/syringe					
21 Label tubes					
22 Check on patient—hemostasis					
23 Apply bandage					
24 Instruct patient in wound care					

Points to Be Awarded:	5 pts	2.5 pts	1 pt	0 pts	total pts
25 Thank patient					
26 Dispose of waste					
27 Package specimen for transport					
28 Remove gloves/wash hands					
29 Document procedure in log book					

Total Points Possible: _____   Total Points Earned: _____

Start Time: _____   End Time: _____

Instructor Signature: _____   Date: _____

Student Signature: _____   Date: _____

Butterfly Infusion Set Venipuncture Competency Check

Given all the equipment and supplies, the student will be required to perform, within 5 minutes a butterfly infusion set venipuncture on a classroom volunteer. A "0" in more than two areas or an overall score of less than 80% will require the procedure to be repeated for competency.

Points to Be Awarded:	5 pts	2.5 pts	1 pt	0 pts	total pts
1 Assemble and prepare equipment and supplies					
2 Wash hands/don PPE					
3 Identify patient					
4 Explain the procedure					
5 Position patient					
6 Apply tourniquet					
7 Select site					
8 Remove tourniquet					
9 Clean site with alcohol					
10 Air-dry site					
11 Reapply tourniquet					
12 Uncoil tubing/inspect needle/ attach syringe of tube holder					
13 Pull patient's skin taut					
14 Insert needle					
15 Fill syringe/evacuated tube					
16 Remove tourniquet					
17 Apply direct pressure					
18 Transfer blood to evacuated tubes in correct order of draw (if syringe is used)					
19 Mix tubes					
20 Dispose of needle/syringe/tube holder					
21 Label tubes					
22 Check on patient—hemostasis					
23 Apply bandage					

Points to Be Awarded:	5 pts	2.5 pts	1 pt	0 pts	total pts
24 Instruct patient in wound care					
25 Thank patient					
26 Dispose of waste					
27 Package specimen for transport					
28 Remove gloves/wash hands					
29 Document procedure in log book					

Total Points Possible: _____ Total Points Earned: _____

Start Time: _____ End Time: _____

Instructor Signature: _____ Date: _____

Student Signature: _____ Date: _____

Centrifuge Red Top Evacuated Tube and Separate Serum into Aliquot Tube Competency Check

Given all the equipment and supplies, the student will be required to perform, within 5 minutes, Centrifugation of Red Top Evacuated Tube and Serum Separation. A "0" in more than two areas or an overall score of less than 80% will require the procedure to be repeated for competency.

Points to Be Awarded:	5 pts	2.5 pts	1 pt	0 pts	total pts
1 Wash hands/don PPE					
2 Upon completion of specimen collection place red top evacuated tube in centrifuge					
3 Balance centrifuge					
4 Set timer					
5 Remove tube from centrifuge					
6 Properly remove stopper or apply transfer device					
7 Separate serum into aliquot tube					
8 Label tubes					
9 Dispose of waste					
10 Package specimen for transport					

Total Points Possible: _____ Total Points Earned: _____

Start Time: _____ End Time: _____

Instructor Signature: _____ Date: _____

Student Signature: _____ Date: _____

STUDY AND REVIEW EXERCISES

Defining Key Terms

Write the definition for each of the following key terms.

1) aliquot _____

2) antecubital _____

3) bevel _____

4) hemoconcentration _____

5) hemolysis _____

6) occluded _____

7) palpate _____

8) periphery _____

9) reflux _____

10) sclerosed _____

11) thrombosed _____

12) venipuncture _____

Reviewing Key Points

1) List the information required on a test requisition.

2) Describe the procedure for applying a tourniquet including the time constraints.

3) Describe a situation that could lead to a "short draw."

4) Describe how to perform a venipuncture when a patient has an IV, and the arm with the IV is the only place you can draw from.

5) List five reasons why a specimen might be rejected.

Sentence Completion

1) _____ is the main method used to obtain a blood sample from a patient for diagnostic testing.

2) When collecting a blood specimen via an evacuated glass tube, you use a _____ needle, 20 to 21 gauge, 1 to $1\frac{1}{2}$ inches long.

3) Patient identification is critical. When verifying information on an inpatient, compare the test requisition slip with the patient's _____.

4) When drawing a patient's blood, gain their cooperation by being _____ and _____.

5) If the phlebotomist forgets to raise the bed rails after specimen collection from an inpatient and the patient falls out of bed, the phlebotomist will be held _____.

6) _____ causes the veins to bulge, which will make them appear more prominent.

7) A _____ vein will feel hard and should not be used as a venipuncture site.

8) Using alcohol preps to clean a puncture site is one method; a second method is to use a(n) _____ prep.

9) Evacuated glass tubes fill approximately _____ of the way full, because of the vacuum contained in the tube.

10) During a venipuncture the phlebotomist notices that the site has begun to swell and turn blue. This is called a(n) _____ and the needle should be removed immediately and pressure applied to the puncture site.

Multiple Choice

1) Additive tubes should be inverted _____ times immediately after being drawn?
   A. 1–2
   B. 3–4
   C. 5–7
   D. 8–10

2) Specimens that must be chilled after collection are all the following *except:*
   A. prothrombin time
   B. CBC
   C. blood gasses
   D. glucagon

3) When collecting a specimen for bilirubin testing, you must protect the specimen from:
   A. heat
   B. cold
   C. light
   D. none of the above

4) Routine specimens must arrive at the laboratory within _____ minute(s) of collection and be centrifuged within _____ hour(s).
   A. 15 minutes; 1 hour
   B. 45 minutes; 1 hour
   C. 30 minutes; 1½ hour
   D. 15 minutes; 2 hours

5) Centrifuge specimens must be allowed to clot for a minimum of _____ prior to centrifugation.
   A. 20 minutes
   B. 30 minutes
   C. 1 hour
   D. 2 hours

6) When a patient has very fragile veins it is best to draw the specimen using the _____ method.
   A. evacuated tube
   B. syringe
   C. butterfly infusion set/with evacuated tube
   D. butterfly infusion set/with syringe

7) Try to keep the patient's arm and the tube in a downward position, with the tube filling from the bottom up. This will prevent _____.
   A. reflux
   B. hemolysis
   C. discomfort to the patient
   D. There is not a specific reason for this—it just looks more professional.

8) When inserting the needle into the patient's arm, typically the angle of insertion should be _____ degrees.
   A. 80 to 90
   B. 30 to 45
   C. 180
   D. 15 to 30

9) A tourniquet must not be left in place for longer than:
   A. 30 seconds
   B. 1 minute
   C. 3 minutes
   D. 5 minutes

10) A patient has been scheduled for blood tests at 8:00 AM and the order states the patient must be NPO. You must verify that the patient has:
   A. not had a bowel movement for 24 hours
   B. not had anything to eat or drink since midnight
   C. not eaten anything containing sugar for 24 hours
   D. not vomited since midnight

Critical Thinking

1) Juanita Chavez, a 53-year-old Hispanic female, has come to the laboratory for outpatient testing. The test requisition from her physician orders a CBC and fasting glucose. Ms. Chavez speaks very little English and seems quite nervous. First describe how you will identify the patient, second how will you explain to Ms. Chavez what the procedures will involve today, and third what if any information you will need to obtain from Ms. Chavez.

2) Thomas Foster is a 28-year-old Caucasian male inpatient. You have orders to draw his blood this morning. Upon examination of his veins you find that his antecubital veins are damaged from scar tissue and the veins in his hands and wrists have been damaged from IV drug use as well. Describe how you will proceed with the collection.

Complications of Blood Collection

KEY TERMS

anaphylactic shock
   (**an**-ah-fi-**LAK**-tik)
anticoagulant
   (**an**-ti-ko-**AG**-u-lant)
hematoma (**hem**-ah-**TOE**-ma)
hemophiliac (**he**-mo-**FIL**-ee-ak)
seizure (**SEE**-zhur)
syncope (**SIN**-ko-pea)
topical (**TOP**-ih-kal)

OBJECTIVES

Upon completion of this chapter the student should be able to:

- Define and correctly spell each of the key terms.
- List possible complications of blood collection.
- Explain how to prevent complications in blood collection and how to effectively handle complications when they occur.

OUTLINE

- Introduction
- Accidental Artery Puncture
- Allergic Response
- Collapsed Vein
- Excessive Bleeding at the Site
- Fainting—Seizures
- Hematoma
- Nerve Damage
- Uncooperative Patient

INTRODUCTION

Complications of blood collections can occur at any time and in a variety of situations. It is extremely important that the phlebotomist is confident in recognizing these situations. Appropriate precautions are the best method of preventing complications from occurring. However, when they do occur, handling them as professionally, quickly, and efficiently as possible is critical.

ACCIDENTAL ARTERY PUNCTURE

If an accidental artery puncture occurs, immediately remove the tourniquet and withdraw the needle from the site. Apply direct pressure for a minimum of 5 minutes and/or until the bleeding has stopped. Bright red blood spurting into the tube is the instant indicator that an artery has been punctured instead of a vein.

ALLERGIC RESPONSE

Allergic responses were discussed in Chapter 8. A quick review is appropriate here as allergic responses qualify as a complication of blood collection. Patients may have an allergy to latex, which would include latex gloves and latex tourniquet tubing. Some patients may be allergic to bandage adhesive or antiseptics such as alcohol or povidone-iodine. Typically patients who know they have an allergy of this type will say so in advance of the collection. Most have had reactions in the past. As a precaution the phlebotomist asks every patient if he or she is allergic to latex, adhesive, or antiseptics. Alternatives such as nonlatex gloves and tourniquets can be used instead. Paper tape and 2 × 2 gauze pads are used in place of adhesive bandages, and patients allergic to isopropyl alcohol can have their skin cleaned with povidone-iodine or with alcohol if allergic to povidone-iodine, in the case of a blood culture collection or blood-alcohol level draw. If, however, the patient is unaware of any previous allergic responses, and a reaction occurs during the collection procedure, complete the procedure as quickly as possible. If an extreme reaction occurs, stop the procedure immediately. Wash the affected area with a non-allergenic soap and running water and report the reaction to the nurse and/or physician immediately.

Most allergic responses are generally mild in nature, and will present as redness or as a rash of the surrounding tissue. They are

TOPICAL

Pertaining to a definite surface area; local. Generally refers to the application of a substance to the skin.

ANAPHYLACTIC SHOCK

An immediate allergic reaction characterized by acute respiratory distress, hypotension, edema, and rash. Anaphylactic shock can be life-threatening.

ANTICOAGULANT

An agent that prevents or delays blood coagulation (clumping).

HEMOPHILIAC

A person afflicted with a hereditary blood disease marked by greatly prolonged blood coagulation time, with consequent failure of the blood to clot and abnormal bleeding, sometimes accompanied by joint swelling.

unpleasant because the tissues will be itchy. Scratching the tissue is the concern, because of the risk of infection. Ointments prescribed by a physician, applied **topically**, will cause the rash to subside and soothe the itching. If the rash is severe a systemic medication can be prescribed for the patient. In extremely severe cases the allergic response can lead to **anaphylactic shock**. In this case the patient will present with acute respiratory distress, hypotension, edema, hives, tachycardia, pale cool skin, convulsions, and cyanosis, which if not treated immediately can cause unconsciousness. Death may result. Edema can compromise the patient's airway if the larynx is involved and in a matter of minutes can cause death. Early recognition and intervention of this complication can save the patient's life. Notify the nurse and/or physician immediately.

COLLAPSED VEIN

The veins of elderly and/or frail patients are often too fragile to withstand the force of the vacuum in the evacuated tube. By using too large an evacuated tube for the patient's vein or exerting too much force when drawing back the plunger of a syringe, the phlebotomist can cause the patient's vein to collapse. A tourniquet tied too tightly or positioned too close to the venipuncture site can also cause a vein to collapse. If a patient tells you that his or her veins "always collapse," pay attention. This is a good indication that alternative collection methods should be used, such as using smaller evacuated tubes (pediatric), a butterfly infusion set, or syringe. Whichever method is used, pull the blood slowly into the tube.

EXCESSIVE BLEEDING AT THE SITE

Usually, bleeding will stop after a venipuncture within a few minutes. Occasionally a patient who is on **anticoagulant** therapy or a patient who is a **hemophiliac** will continue to bleed. If bleeding does not stop after a few minutes, apply direct pressure over the site and raise the patient's arm above heart level. Pressure must be maintained over the venipuncture site until the bleeding has stopped, by either the patient or the phlebotomist. If the bleeding does not stop after 5 minutes, notify the nurse and/or physician. Do *not* leave the patient unattended at *any* time during this situation until the nurse or physician assumes responsibility for the patient.

FAINTING—SEIZURES

Fainting or **syncope** is a common complication of blood collection. Patients often feel faint just thinking about having their blood drawn. Some patients have a tremendous fear of needles, and the fear of being in pain can lead to a syncopal episode. For other patients it is the sight of blood that makes them feel faint.

Box 11-1: Needle Phobia

Needle Phobia Is for Real

(*Health News* from the publishers of the *New England Journal of Medicine,* September 1995)

Several million Americans fear needles so intensely that being stuck with one for an injection or a blood test can trigger fainting, convulsions, and, in 23 reported cases, death.

Such "needle phobia"—a medical condition formally recognized last year—isn't all in one's head, explains James Hamilton, MD, in the *August Journal of Family Practice.* (He dedicates the paper to his father, who died in 1977 apparently from a heart attack triggered by a needle stick.) The condition runs in some families, suggesting that an inherited trait plays a role. But most people probably acquire their morbid fear of needles through a painful or unpleasant association.

As people with needle phobia steel themselves for an injection (or blood draw), their blood pressure rises. When the needle punctures the skin, a physiological reaction called the vasovagal response kicks in, causing stress hormones to flood the bloodstream and blood pressure to plummet. Many faint and some lose control of their bladders or have small seizures. In people with heart disease, the abrupt drop in blood pressure can be very dangerous.

Several strategies may help needlephobes get through an injection or blood test. Lying with the legs elevated and tensing the muscles during an injection can maintain blood pressure. Sedatives help, as do anesthetics to numb the skin.

The feeling starts with increased nervousness, increased respirations, a slow and weak pulse, decreased blood pressure, pallor and mild sweating, and possibly nausea and vomiting. The feeling may progress to periods of unconsciousness and in extreme cases may include **seizures**.

Patients may tell you in advance that they faint every time their blood is drawn. Listen to them. When so advised, ask the patient to lie down prior to drawing their blood. This is often enough to prevent the patient from fainting. Most laboratories are equipped with a bed or reclining chair to accommodate this situation.

If the patient tells you he feels faint or starts to faint during the procedure, take the following steps:

● Remove the tourniquet and withdraw the needle as quickly as possible.
● Talk to the patient to divert attention. This helps the patient to stay alert and retain consciousness.
● Ask and assist the patient to lower the head between the knees. Ask the patient to breathe slowly and deeply (Figure 11-1).

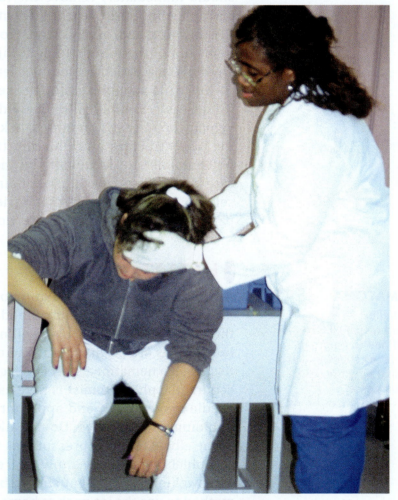

FIGURE 11-1: Patient being treated for fainting

● Physically support the patient to prevent further injury.
● Loosen any tight clothing, such as collars or ties.
● Apply a cold compress or washcloth to the forehead and back of the neck.

- If necessary, use an ammonia inhalant to bring the patient "back around." *Note:* Alcohol wipes work just as well as ammonia inhalants and are generally quicker to procure.
- Alert the nurse and/or physician as quickly as possible.
- Monitor the patient's vital signs until they return to normal or a nurse or physician assumes responsibility for the patient.

Seizures are a rare occurrence. However, if a patient has a seizure while the phlebotomist is drawing blood, the phlebotomist should immediately remove the tourniquet, withdraw the needle, and apply pressure over the site without restricting the patient. Notify the nurse and/or physician. Protect the patient's head and move items out of the way that might injure the patient and *never* place anything in a patient's mouth or leave the patient unattended.

Once the patient has stopped seizing, he should stay in the area for at least 15 minutes. He should be instructed not to operate a vehicle for at least 30 minutes. Ask the nurse or physician to check the patient before allowing him to leave. It is important for the phlebotomist to document the incident according to the health care facility's protocol. Depending on the seriousness of the seizure, it is recommend that a friend or family member drive the patient home based on the directions of a physician.

❚ HEMATOMA

HEMATOMA

A swelling or mass of blood (usually clotted), confined to an organ, tissue, or space that is caused by a break in a blood vessel.

A **hematoma** is an accumulation of blood at the venipuncture site (Figure 11-2). It is caused by blood leaking into the tissues around the site and identified by swelling and discoloration (bruising). Hematomas are often painful and can cause damage to underlying tissues. If a hematoma starts to occur during the venipuncture procedure, the phlebotomist is to release the tourniquet, withdraw the needle immediately, and apply direct pressure over the site for a minimum of 5 minutes. Do not allow the patient to bend the arm at the elbow to apply pressure, as this will cause further bruising. The phlebotomist may apply an ice pack to the site to reduce pain and swelling. The patient should be instructed on the appropriate method to use the ice pack at home. (Apply ice pack for 20 minutes, then remove for 20 minutes.) Do not apply a cold pack directly on the patient's skin. Drape a towel or sheet over the injured area, then apply the ice pack.

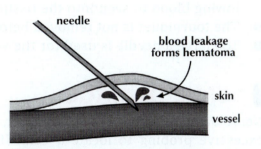
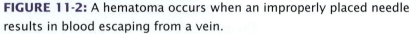

FIGURE 11-2: A hematoma occurs when an improperly placed needle results in blood escaping from a vein.

The following are reasons why a hematoma may occur:

● Inadequate pressure is applied to the venipuncture site for an inadequate amount of time.
● Excessive probing is used to locate a vein.
● The needle is only partially in the vein, thereby allowing blood to seep into the tissue.

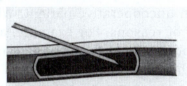

Correct — blood flows freely into the needle

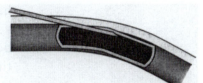

Incorrect — bevel against the upper wall impedes flow

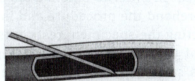

Incorrect — bevel against the lower wall impedes flow

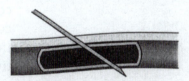

Incorrect — needle is inserted too far

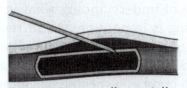

Incorrect — needle partially inserted, causing hematoma

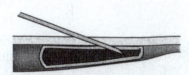

Incorrect — a collapsed vein

FIGURE 11-3: Improperly placed needles

- The needle penetrates all the way through the vein, thereby allowing blood to seep into the tissue.
- The tourniquet is not removed before the needle is withdrawn.
- Too large a needle is used for the vein size.

NERVE DAMAGE

Nerve damage is rare but it can occur, and is generally caused by excessive probing to locate a vein. If the phlebotomist "hits" a nerve during the draw, it will cause a painful burning sensation in the patient's arm. The phlebotomist should remove the tourniquet and withdraw the needle immediately. "Hitting" a nerve is painful and can cause permanent damage. To eliminate this risk, avoid excessive probing for the vein. If you cannot locate a vein, ask another phlebotomist to do the draw.

UNCOOPERATIVE PATIENT

At some time in your career as a phlebotomy technician you will have an uncooperative patient. While uncommon, it occurs for a variety of reasons. For example, a young child who does not understand the procedure and is afraid of being hurt; a very ill patient who is tired of being "poked and prodded"; or a patient who is in the emergency room for a drug overdose. Although occurring only as a last resort, the phlebotomist may be required to restrain a patient in order to obtain a specimen. If the patient is unable to comprehend the procedure and is physically preventing you from collecting the specimen, restraints may be necessary. Immobilization of the patient before you begin the collection is for the patient's safety. Always request the assistance of a second person when a collection is performed on a restrained patient.

Typically the only time restraint of a patient is required is in the case of very small children and infants, when the patient is incapable of understanding what is happening, and cooperation by reasoning is impossible. Adult restraint is extremely rare. The restraint of an adult patient for collection of a specimen must be requested in writing by the physician, and is performed only when the collection of a specimen is imperative to the health and welfare of the patient.

When patients are ill and have been through numerous procedures, they may be very resistant and deny that the procedure be performed. This is where the phlebotomist's interpersonal skills are of great importance. Remain calm, confident, and friendly without being condescending. Take your time. Talk with the patient for a few minutes; communicate that you understand his or her reluctance. Be sincere and appreciate the patient's anxiety. Explain exactly what you are going to do step by step. Explain how important it is that the procedure be performed. If you still have not gained the patient's confidence and permission to do the procedure, notify the nurse and/or physician. Patients have the right to refuse any procedure. If this should occur, thoroughly document the refusal on the requisition form and/or the patient's chart. Notify the nurse. Perhaps another person can persuade the patient to cooperate or perhaps later in the shift the patient will feel more comfortable and cooperative. Do not give up nor take it personally.

SUMMARY

Every phlebotomist will encounter one or more complications at some point in his or her career. It is important to remember how to recognize the situation and how to deal with it. Acting professionally and following emergency procedures should become second nature because there may be no time to stop and check a procedure manual when a patient has fainted, or a hematoma is forming at a venipuncture site.

STUDY AND REVIEW EXERCISES
Defining Key Terms

Write the definition for each of the following key terms.

1) anaphylactic shock_____

2) anticoagulant _____

3) hematoma_____

4) hemophiliac_____

5) seizure_____

6) syncope_____

7) topical _____

Reviewing Key Points

1) List eight possible complications of blood collections.

2) Describe how to identify if an artery has been punctured instead of a vein.

3) Identify the causes of collapsed veins.

4) List two conditions that could lead to excessive bleeding at a venipuncture site.

5) List six reasons that a hematoma may occur.

Sentence Completion

1) _____ can be caused by a severe allergic reaction to latex.

2) Ointments prescribed by a physician, applied _____, will cause an allergic rash to subside.

3) Symptoms of the complication of _____ are: increased nervousness, increased respirations, a slow and weak pulse, and decreased blood pressure.

4) A _____ is an accumulation of blood at the venipuncture site.

5) Never place anything in the mouth of a patient who is having a(n) _____.

Multiple Choice

1) A hereditary blood disease marked by greatly prolonged coagulation time.
   A. Anaphylactic shock
   B. Sickle cell
   C. Anemia
   D. Hemophilia

2) If an artery is accidentally punctured the phlebotomist should apply pressure for a minimum of:
   A. 2 minutes
   B. 5 minutes
   C. 10 minutes
   D. 15 minutes

3) If a patient is allergic to alcohol, _____ should be used instead.
   A. Cidex
   B. povidone-iodine
   C. Zephiran
   D. sodium chloride

4) Which one of the following is not a means of collapsing a vein?
   A. Too small a needle
   B. Too much force pulling back plunger
   C. Tying tourniquet too tight
   D. Force of vacuum in evacuated tube

5) If a hematoma starts to form during a venipuncture, the phlebotomist should *not* do which one of the following?
   A. Continue the draw as quickly as possible
   B. Withdraw the needle
   C. Apply direct pressure over the site
   D. Apply an ice pack

Critical Thinking

1) Mr. Hamilton is deathly afraid of needles. Just the thought of having his blood drawn makes him feel dizzy. Describe how best to accommodate this patient.

2) Ms. Alexander is having a CBC and Chem panel drawn today. Her veins are difficult to draw from, but the new phlebotomist "dug" around a bit to find one. During the venipuncture the new phlebotomist "hit" a nerve in Ms. Alexander's arm. Ms. Alexander told the phlebotomist that she had a burning pain in her arm and to please take the needle out. The new phlebotomist told Ms. Alexander to sit very still as he was almost done with the collection. He finished drawing the required tubes. Ms. Alexander was in extreme pain and her fingers were feeling numb when she demanded to speak to the new phlebotomist's supervisor. How would you have handled this situation differently?

Specialized Phlebotomy Techniques

OBJECTIVES

Upon completion of this chapter the student should be able to:

- Define and correctly spell each of the key terms.
- Identify the challenges associated with the collection of specimens from pediatric patients.
- Describe the methods used to interact effectively with pediatric patients and their parents or guardians.
- Describe and demonstrate the ways in which a pediatric patient can be restrained.
- Identify the equipment and supplies used for a pediatric collection.
- Define arterial blood gases and describe the collection procedures, equipment, and supplies required to perform arterial blood gases and, finally, demonstrate the ability to perform arterial blood gases.
- Describe and demonstrate the Allen test for collateral circulation.
- Identify potential complications of arterial blood collection and reasons why the laboratory may reject a specimen.
- Explain and state the reasons for sterile techniques in the collection of blood cultures, and why a physician might order them.
- Identify the equipment and supplies required for blood culture collection and demonstrate the procedure.

(continues)

● Identify and describe the collection of nonblood specimens to include: throat cultures, fecal specimens, semen specimens, gastrointestinal secretions, amniotic fluid, cerebrospinal fluid, nasopharyngeal specimens, and urine.
● Identify the types of urine specimens and the methods of collection.
● Describe the collection process of blood donor collections.
● Describe the rationale for type and crossmatch.
● Identify and describe "special" collection procedures to include indwelling catheters and the various types of vascular access devices.

OUTLINE

● Pediatric Collection
● Arterial Blood Gases
● Blood Cultures
● Collection of Nonblood Specimens
● Blood Donor Collections
● Special Situations

PEDIATRIC COLLECTION

Collecting blood specimens from children often presents the phlebotomist with unique challenges. Given that children's blood vessels are smaller and, thus, more difficult to visualize and palpate, the process of collecting blood is not the only concern or consideration of the phlebotomist. Young children do not have the same skills for logical and emotional reasoning as adults. Explaining the procedure to a child may be difficult. Children have been conditioned to understand that needles hurt. They will have a hard time separating their anxiety of pain from their fear of needles. It is critical to gain the cooperation and trust of not only the pediatric patient, but also the child's parent or guardian, when present. Cooperation and trust are best gained by introducing yourself in a warm, friendly, and confident manner. Explain the procedure to the adult and child each step of the way. Taking a few extra minutes with the patient to ensure cooperation will greatly increase chances of a successful blood draw and also promote a healthier relationship between the patient and health care provider. Older children respond more easily to the phlebotomist who takes time to get to know the patient before beginning a procedure. Talk with the child and establish a positive rapport even before looking at the child's arm or touching any equipment. Never tell a child that the procedure is not going to hurt. Even the most skilled phlebotomist may cause the patient some discomfort when inserting a needle. If a child is told it will not hurt and then it does, the child may learn to distrust health care providers, which may be quite traumatic to the patient over time. A skilled and patient phlebotomist can contribute immensely to preventing this fear by taking the time to explain the procedures thoroughly.

Ask the parent or guardian if he or she wishes to remain in the room during the procedure. Some adults will be uncomfortable and will not want to stay; this is perfectly acceptable. If the adult leaves the room, the help of another health care professional may be required. If the adult prefers to stay with the patient, the phlebotomist may ask for assistance in one or more ways, such as holding the child on the lap, helping to restrain a small child, distracting the child during the procedure, or offering encouragement and reassurance. There are two schools of thought about the parent remaining during the procedure. One view is that the adults should not be present because they will transmit their own fears to the child, or the child will associate pain with a parent. A second view, and this author's personal preference, is to ask the adult to remain with the patient, whenever possible, as a means of comfort. Skilled phlebotomists are trained to perform blood collecting as painlessly and nontraumatically as possible.

Involve the older child in the procedure. Ask the child to hold the adhesive bandage or gauze pads. Ask the child to tell you exactly when it is he or she feels pain; this focuses attention away from fear of the needle and back to the actual physical pain involved, which is usually minimal. Use a doll, puppet, or stuffed animal to demonstrate to the child exactly what the venipuncture procedure involves. If the child has a favorite comfort item, such as a blanket or stuffed animal, encourage the child to hug the item for comfort during the procedure.

It is imperative that all supplies are gathered and assembled prior to the "stick." If the child is an inpatient and it is at all possible, the procedure should take place in a treatment room rather than in the child's bed. The child's bed should be a "safe" place, free from pain and anxiety, to promote the healing process.

Another challenge when collecting blood from a child is the requirement of drawing the least amount of blood possible to perform the ordered tests, as children have a smaller ratio of blood to body mass and cannot maintain homeostasis if large quantities are removed. Removal of large quantities of blood over long periods of time can cause the child to become anemic. Removal of over 10% of an infant's blood volume can cause cardiac arrest.

Restraining the Child Patient

The phlebotomist may be required to restrain a pediatric patient. This occurs mainly with infants and very young children. Restraining the patient is often the safest and most nontraumatic method of obtaining a specimen. Young children can easily be restrained by sitting them on a parent's lap (Figure 12-1). The parent helps the child extend his or her arm on the table and then wraps his or her arms around the child's free arm and torso. To help steady the patient's arm the parent should grasp the child's arm just behind the bend of the elbow. This will prevent the child from pulling it away during the needle stick.

Very young children and infants can be restrained by using a "papoose." A papoose is a specially designed board with attached canvas flaps. The child is positioned in the center of the device and the flaps are wrapped around the infant and securely fastened, leaving the extremity being drawn exposed. Some health care providers feel that using a "papoose" to restrain a child is more traumatic than the actual blood draw itself. The safety of the child is the primary concern. If the sample can be collected without using a "papoose" to restrain the child, then select the alternative method first.

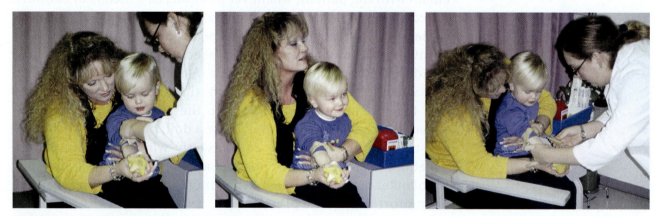

FIGURE 12-1: Restraint of a child in parent's arms

Older children can sit in the phlebotomy chair by themselves with the parent standing behind the chair helping to steady the child's arm. The child may also be placed in a supine position with the parent or another health care provider leaning over the child from the opposite side of the bed, grasping the child's arm being drawn on from behind, and holding the free arm close to the patient's body (Figure 12-2).

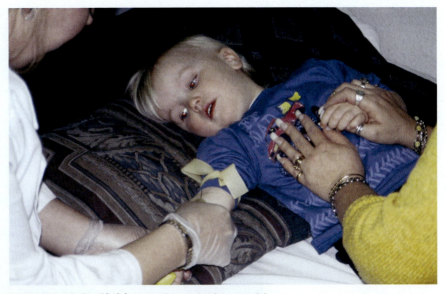

FIGURE 12-2: Child restraint—supine position

Another fact that must be taken into consideration is that a child or infant's blood vessels are significantly smaller than that of an adult. This means that the phlebotomist must use smaller tubes and needles for the collection process. The 23 gauge butterfly infusion set with a 2 to 3 mL evacuated tube typically provides the best results at an antecubital site. Because children may struggle and twist during the procedure, a butterfly infusion set provides the phlebotomist with more flexibility because of the length of the tubing between the needle and the tube holder. Tourniquets are also available in pediatric sizes. Because a child's veins are small, they are not able to withstand the same amount of vacuum from an evacuated tube as an adult. By using smaller tubes, the vacuum pressure is lower and will cause less damage and less chance of the vessel collapsing (Figure 12-3).

Collecting blood specimens from the antecubital veins is the preferred method. However, the dorsal hand veins are excellent sites for drawing labs on neonates and children under the age of two. The dorsal hand vein as a collection site on infants is preferred over capillary puncture collection because it is much more efficient and less time consuming, and the phlebotomist can collect a sufficient amount of blood for testing. When the capillary puncture method is used, the phlebotomist will often need to perform several punctures to obtain enough blood for the ordered tests.

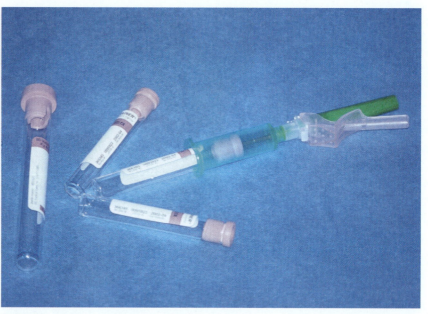

FIGURE 12-3: Comparison of pediatric evacuated blood collection tubes to an adult-size evacuated tube (left)

Box 12-1: Take Care When Using Tourniquets and Adhesive Bandages on Infants and Small Children

An infant's skin is extremely fragile. Using tourniquets and adhesive bandages can tear the skin. When drawing blood from an infant use the dorsal hand vein. Encircle the infant's wrist with your thumb underneath and index finger on top. Apply pressure; a tourniquet will not be necessary. Not only can adhesive bandages tear an infant or small child's skin upon removal, but it is also possible that the child may swallow the adhesive bandage and choke.

ARTERIAL BLOOD GASES (ABGs)

Literally, any of the gases present in blood. Clinically, the determination of levels in the blood of oxygen and carbon dioxide.

ACID-BASE BALANCE

The mechanisms by which the acidity and alkalinity of body fluids are kept in a state of equilibrium so that arterial blood is maintained at approximately a 7.35 to 7.45 pH level.

ARTERIAL BLOOD GASES

Arterial blood gases (ABGs) are performed to provide valuable information regarding the status of the patient's oxygenation, ventilation, and **acid-base balance**. Arterial blood is used for these determinations because it is relatively consistent in composition throughout the body, whereas venous blood fluctuates in composition with the metabolic needs of the body tissues surrounding the vein.

If an arterial blood gas collection is performed incorrectly, the patient can be seriously injured. Therefore, personnel who are required to perform ABGs must be specially trained and, as a rule, are certified by their health care institution as having met the qualifications to perform this advanced procedure. NCCLS has determined the criteria for meeting these qualifications to be didactic (theory) training, observation of a demonstration of the technique, and performance of the procedure under the supervision of qualified personnel.

Selection of Arterial Puncture Site

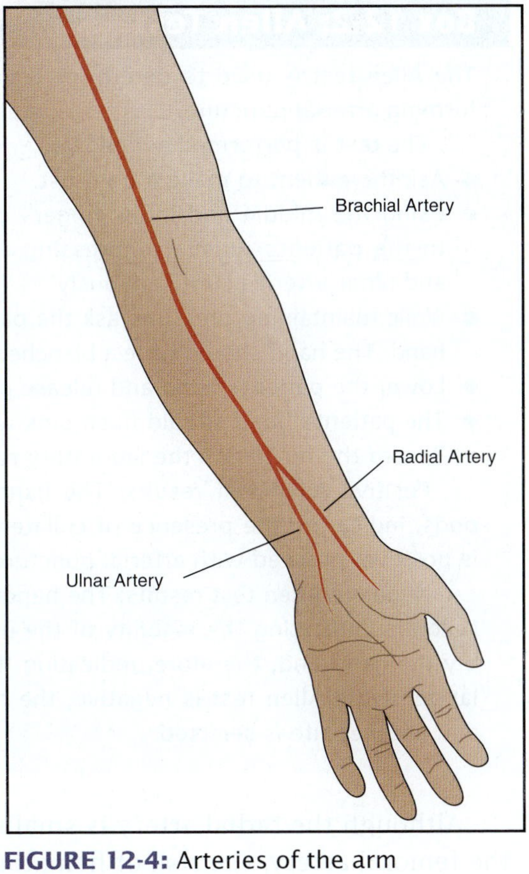

FIGURE 12-4: Arteries of the arm

COLLATERAL CIRCULATION

A process allowing tissue to be supplied with blood from an accessory vessel.

Several arterial sites may be used for the arterial puncture. Selection of the site will depend on the size and accessibility of the artery, the stability of the tissue surrounding the site, and **collateral circulation**. The site selected should not be inflamed or in close proximity to a wound, nor should the phlebotomist ever select a limb with an AV shunt or fistula. Sites that are preferred are the radial artery, the brachial artery, and the femoral artery. The radial artery is the site most commonly selected because it typically has the best collateral circulation (Figure 12-4). Collateral circulation means that blood is supplied to the area by more than one artery. Under normal circumstances the hand and wrist, which are preferred sites, are supplied blood via the radial artery and the ulnar artery. This is important because if the radial artery were damaged during the arterial puncture, the ulnar artery would continue to supply blood to the area. Collateral circulation of the hand and wrist can be determined by the use of a Doppler ultrasonic flow indicator or by performing a modified Allen test (Box 12-2). If collateral circulation is absent the radial artery should not be punctured.

Box 12-2: Allen Test

The Allen test is used to determine collateral circulation prior to performing arterial puncture.

The test is performed as follows:
● Ask the patient to make a tight fist.
● Using the middle and index fingers of both hands, apply pressure to the patient's wrist, compressing and occluding both the radial and ulnar arteries simultaneously.
● While maintaining pressure, ask the patient to slowly open his or her hand. The hand should have a blanched appearance, drained of color.
● Lower the patient's hand and release pressure on the ulnar artery.
● The patient's hand should flush pink within 15 seconds.
● Record the results on the laboratory requisition form.

Positive Allen test results: The hand flushed pink within 15 seconds, indicating the presence of collateral circulation. If the Allen test is positive, proceed with arterial puncture.

Negative Allen test results: The hand does not flush pink within 15 seconds, indicating the inability of the ulnar artery to adequately supply the hand and, therefore, indicating the absence of collateral circulation. If the Allen test is negative, the radial artery is not to be used and another site is selected.

Although the radial artery is smaller than the brachial artery or the femoral artery, the risk of hematoma is considerably less. This is because the radial artery can easily be compressed against the ligaments and bones of the wrist. The brachial artery is the second choice. The brachial artery is larger and more easily palpated than the radial artery. The brachial artery also has sufficient collateral circulation, but not as much as the radial artery. The brachial artery is located deeper in the tissue than the radial artery and lies next to the brachial vein and the median nerve, both of which might be inadvertently punctured instead of the brachial artery. The brachial artery does not have underlying ligaments or bone to support compression of the artery, which increases the risk of hematoma.

The femoral artery is the third choice. It is a large artery located superficially in the groin area and can be easily palpated. Physicians or specially trained emergency room personnel are typically the only health care professionals who puncture the femoral artery. Collateral circulation is not as optimal in this area as it is in the two previous sites. The risk of infection also increases when puncturing the femoral artery, because of pubic hair. The femoral vein lies in close proximity to the femoral artery, which can be punctured instead of the artery. The femoral artery is used mainly as a last resort when other sites cannot be used.

There are other sites where arterial punctures can be performed, such as the umbilicus of the newborn and the dorsalis pedis arteries of an adult patient. As with draws using the femoral artery, a physician or specifically trained emergency room personnel will perform this procedure. A phlebotomist is not trained to perform these collections.

Equipment and Supplies

The phlebotomist must gather and assemble the following equipment and supplies prior to the arterial puncture:

- Safety equipment: Personal protective equipment (PPE) includes the following when collecting ABGs: Fluid-resistant lab coat, gown, or aprons, gloves, face protection (arterial punctures have a higher risk of splattering blood), puncture-resistant sharps container.
- Antiseptic solution: Povidone-iodine (Betadine) solution or chlorhexidine is used to clean the site.
- Local anesthetic solution: 0.5% to 1% lidocaine solution is used to numb the site. *(Phlebotomists must check the facility's regulations regarding the phlebotomist use of lidocaine.)*
- Hypodermic needles: Size and length vary depending on site location used, but will be selected from 20 to 25 gauge, 5/8 to 1½ inches in length. The most commonly used needle is a 22 gauge, 1 inch for radial and brachial punctures and a 22 gauge, 1½ inch for femoral punctures. A 25 to 26 gauge needle is used for administration of an anesthetic.
- Syringes: ABGs are collected in 1 to 5 mL syringes depending on the amount of blood required. ABG kits contain a special glass or plastic syringe that is prefilled with heparin and designed to fill spontaneously upon puncture of the artery. A 1 or 2 mL syringe is used for administration of an anesthetic.

Glass syringes have traditionally been used for the collection of blood gases because of the limited exchange of gas through the glass and the ease with which the arterial pressure fills the syringe. However, plastic syringes have become much more efficient. They are prefilled with heparin and can also fill without manual aspiration. The exchange of gas has become less of a factor with the new plastics. Evacuated tubes should not be used for collection of ABGs because the tubes alter the partial pressure of the gas in the blood sample.

The Luer-tip cap that is removed from the syringe to attach the needle should be saved so that after the collection when the needle is removed from the syringe, the cap can be replaced for maintenance of anaerobic conditions during transportation of the specimen to the lab.

● A small block of latex or rubber, or other similar device to insert the needle in immediately after collection, to prevent air from entering the syringe.

● Lithium (or sodium) heparin solution, 1000 units/mL. Heparin is used to prevent the specimen from clotting. Typically the syringes used are prefilled with heparin.

● Coolant: Plastic bag or cup with crushed ice and water. A coolant that can maintain a temperature of 1° C to 5° C is required to prevent gases from escaping into the atmosphere and to slow the metabolism of white blood cells, which consume oxygen. The collection syringe must be fully submerged in ice water, which is the typical coolant.

● Gauze: 2 × 2 gauze pads used to hold pressure over the puncture site.

● Patient identification label.

● Waterproof marker or pen.

● Alcohol pad.

● Adhesive bandage or tape.

● Oxygen measuring device: Used for patients who are on oxygen-enriched gases instead of room air. The oxygen concentration is recorded on the laboratory requisition slip. This measurement is taken prior to the collection of the specimen.

● Thermometer: Patient's temperature is recorded on the laboratory requisition slip.

● Puncture-resistant sharps container: To properly dispose of needles.

Preparation and Procedure

A physician requests arterial blood gases to be drawn using a laboratory requisition form, as with all other laboratory tests. Once the procedure has been ordered, the phlebotomist properly identifies the patient, explains the procedure, and obtains the patient's consent. The phlebotomist also determines if the patient has allergies (e.g., latex, alcohol, anesthetics), or is on anticoagulant therapy.

First, calm the patient. A patient who is anxious or excited will have altered breathing patterns and an increased body temperature, which will compromise test results. The patient must be in a "steady state." This means the patient has been resting comfortably for a minimum of 30 minutes with no exercise, treatments, or respirator changes. A patient who is afraid of needles or the pain that is associated with arterial blood collection will quickly move out of a steady state.

Complications of Arterial Punctures

Arterial punctures can cause the patient discomfort, even with the use of anesthesia. The phlebotomist must demonstrate confidence and efficiency during the procedure so that the discomfort is not prolonged or repeated unnecessarily. Arterial punctures, as with any other invasive procedure, run the risk of infection. Proper antiseptic procedures minimize this risk. The chance of a hematoma is increased in arterial puncture because the blood in the arteries is under great pressure. This tends to cause blood to leak into the tissues surrounding the puncture site. This is further increased in older patients by the loss of elasticity of the arteries that occurs with age. The risk of a hematoma is also increased in patients on anticoagulation therapy. Another complication of arterial puncture is the risk of an **arteriospasm**. Arteriospasms may occur when the insertion of the needle into the artery causes irritation of the arterial muscle. The artery will reflexively contract. This condition is usually temporary, but it does make collection of a specimen difficult. Thrombus formation is also a risk with arterial punctures. Injury to the lining of the artery can cause a thrombus to form, which can obstruct the flow of blood and impair circulation.

ARTERIOSPASM

arteria (artery) + *spasmos* (convulsion) = arterial spasm.

Errors and Specimen Rejection

There are several situations or conditions that can cause an arterial blood sample to render inaccurate test results or to be rejected by the laboratory:

● Air bubbles in the specimen.
● Inadequate amount of blood collected.
● Improperly cooled specimen.
● Venous sample collected instead of arterial sample.
● Incorrect anticoagulant used.
● Too much or not enough anticoagulant used.
● Specimen improperly mixed.

Procedure 12-1

Collection of Arterial Blood Gases

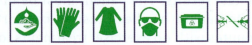

Equipment/Supplies

- Safety equipment
- Prepackaged ABG kit

OR

- Povidone-iodine (Betadine) solution or chlorhexidine
- Local anesthetic solution: 0.5% to 1 % lidocaine
- Hypodermic needles: 22 gauge, 1 inch for ABG; 25 gauge, ½ inch for anesthesia
- Syringes: 1 to 5 mL for ABG/1 or 2 mL syringe for anesthesia
- A small block of latex or rubber
- Lithium (or sodium) heparin solution, 1000 units/mL, 0.5 mL
- Plastic bag or cup with crushed ice and water
- Gauze: 2 × 2 gauze pads
- Patient identification label
- Waterproof marker or pen
- Alcohol pad
- Adhesive bandage or tape
- Oxygen measuring device
- Thermometer
- Puncture-resistant sharps container

Method/*Rationale*

1. Review physician's order and note time ABGs are to be drawn.

2. Gather equipment and supplies. Transport equipment and supplies to patient's bedside or examination table.

   Ensures everything is available to perform the procedure.

3. Identify the patient.

   Ensures the procedure is performed on the correct patient.

4. Wash hands/don personal protective equipment.

   Thorough handwashing aids in controlling the spread of infection. Remember, you must comply with Standard Precautions whenever you may come in contact with any body fluids. Because there is pressure behind the arteries, it is important that the phlebotomist wear face/eye protection.

5. Obtain and record the patient's temperature, respiratory rate, and breathing mixture (e.g., room air) on the laboratory slip.

   Remember that changes in the patient's temperature and respiration change the composition of the patient's blood, thereby compromising the test results.

6. Open the ABG kit or prepare the syringe with heparin.

7. To prepare the syringe:

   1. Check the syringe for free movement of the plunger and attach with a 20 gauge needle.

   2. Clean the top of the heparin bottle with an alcohol pad.

   3. Draw 0.5 mL heparin into the syringe. While pulling back on the plunger, rotate the syringe to wet the barrel.

   4. Holding the syringe vertically, expel the excess heparin.

   5. Remove the 20 gauge needle and replace it with the appropriate needle for the arterial puncture.

   Coating the syringe with heparin prevents the clotting of arterial blood.

8. Prepare the anesthetic: Clean the top of the bottle; draw 0.5 mL of anesthetic into a 1 mL syringe using a 25 gauge, ½ needle. Carefully recap the needle using the one-handed scoop method.

9. Position the patient's arm with the palm facing up. A rolled towel may be placed under the wrist for support.

   This position adequately exposes the patient's wrist.

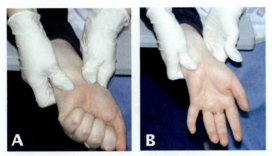

FIGURE 12-5 (A AND B): Checking for collateral circulation

10. Assess collateral circulation using the Allen test or a Doppler ultrasonic flow indicator. If collateral circulation is present, continue with the procedure. If collateral circulation is absent, then select another site.

    1. Position the patent's arm wrist-up and support with a rolled towel. Ask the patient to make a fist.

    2. Occlude the radial and ulnar arteries simultaneously (Figure 12-5A).

    3. Ask the patient to unclench his or her fist. Observe blanched appearance.

    4. Release pressure on ulnar artery. The patient's hand should flush pink as circulation returns (Figure 12-5B).

       Remember that collateral circulation is important because if damage is done to the artery, another artery will supply the area with blood.

11. With the patient's palm still facing up, ask the patient to flex the wrist at a 30 to 45-degree angle.

    This fixes the soft tissues over the firm ligaments and bone.

12. Locate the radial artery on the thumb side of the wrist using the index and middle fingers of the left hand. Palpate the artery to determine its size, depth, and direction.

    Never use the thumb to palpate the pulse as the thumb has a pulse of its own and it may be confused with the patient's.

13. Prepare the site by first cleaning with an alcohol pad in a circular motion, starting from the site outward. Allow the alcohol to air dry. If anesthesia is to be used, anesthetize the skin. Infiltrate the skin over the puncture site, inserting the needle at approximately a 10-degree angle. Pull back on the plunger to ensure that a vein has not been punctured. If blood appears in the syringe, withdraw the needle, prepare a new syringe and needle, and repeat the procedure in an area close to the last puncture. If no blood appears in the syringe, slowly inject enough of the anesthesia into the skin to form a raised **wheal**. Wait approximately 1 to 2 minutes for the anesthesia to take effect before proceeding with the arterial puncture. Note on the lab request form that anesthesia was administered. Note the type and amount.

WHEAL

A more or less round and evanescent elevation of the skin, white in the center with a pale-red periphery.

If anesthesia is not administered, clean with alcohol in the above manner and proceed to the next step.

(continues)

Procedure 12-1 *(continued)*

14. Clean the site with povidone-iodine in the same manner as the alcohol. Allow to air dry.

    The fingers that will be used to palpate for the artery may also be cleaned with povidone-iodine if they are to be used to palpate for the artery. Take care not to contaminate the site or fingers once they have been cleaned.

15. Relocate the artery.

    A tourniquet will not be necessary to help locate the artery.

16. Holding the syringe in the dominant hand as you would a dart, uncap the needle. Be careful not to draw air into the syringe.

    If air is drawn into the syringe inadvertently, the ABG results will be altered.

17. Signal the patient that you are about to stick. Place your cleaned fingers on the pulse over the site where you want the needle to be after insertion. Puncture the skin 5 to 10 mm lower on the artery towards the palm, from the point you feel the pulsating artery. Insert the needle at a 45-degree angle (femoral ABGs will require a 90-degree angle) with the bevel of needle facing the direction of the blood flow (Figure 12-6). This will place the bevel of the needle directly under the finger that is feeling the pulsating artery.

    Give the patient notice that you are going to "stick" so that it does not come as a surprise. Remember that your finger is in close proximity to the needle. Surprising the patient may cause the patient to quickly pull away. The needle may be hit in the process, sticking the patient and then you, and causing a contaminated needle stick.

18. Advance the needle until the artery is punctured. Once this occurs, a "flash" of blood will appear in the hub of the needle. When the flash appears, stop advancing the needle. Blood will fill the syringe without the phlebotomist pulling back on the plunger.

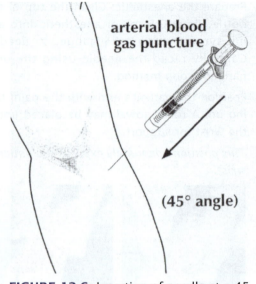

arterial blood gas puncture

(45° angle)

FIGURE 12-6: Insertion of needle at a 45-degree angle

If blood does not "flash" into the hub of the needle, slowly withdraw the needle until the bevel is just beneath the surface of the skin and redirect the needle into the artery as described above. Never probe for an artery; it is extremely painful and may cause a hematoma or thrombus formation or permanently damage the artery.

19. When the desired amount of blood has been collected, quickly withdraw the needle and immediately apply pressure over the puncture site with a clean 2 × 2 gauze pad. Pressure must be applied for a minimum of 5 minutes. If the patient is on anticoagulation therapy, pressure must be applied for approximately 20 minutes. Do not allow the patient to apply the direct pressure.

    Patients who are on anticoagulation therapy have blood that has been thinned and will take longer for the puncture site to form a clot and stop bleeding. Patients should not be asked to apply the pressure themselves because they typically will not apply firm enough pressure.

20. Once the needle has been removed from the patient's arm, immediately expel any air bubbles from the specimen and insert the needle into the latex cube.

    Air bubbles may have been drawn into the syringe inadvertently as the needle was removed from the patient's arm. This will alter the test results and must be avoided. By inserting the needle into the latex cube, the phlebotomist prevents any further contamination of the specimen from outside air.

21. While maintaining pressure on the puncture site, mix the collected specimen by gently inverting the syringe in a rolling figure eight.

    The collected specimen must be mixed with the heparin that is coating the syringe to prevent coagulation of the specimen. The phlebotomist must take care to mix the specimen gently; vigorous shaking will cause the cells to lyse, rendering the test results inaccurate.

22. Remove the needle from the latex cube, carefully avoiding the introduction of air into the syringe. Discard the needle in the appropriate sharps container and replace the Luer cap onto the syringe.

23. Label the specimen and place in the bag or container of crushed ice and water.

    Arterial blood specimens must be kept at a temperature of 1 to 5˚C. Samples kept at this temperature are accurate for 1 to 2 hours; at room temperature they are accurate for 5 to 10 minutes. Samples must be immersed in ice water prior to terminating pressure on the puncture site. Waiting will invalidate the test.

24. After pressure has been applied for 5 minutes, check the puncture site for swelling, bruising, and bleeding. If none, clean the site with an alcohol pad to remove any remaining povidone-iodine. Check the pulse distal to the site. If it is absent or faint, notify the patient's nurse or physician immediately. If the site appears normal, apply a pressure dressing.

    If the site is still bleeding or is swollen, before proceeding, reapply pressure and check the site every 2 minutes until the bleeding has stopped.

25. Dispose of used equipment and supplies appropriately. Remove gloves and wash your hands. Thank the patient. Transport the specimen to the lab immediately.

● Improper syringe used. (If a plastic syringe is used it must be designed especially for ABG collection. Regular plastic syringes alter test results).
● Improper labeling of specimen.
● Too long of a delay transporting specimen to the laboratory.

BACTERIEMIA

Bacteria in the blood.

SEPTICEMIA

The presence of pathogenic microorganisms in the blood.

BLOOD CULTURES

A physician often orders blood cultures when a patient has a fever of unknown origin (FUO) or when the physician suspects **bacteriemia** or **septicemia**. Blood cultures can provide the physician with information regarding the presence of infection, the extent of the infection the organism is causing, and the antibiotics the organism is most susceptible to. Once a diagnosis has been made, blood cultures can provide valuable information to the physician regarding the progress of the patient and the effectiveness of the antibiotic therapy.

The collection of blood cultures is often a timed procedure. The specimens are collected from a patient with an FUO at the height of the fever when the microorganisms are thought to be most plentiful in the blood. With new technology and improvement of collection procedures, this is not as critical as it once was.

If blood cultures are to be drawn to monitor antimicrobial therapy, they will be drawn in special collection bottles, which contain a resin solution to inactivate the antimicrobial agent. This allows the bacteria to grow. The collection bottles containing resin are called antibiotic removal device (ARD) bottles. The resin removes the antimicrobial agent from the blood. Specimens collected in ARD bottles must be submitted to the laboratory as soon as possible for processing, as blood should not be exposed to the device for more than 2 hours.

Blood cultures that are drawn prior to antimicrobial therapy are collected in special tubes or bottles containing a nutrient media that promotes the growth of microorganisms present in blood. Two different collection bottles are used. One is an **anaerobic** bottle that is designed specifically for organisms that grow best when oxygen is not present, while the second bottle is **aerobic**. If the collection of blood is performed using a syringe, the anaerobic bottle is filled first. If a butterfly collection kit is used, the aerobic bottle is filled first, so that any air in the tubing is released into the oxygen-containing bottle.

Specially designed blood culture collection bottles eliminate the need for either the syringe or butterfly collection method. These specially designed bottles have long necks that fit into the evacuated tube holders that are used for regular venipuncture collection. The use of these bottles also allows for collection of other blood specimens via evacuated tubes, to be collected without an additional venipuncture.

The amount of blood that is collected is critical for the optimal recovery of microorganisms. Up to 10 mL of blood is typical, but can vary according to the recommendations of the manufacturer of the collection bottle. Collections from infants and children are 1 to 5 mL. If too little blood is collected, the ratio of blood-to-nutrient broth will inhibit the growth of microorganisms. If too much blood is collected from a patient, the patient risks a hospital-induced anemia and the ratio of blood-to-nutrient broth will tilt in the opposite direction, which also is not conducive to optimal growth.

ANAEROBIC

Pertaining to an anaerobe; able to live without oxygen.

AEROBIC

Living only in the presence of oxygen. Concerning an organism living only in the presence of oxygen.

Blood cultures are often ordered in sets. Collection of sets can occur in two ways. First, both sets can be collected at the same time from different sites (i.e., right arm, left arm) or they can be collected 30 minutes apart. If the timing method is not noted on the order, follow laboratory protocol. Correct labeling of the bottles is imperative.

The most critical factor in collecting blood cultures is antisepsis of the patient's skin. The site must be as clean as possible to avoid contamination of the specimen with surface microorganisms, which will produce a false-positive blood culture. Every microorganism that is found must be reported. It is then up to the patient's physician to interpret whether the microorganism is clinically significant. If the pathogen is determined clinically significant and it was introduced as a result of inaccurate antiseptic procedures, inappropriate treatment can be ordered and the patient may suffer.

COLLECTION OF NONBLOOD SPECIMENS

Laboratories process many types of specimens and the multiskilled phlebotomist will receive laboratory requests ordering collection of specimens other than blood. These nonblood specimen requests might include throat cultures, urine, fecal, or semen specimens, gastric secretions, amniotic fluid, cerebrospinal fluid, or nasopharyngeal culture collections. A multiskilled phlebotomist can collect some of these specimens from the patient, such as a urine specimen or throat culture. Other nonblood specimens are collected by a nurse or physician and the phlebotomist may simply transport them to the laboratory for processing and testing. The phlebotomist may also perform CLIA-waived point-of-care testing on collected specimens as described below.

All nonblood specimens must be labeled with the same patient identification information as blood specimens. Most laboratories require that the type of specimen and the source of the specimen be included on the label. Handling nonblood specimens requires the same use of Standard Precautions as if handling blood specimens. Nonblood specimens may be a body fluid or may contain a body fluid that may cause the phlebotomist risk of contamination.

Throat Cultures

Throat cultures are ordered by physicians to aid in the diagnosis of streptococcal infections (strep throat). In an office or clinical

Procedure 12-2

Collection of Blood Cultures

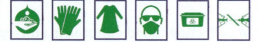

Equipment/Supplies

- Personal protective equipment
- Alcohol prep swabstick, alcohol prep pads
- Povidone-iodine swabsticks or blood culture prep kit
- 2 × 2 gauze pads
- Adhesive dressing or adhesive tape
- Tourniquet
- Evacuated tube holder and needle, or syringe and needle, or butterfly collection kit and blood culture bottle adapter (equipment depends on the method of collection)
- Blood culture bottles: 1 anaerobic, 1 aerobic; ARD if applicable
- Puncture-resistant sharps container

Method/*Rationale*

1. Gather equipment and supplies. Transport equipment and supplies to patient's bedside.

   Ensures everything is available to perform the procedure.

2. Identify the patient.

   Ensures that the procedure is performed on the correct patient.

3. Wash hands/don personal protective equipment.

   Thorough handwashing aids in controlling the spread of infection. Remember, you must comply with Standard Precautions whenever you may come in contact with any body fluids.

4. Select the venipuncture site. Release tourniquet if applicable.

   Select the site as if performing a routine venipuncture.

5. Clean the site initially with an alcohol pad to remove excess dirt and surface debris such as lotions and oils. Next, scrub the site for a minimum of 2 minutes, using a povidone-iodine swabstick, covering an area of 3 to 4 inches surrounding the puncture site.

   Cleaning an area of 3 to 4 inches surrounding the site lessens the risk of accidental contamination of the site by surface microorganisms (Figure 12-7).

6. Clean the site again using a new povidone-iodine swabstick. This time start at the puncture site and in a circular motion "paint" the area, moving outward without going over any area more than once. Allow the site to air dry.

   Going over the site more than once increases the risk of extraneous contamination. Povidone-iodine is only an effective antiseptic if it is allowed to air dry. If the patient is allergic to iodine, 70% isopropyl alcohol must be used.

7. While the site is drying, clean the tops of the blood culture bottles with a third povidone-iodine swabstick. Use one side of the swab for one bottle and the other side of the swab for the other bottle. Lay clean alcohol prep pads on top of each bottle until ready to use.

   The alcohol pads reduce the risk of contamination by extraneous microorganisms. Bottles that are covered by a protective plastic cap from the manufacturer, may be prepared in the following manner: Break the seal of the plastic cap, remove, clean the top of the bottle with an alcohol prep pad, and leave in place.

8. Prepare venipuncture equipment as required for method selected (i.e., syringe, butterfly infusion set, evacuated tube equipment).

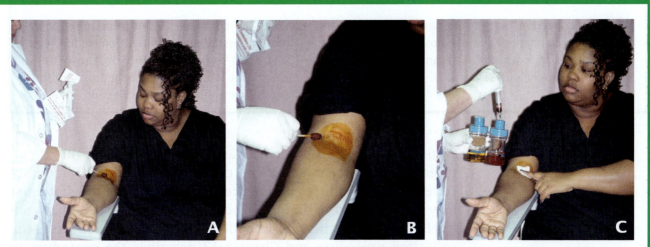

FIGURE 12-7: (A) Cleansing antecubital space with povidone-iodine in preparation of blood culture collection; (B) Second cleansing in concentric circles; (C) Evacuation of blood specimen from syringe into aerobic and anaerobic blood culture bottles

9. Reapply tourniquet.

   Take care not to touch the prepped collection site. If this occurs, then the process must begin again.

10. Perform the venipuncture.

11. Before introduction of blood into the culture bottle, wipe the top with an alcohol prep pad to remove any residual povidone-iodine.

    If povidone-iodine is introduced into the specimen bottle it will inhibit the growth of microorganisms.

12. When using the specially designed collection bottles that fit directly into the evacuated tube holder, keep the culture bottles lower than the collection site to prevent back flow. This prevents the culture media from contacting the stopper or needle during the collection process and contaminating the patient's blood.

13. Mix the container after removing it from the needle holder. After both containers have been filled, remove the needle from the patient's arm and hold pressure over the site.

The blood must be mixed gently with the nutrient broth to promote the growth of microorganisms.

14. When the syringe method is used, blood must be transferred to the culture bottles after the draw is complete. Changing needles on the syringe is no longer necessary prior to introduction of blood into the culture bottle. It has been determined that using the needle that was in the patient's arm does not reduce the risk of extraneous contamination. It does, however, increase the risk of accidental contaminated needlestick injury to the phlebotomist. When introducing blood into the culture bottle, direct the flow of blood to the side of the bottle. Allow the vacuum of the container to fill the bottle and never push on the plunger of the syringe to expel the blood into the bottle.

Pushing on the plunger can hemolyze the specimen and cause aerosol formation when the needle is removed from the stopper.

(continues)

P r o c e d u r e 1 2 - 2 *(continued)*

15. After collection procedures have been completed, clean the residual povidone-iodine from the patient's skin with an alcohol prep pad and apply a dressing.

16. Label the containers with the required information, including the site of collection (e.g., left arm) and depending on the orders, which set it is: 1st set collection, 2nd site set, or same site $1/2$-hour collection.

setting, nursing staff or medical assistants both collect throat cultures. In a hospital environment, the nursing staff most frequently collects throat cultures on inpatients. However, the phlebotomist may also be asked to do the collection on inpatients and may routinely do the collection on outpatients. This chapter addresses the collection procedure and Chapter 13 describes the procedure to perform the CLIA-waived strep test.

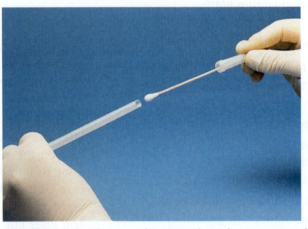

FIGURE 12-8: Throat culture swab and transport tube

Fecal (Stool) Specimens

Fecal specimens are examined to help evaluate gastrointestinal disorders and conditions. Specimens are evaluated for the presence of intestinal parasites and their eggs (Ova and Parasite, O&P), occult (hidden) blood (guaiac test), fat, and urobilinogen content. It can also be cultured to determine the presence of enteric bacteria such as *Salmonella*, *Shigella*, *Staphylococcus aureus*, or enteric viruses.

Fecal specimens are collected in clean, dry containers and must be kept at body temperature, especially those to be used for parasite testing. Special containers, containing a preservative for O&P collections, are provided to the patient. Patients requested to provide a 24, 48, or 72-hour stool collection for the determinations of

Procedure 12-3

Throat Culture Collection

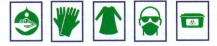

Equipment/Supplies

- Personal protective equipment
- Throat culture kit containing a sterile polyester-tipped swab; plastic transport tube containing transport media (Figure 12-8)
- Tongue depressor
- Pen light or small flashlight (optional)

Method/*Rationale*

1. Gather equipment and supplies.

   Ensures everything is available to perform the procedure.

2. Identify the patient.

   Ensures the procedure is performed on the correct patient.

3. Wash hands/don personal protective equipment.

   Thorough handwashing aids in controlling the spread of infection. Remember, you must comply with Standard Precautions whenever you may come in contact with a body fluid.

4. With the patient seated, instruct the patient to open his or her mouth wide and tilt the head back.

   Allows for visualization of the throat. A small flashlight may be used to further illuminate the back of the throat. A tongue depressor may be used to depress the tongue. Asking the patient to say "aah" depresses the tongue as well.

5. Brush the sterile swab over the back of throat. Both tonsils (if present), any areas with **exudation**, ulcerations, or inflammation should also be swabbed.

   Care should be taken to avoid brushing the tongue or lips with the sterile swab, as this will contaminate the specimen.

   EXUDATION

   Pathological oozing of fluids, usually the result of inflammation.

6. This procedure may cause the patient to gag and cough. Either wear a protective mask or stand off to the side of the patient to prevent the patient from contaminating you.

   This procedure should be completed in an efficient and timely manner to prevent discomfort to the patient.

7. Once the specimen has been collected, place the swab into the plastic transport tube. Break the ampule in the bottom of the tube by squeezing with the thumb and first finger to release the transport medium.

8. Label the specimen and transport to the lab immediately.

fat and urobilinogen content are provided with large gallon containers resembling paint cans. These types of specimens must be kept refrigerated throughout the collection period.

Guaiac test cards used to determine occult blood are given to outpatients to collect stool specimens at home. The patient is typically instructed to eat a meat-free diet for 3 days prior to collecting of the specimen. Patients are then instructed to collect specimens for 3 consecutive days. Cards can either be mailed or delivered to the lab after the collection.

Semen Specimens

A patient may be requested to provide a semen sample for the determination of fertility, the effectiveness of a sterilization procedure (vasectomy), or criminal investigation of sexual assault. The specimen may be collected in a sterile urine container. Semen specimens are never to be collected in a condom. Condoms often contain spermicides which will kill living sperm and render the test invalid. Semen specimens are to be kept warm and delivered to the lab immediately.

Gastrointestinal Secretions, Amniotic Fluid, Cerebrospinal Fluid, and Nasopharyngeal Specimens

These procedures are performed by a physician. The phlebotomist's role in the collection of these specimens is to label the specimen and transport it to the laboratory.

The gastrointestinal analysis test is performed to determine the function of gastric secretions in terms of acid production. These secretions are aspirated by passing a tube through the mouth or nose through the throat and into the stomach.

Amniotic fluid surrounds a fetus in utero. It is normally a clear, pale yellow fluid that is aspirated by inserting a needle through the abdominal wall of the mother into the uterus. A physician performs this procedure to determine fetal abnormalities that can be detected through chromosomal analysis and chemical tests at approximately 16 weeks gestation. This specimen is to be protected from light and extremes in temperature fluctuations and must be delivered to the laboratory ASAP.

Cerebrospinal fluid (CSF) is a clear, colorless liquid that circulates in the cavities of the brain and spinal cord. The constituents of CSF closely resemble those of blood plasma. To obtain a sample of CSF, the physician must insert a needle into the lumbar spine. The fluid is generally collected in three sterile containers numbered in the order in which they are collected. As the first tube is usually contaminated with blood, the second and third tubes are the specimens used for analysis. Tests might include total protein level, glucose level, cell count, microbiologic evaluations, or chloride levels. CSF must be transported immediately to the laboratory.

Nasopharyngeal (NP) cultures are collected to determine the presence of microorganisms that cause diphtheria, meningitis, pertussis, and pneumonia. NP specimens are collected using a sterile Dacron or cotton-tipped flexible wire swab which is inserted into the nasopharynx and gently rotated. Once removed from the NP cavity, the swab is placed in transport media and transported to the lab.

Urine

Urine specimens provide the physician with a valuable diagnostic tool. The physician can make several determinations of the patient's health status based on this nonblood specimen from urinary tract infections to metabolic disorders such as diabetes. Urine specimens collected from a patient at any time throughout the day are called random specimens. Specimens can also be collected at specifically ordered times of the day, such as a first morning specimen. The first morning specimen is often favored because the urine is at its highest concentration as it has been "incubating" in the bladder while the patient has been sleeping. Although nursing staff typically collect specimens from inpatients, the phlebotomist working with outpatients is required to instruct patients on the procedure for urine collection. Instructions are generally given verbally by the phlebotomist but should also be given to the patient in writing, preferably with illustrations. In an outpatient setting, the instructions may be printed on a chart that is posted in the laboratory's bathroom facilities. The phlebotomist must present this information in a concise and tactful manner, as the discussion has the potential to be embarrassing for the patient.

Correct urine collection procedures are essential to the integrity of the specimen. The properties of the specimen can be greatly altered if the collection process is not followed as ordered. Types of urine specimens refer to the time the specimen is collected (i.e., random, fasting, first morning) while the collection method refers to how the specimen is collected (i.e., clean-catch, midstream, regular voided).

ANALYTE

A substance being analyzed, especially the method of chemical analysis.

SPECIFIC GRAVITY

The weight of a substance compared with the weight of an equal volume of water. The specific gravity of water is 1.000.

VOID

To evacuate the bowels or bladder.

Types of Urine Specimens

● Random: Urine can be collected at any time. Random specimens are used for routine urinalysis (UA) and for screening tests.

● First morning: The specimen is collected immediately after the patient wakes, either first thing in the morning or after approximately 8 hours of sleep. This type of specimen has a higher concentration of **analytes**, with a higher **specific gravity**. First morning specimens are requested for routine urinalysis, confirmation of random test results, or when higher concentrations of analytes are required, such as for pregnancy testing, protein, nitrites, and microscope evaluations.

● Timed collections (e.g., 2-hour, 4-hour, 24-hour): Some tests require that the patient **void** at specific time intervals, such as when an excretion rate of an analyte is to be measured. Tolerance testing, like the glucose tolerance test (GTT), requires the patient to provide urine specimens at regular intervals that correspond to blood collection intervals, such as fasting $\frac{1}{2}$ hour, 1 hour, and so forth. The timing of these collections is critical for accurate determination of disorders. The specimens must be collected as closely as possible to the required time, and each specimen is labeled clearly with the time of the collection and the type of specimen (e.g., clean-catch, fasting, $\frac{1}{2}$-hour).

● 24-hour collections: This is also a timed collection but warrants a separate discussion. 24-hour collections are requested when a quantitative analysis of an analyte is needed. All urine voided within a 24-hour period is collected. The patient starts by voiding the first morning specimen of the first day into the toilet as usual, noting the time and date on the specimen container. Every specimen thereafter, including the first morning specimen of the second day, is collected. The patient must avoid contaminating the specimen with fecal matter by urinating first, transferring the urine into the collection container, and then proceeding with a bowel movement. Generally the specimen is refrigerated unless the specimen is being collected for urate testing. Refrigeration can be accomplished by placing the collection container in an ice chest. Urine specimens must *not* be placed in a refrigerator used to contain food. Specimens not refrigerated require the use of a preservative that can be added to the specimen collection container.

Special containers are used for the collection of 24-hour collections. Patients are provided with a special device that fits over the toilet and resembles an upside-down hat. This means of collecting the specimen is much easier for the patient when quantities are required. The toilet hat has graduated markings that can measure output amounts as well. Along with the required patient identification information, the specimen must be labeled as a 24-hour collection, the time the collection started and the date, and if applicable, the preservative that was added.

● Fractional or double void specimen: This type of specimen is used to compare concentrations of analytes, such as glucose and ketones. The patient first collects a urine specimen, emptying the bladder completely. The time is recorded and the specimen is tested for the analyte. The patient is then requested to drink approximately 200 mL of water. The patient waits a required amount of time (typically a half-hour) while the urine has time to accumulate in the bladder. The patient then collects another urine specimen, which is tested for the analyte, and the results are compared. Most tolerance tests are fractional specimens.

Collection Methods

● Regular void: There is no special patient preparation. The urine is simply collected in a clean, wide-mouthed container.

● Midstream: This method is used to ensure that the urinary opening is free from contaminates, such as genital secretions, pubic hair, and bacteria. The patient is instructed to void the initial flow into the toilet; the flow is then momentarily stopped, the specimen is collected, and the remainder of the urine is voided into the toilet.

● Midstream clean-catch: A clean-catch specimen (Figure 12-9) allows for a specimen that is free from contaminates from the external genitalia. This type of specimen is requested when microbial analysis or culture and sensitivity testing is to be done. This specimen is collected in a sterile container. Special cleaning procedures must be explained to the patient by the phlebotomist or given in writing. The procedure varies between male and female patients.

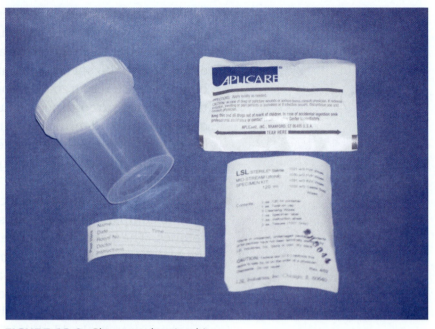

FIGURE 12-9: Clean-catch urine kit

Box 12-3: Clean-Catch Collection Procedure—Female Patient

● Stand in a squatting position over the toilet.
● Open three prepackaged Towelettes or prepare a sterile 2 × 2 gauze pad with soapy water.
● Separate the folds of the skin around the urinary opening.
● With one towelette, cleanse from front to back, wiping once down the right side; with the second towelette follow the same procedure front to back on the left side. With the third towelette wipe from front to back down the center.
● Void the first portion of urine into the toilet (midstream). Stop the flow and void the next portion of urine into a sterile collection cup, making sure that the inside or lip of the cup does not touch any part of the body including the hands.
● Void the remainder of urine into the toilet.
● Cover the specimen with the lid provided, touching only the outside surfaces of the lid and container.
● Wipe excess urine from the outside of the container.
● Wash hands.

Box 12-4: Clean-Catch Collection Procedure—Male Patient

- Wash hands thoroughly.
- Cleanse the end of the penis with special Towelettes or sterile, soapy 2 × 2 gauze pad beginning at the urethral opening and working away from it. (Patients who are not circumcised must retract the foreskin prior to cleaning.)
- Repeat the cleansing process twice more with new Towelettes.
- Void the first portion of urine into the toilet. Stop the urine flow, then resume the flow into the sterile collection container, being careful not to touch the lip or inside of the container with the hands or any other part of the body.
- Void the remainder of urine into the toilet.
- Cover the specimen with the lid provided, touching only the outside surfaces of the lid and container.
- Wash hands.

CATHETERIZATION

Use or passage of a catheter into a part, chamber, or cavity.

SUPRAPUBIC

Located above the pubic arch.

- **Catheterization**: A catheterized specimen is collected by inserting a sterile catheter through the patient's urethra into the bladder. This specimen is collected when a patient is having trouble voiding, is already catheterized, or when analysis must be done on the urine directly from the bladder, which is free from urethral and external genitalia contaminates.
- **Suprapubic**: A suprapubic specimen is collected in a sterile syringe by inserting the needle directly into the bladder and aspirating urine. This procedure is performed by a physician, typically with the use of a local anesthetic. The urine, once collected, is transferred into a sterile container or tube. This type of specimen is collected for evaluation of microbial analysis or cytology studies. This type of collection is sometimes performed on infants and small children to obtain an uncontaminated sample.
- Pediatric specimens: Young children and infants present a special challenge when a urine specimen is requested. A specially designed plastic urine collection bag with hypoallergenic skin adhesive is used. The patient's genital area is cleaned and dried. The bag is then placed around the urethral opening of a female or over the penis of a male. A diaper is then placed over the collection bag. The patient is checked every 15 minutes until an adequate specimen has been collected. The bag is removed, sealed, labeled, and then sent to the laboratory as soon as possible. 24-hour specimens can be collected in the same manner by using a bag with a tube attached that allows for periodic drainage of the specimen into a collection container.

A complete urinalysis includes physical, chemical, and microscopic examination of the specimen. The phlebotomist may be responsible for not only collecting the specimen, but for the physical and chemical examination. Examination techniques are described in Chapter 13.

BLOOD DONOR COLLECTIONS

BLOOD BANKING

The process of collecting whole blood and certain derived components for processing, typing, and storing until needed for transfusion.

There are several specific requirements the phlebotomist must follow when performing **blood-banking** procedures. Almost every blood bank test requires a large, plain, red top evacuated tube or a large, lavender top EDTA evacuated tube. Identification of the patient and the labeling of the specimen must be completed with the utmost care. The laboratory will reject specimens that are mislabeled or incomplete.

Blood bank specimens require the following information:
● Patient's full name, including middle initial
● Patient's hospital identification number or social security number if an outpatient
● Patient's date of birth
● Date and time of collection
● Phlebotomist's initials
● Room number and bed number (optional)

One of the most common blood-banking tests performed is a Type and Crossmatch. Blood type and crossmatch is performed to determine the compatibility of blood to be used for a transfusion. As discussed in Chapter 3, every patient has a particular blood type and may only receive blood from a donor with a compatible blood type. If blood that is transfused is incompatible, it could prove fatal because of agglutination (clumping) or lysing of red blood cells. Therefore, whenever there is a chance that a blood transfusion might be required, a type and crossmatch must be completed using strict identification and labeling guidelines.

Box 12-5: Blood Transfusions

Blood transfusion is the procedure of introducing the blood of a donor or blood predonated by the recipient (autologous transfusion) into the bloodstream. It is a highly effective form of therapy and has saved the lives of incalculable numbers of people suffering from shock, hemorrhage, or blood diseases. Blood transfusions are employed routinely in cases of surgery, trauma, gastrointestinal bleeding, and in childbirths involving great loss of blood.

In the 17th century, the French physician Jean Baptiste Denis performed the first recorded transfusion by infusing sheep's blood into a human. Later, most attempts were unsuccessful. Even when human blood was used, the majority of recipients died because of blood incompatibility. With the discovery of the major blood groups and the introduction of blood typing in the 20th century, transfusion became routinely successful.

Transfusions still tend to cause the development of sensitivity and increase the possibility that the recipient will react to later transfusions. Transmission of viral hepatitis was a major risk until a method of screening blood for infectivity was developed in the 1960s; some other forms of hepatitis, however, were not detected by this test. In 1985 a test was introduced to screen donated blood for an antigen associated with AIDS.

For most of the 20th century, transfusion was accomplished with whole blood. Methods of separating blood into its components were devised during the 1960s. Between 1970 and 1980, the use of these blood components became more frequent than the use of whole blood. Replacement with packed red blood cells (concentrated blood cells that have been separated from the blood plasma) is now the preferred treatment for most blood loss caused by injury or surgery.

Hospitals use blood that has been collected earlier and stored in blood banks. The use of stored blood began during World War I (1914–1918), but the first large-scale blood bank was not created until 1937 in Chicago. Many health care centers now maintain their own blood banks.

"Blood Transfusion," Microsoft® Encarta® Online Encyclopedia 2000.

http://encarta.msn.com © Microsoft Corporation. All rights reserved.

Collecting blood from a volunteer blood donor requires a properly trained health care individual, such as a certified phlebotomist, laboratory technologist, or nurse. Blood donor collections are performed as a division of blood-banking procedures and may be a part of a regional blood bank or hospital. All blood donor facilities must follow the guidelines of the American Association of Blood Banks (AABB).

Blood donor collections require the donor to meet certain criteria. The individual must be at least 17 years of age (some states permit younger persons to donate with permission of a parent or guardian), be in generally good health, and weigh at least 110 pounds. Most blood banks do not have upper age limits. All donors must pass the physical and health history examination given prior to donation. The physical includes checking the blood pressure, pulse, and temperature. A few drops of blood are taken from a capillary puncture to ensure that anemia is not present. Abnormalities found in any part of the physical examination may be a cause for deferral. The health history includes questions that are designed to protect the health of both the donor and the recipient. To ensure that every donor is asked the same questions, the AABB recommends use of a uniform donor history questionnaire. However, donor centers often create their own questionnaires using the same general guidelines. In addition to questions about transfusion-transmissible diseases, prospective donors are asked questions to determine whether donating blood might endanger their health. If a prospective donor responds positively to any of these questions, he or she will be deferred or asked not to donate. The health history and physical are required every time a person donates, regardless of how many previous times they have donated. All donor information is kept confidential. The donor is also required to sign a release, giving permission for his or her blood to be used.

Once the prospective donor has successfully passed the physical and health history, the actual collection can take place. The collection process takes approximately 20 minutes. The donor sits in a recumbent position or lies down. **Donor units** are typically collected from a large antecubital vein and are selected in the same manner as for routine venipuncture. The antecubital area is cleaned in a two-step cleaning procedure with alcohol and povidone-iodine in much the same way as for blood cultures. A blood pressure cuff or a tourniquet may be used. Typically a tourniquet is used for regular blood draws, and a blood pressure cuff pumped to 120 mm Hg is used for blood donations. Equipment and supplies are gathered and assembled. The collection unit is a sterile, closed system consisting of a bag containing an anticoagulant to collect the blood, connected to a length of tubing to a sterile needle. The needle most commonly used is 16 gauge and coated with an anticoagulant. The donor is asked to make a fist around a small ball and periodically squeeze his hand to help blood flow from the vein into the collection bag. Typically one unit of blood is collected, which is approximately the equivalent of one pint. As blood fills the bag by the pull of gravity, the bag must be placed lower than the patient's arm. The bag is placed on a mixing device, or "rocker." Only one puncture is allowed to fill a bag. If the bag does not fill completely and another puncture must be performed, the procedure must be repeated completely using a new collection unit. It takes approximately 7 minutes to fill a bag. After the collection is completed, the blood pressure cuff is released, the needle is removed, and pressure is applied over the puncture site until the puncture site has stopped bleeding. A pressure dressing is applied, and the donor is returned to a full-

DONOR UNIT

A specific amount of blood, approximately 1 pint, supplied by a volunteer as part of a blood-banking procedure.

sitting position. If the donor feels faint or light-headed, he is returned to a recumbent position. If the donor feels fine, he is offered a light refreshment such as juice and cookies and escorted to an observation area where he can rest for a few minutes. The collected blood is sent to the laboratory for testing and component preparation.

Autologous Blood Donation

Autologous transfusions refers to those transfusions in which the blood donor and transfusion recipient are the same. In other words, a person donates blood for his or her own use. This may be done prior to elective surgeries or when an anticipated transfusion will be required. A person may donate one unit of blood each week for up to 6 weeks before surgery. Blood can be stored in its liquid form for up to 42 days. Preoperative autologous donations may not be made within 72 hours of surgery. Using one's own blood for transfusion eliminates numerous risks associated with donor transfusions, such as disease transmission and incompatibilities. If the blood is not required for transfusion, it may be used for the general population with the donor's permission.

Intraoperative Blood Collection

In an intraoperative blood collection, blood lost by the patient during surgery is recovered and recycled throughout the surgery. Most intraoperative blood collection programs use machines in which shed blood is collected and the red blood cells are concentrated and washed prior to transfusion. This procedure is widely used for surgical procedures, such as cardiac, vascular, orthopedic, urologic, trauma, gynecologic, and transplant surgery. In these surgeries, the anticipated blood loss is 20% or more of the patient's estimated blood volume and there is no contamination of the area by bacteria or cancer cells. This procedure is generally not used in cancer surgery or surgery of the lower gastrointestinal tract.

● SPECIAL SITUATIONS

Advanced training is required for the following blood collections. Many hospitals permit only the nursing staff to perform blood collection from indwelling catheters. However, it is important that the phlebotomist be familiar with these procedures as they may be required to assist or have the opportunity for further on-site training.

AUTOLOGOUS TRANSFUSION
Transfusion of blood donated by a patient before surgery or collected from a patient during surgery.

Indwelling Catheters

Indwelling catheters are also called **vascular access devices (VADs)**. Drawing blood specimens from VADs requires special techniques, special training, and experience. VADs consist mainly of tubing inserted into a main artery or vein (Figure 12-10). This main vein or artery is customarily the subclavian, which is located in the chest below the clavicle. VADs are most generally inserted for administering fluids and medications, monitoring pressures, and drawing blood. A patient who is severely burned or terminally ill often has an indwelling catheter implanted to provide access for medications and blood draws.

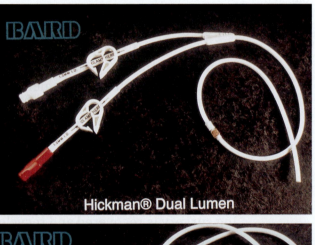

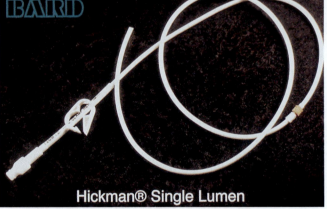

FIGURE 12-10: Hickman® Catheter (Photo provided by Bard Access Systems. Hickman is a registered trademark of Bard Access Systems.)

CENTRAL VENOUS CATHETER (CVC)

A catheter inserted into the superior vena cava to permit intermittent or continuous monitoring of central venous pressure and to facilitate collecting blood samples for chemical analysis.

PERIPHERALLY INSERTED CENTRAL CATHETER (PICC)

Catheter inserted into the peripheral venous system (veins of an extremity) and then threaded into the central venous system.

ARTERIAL LINE

A hemodynamic monitoring system consisting of a catheter in an artery connected to pressure tubing, a transducer, and an electronic monitor. It is used to measure systemic blood pressure and to provide ease of access for the drawing of blood for study of gases present.

Types of VADs

- **Central venous catheters (CVCs)** or central venous lines are inserted into a large vein such as the subclavian and advanced into the superior vena cava, proximal to the right atrium. Several inches of tubing protrude from the exit site, and are normally covered by a transparent dressing.

- **Peripherally inserted central catheters (PICCs)** are inserted into the peripheral venous system (veins of an extremity) and are then threaded into the central venous system (main veins leading to the heart). PICCs do not require surgical insertion and are most commonly placed into the basilic or cephalic vein with the exit in the antecubital space. PICCs tend to collapse on aspiration; drawing blood from a PICC is not recommended.

- Implanted port is a small chamber that is attached to an indwelling line. It is surgically implanted under the skin. The device can be located by palpating the skin. A special noncoring needle is inserted into the self-sealing septum of the chamber. The site is not normally covered with a bandage.

- An **arterial line** is most commonly located in the radial artery and is used to provide continuous monitoring of a patient's blood pressure. It can also be used for the collection of arterial blood gases.

- Heparin or saline locks are special winged needle sets or cannulas that can be left in a patient's vein for up to 48 hours (Figure 12-11). They are typically inserted into the lower arm above the wrist and are used to administer medication or to draw blood. Because a heparin lock is periodically flushed with heparin or saline to keep it from clotting, a 5 mL tube is drawn and discarded prior to collection of a specimen when drawing blood from a heparin lock. Coagulation studies are not to be drawn from a heparin or saline lock.

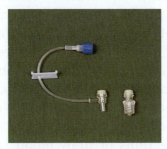

FIGURE 12-11: Heparin-locking device

● Arteriovenous (AV) shunts are an artificially created connection between a vein and an artery. They are typically created to provide access for dialysis. Venipuncture or blood pressures are not to be performed on an arm with an AV shunt.

● An external AV shunt or cannula is a temporary external connection between a vein and artery used for dialysis and for drawing blood. The tubing of the cannula extends to the outside surface of the arm and is capped by a small rubber diaphragm in which a needle can be inserted and blood drawn. Drawing blood through a cannula must be performed by specially trained professionals and may be performed only with permission from the patient's physician.

● An internal AV shunt or fistula is created by a surgical procedure, which permanently fuses a vein and artery together. The connection is made close to the surface of the skin and it can easily be seen and felt. It is used for dialysis and should never be used for phlebotomy. Blood specimens must be drawn from the patient's other arm or other acceptable location.

● SUMMARY

There are many variables that play an important role in the collection of blood and nonblood specimens. The phlebotomist must take into consideration each patient's individual needs. When performing the collection of a specimen the phlebotomist must work within the parameters of existing situations, whether the patient is an infant, child, or adult.

Performing specialized phlebotomy techniques requires the phlebotomist to have a thorough understanding of skills beyond those of routine blood drawing. For example, if arterial blood gases are performed incorrectly, they can be very painful and may cause severe damage of an artery. Collection of blood cultures can provide the physician with valuable information regarding the progress of the patient and the effectiveness of antibiotic therapy, but only if the collection procedure is performed and documented correctly. Although the phlebotomist may transport some nonblood specimens to the laboratory, he or she may be requested to collect other nonblood specimens and perform CLIA-waived tests. The phlebotomist may have the opportunity to perform donor blood collections or draw blood specimens from vascular access devices. In performing any of these specialized phlebotomy techniques, the phlebotomist must perform these skills with confidence and ease. Confidence is acquired through a solid knowledge base and practice through repetition.

● COMPETENCY CHECK-OFF SHEETS
Arterial Blood Gas Collection Competency Check

Given all the equipment and supplies, the student will be required to perform, within 10 minutes, an arterial blood gas collection on a mannequin arm. A "0" in more than two areas or an overall score of less than 80% will require the procedure to be repeated for competency.

Points to Be Awarded:	5 pts	2.5 pts	1 pt	0 pts	total pts
1 Assemble and prepare equipment and supplies					
2 Identify the patient					
3 Explain the procedure					
4 Wash hands/don PPE					
5 Obtain and record TPR and breathing mixture					
6 Open ABG kit or prepare syringe with heparin					
7 Prepare anesthesia					
8 Assess collateral circulation					
9 Position patient					
10 Locate radial artery					
11 Prepare/clean site					
12 Relocate artery					
13 Warm patient prior to stick					
14 Perform the puncture					
15 Apply direct pressure for 5 minutes					
16 Expel air bubbles from syringe					
17 Insert needle into latex cube					
18 Mix specimen					
19 After 5 minutes check puncture site					
20 Apply pressure dressing					
21 Dispose of used equipment and supplies					

Points to Be Awarded:	5 pts	2.5 pts	1 pt	0 pts	total pts
22 Label specimen					
23 Remove gloves					
24 Wash hands					
25 Transport specimen to lab					

Total Points Possible: _____ Total Points Earned: _____

Start Time: _____ End Time: _____

Instructor Signature: _____ Date: _____

Student Signature: _____ Date: _____

Collection of Blood Cultures Competency Check

Given all the equipment and supplies, the student will be required to perform, within 10 minutes, a blood culture collection on a classmate/patient. A "0" in more than two areas or an overall score of less than 80% will require the procedure to be repeated for competency.

Points to Be Awarded:	5 pts	2.5 pts	1 pt	0 pts	total pts
1 Assemble and prepare equipment and supplies					
2 Identify the patient					
3 Explain the procedure					
4 Wash hands/don PPE					
5 Select venipuncture site					
6 Clean site with alcohol					
7 Scrub site with povidone-iodine for 2 minutes					
8 Clean site 2nd time with povidone-iodine					
9 Clean tops of collection bottles					
10 Prepare venipuncture equipment					
11 Apply tourniquet					
12 Perform puncture					
13 Remove needle; apply direct pressure					
14 Mix specimens					
15 Clean residual povidone-iodine from site					
16 Dispose of any contaminated materials					
17 Remove gloves					
18 Wash hands					
19 Transport specimen to lab					

Total Points Possible: _____ Total Points Earned: _____

Start Time: _____ End Time: _____

Instructor Signature: _____ Date: _____

Student Signature: _____ Date: _____

STUDY AND REVIEW EXERCISES

Defining Key Terms

Write the definition for each of the following key terms.

1) acid-base balance _____

2) aerobic_____

3) anaerobic _____

4) analyte_____

5) arterial blood gases _____

7) arterial line _____

6) arteriospasm_____

8) autologous transfusion_____

9) bacteriemia _____

10) blood banking_____

11) catheterization_____

12) central venous catheter _____

13) collateral circulation _____

14) donor unit _____

15) exudation _____

16) peripherally inserted central catheter (PICC)_____

_____

17) septicemia _____

18) specific gravity_____

19) suprapubic_____

20) vascular access device _____

21) void_____

22) wheal _____

Reviewing Key Points

1) Describe the procedure for assessing collateral circulation, the Allen test.

2) Describe two methods for restraining an infant.

3) List three reasons that the laboratory would reject an arterial blood gas specimen.

4) Describe how to collect a clean-catch urine specimen to a female patient.

5) List the equipment and supplies required for a blood culture collection.

Sentence Completion

1) Withdrawal of large quantities of blood over long periods of time can cause a pediatric patient to become _____.

2) A _____, with a 2 to 3 mL evacuated tube, typically provides the best results at an antecubital site of a pediatric patient.

3) _____ are performed to provide valuable information regarding the status of a patient's oxygenation, ventilation, and acid-base balance.

4) When performing an arterial blood collection, the patient's wrist should be flexed at approximately a _____ to _____ -degree angle.

5) When an artery has been effectively entered a _____ of blood will appear in the hub of the needle.

6) Patients who are on _____ have blood that has been "thinned," and therefore take longer for an arterial puncture site to form a clot and stop bleeding.

7) The most critical factor in collecting blood culture specimens is _____ of the patient's skin.

8) _____ are ordered by physicians to aid in the diagnosis of streptococcal infections of the throat.

9) _____ are used to determine if occult blood is in the stool.

10) One of the most common blood-banking tests performed is a _____.

Multiple Choice

1) Individuals donating blood must be at least _____ years old.
   A. 15
   B. 17
   C. 19
   D. 21

2) VADs are inserted for all the following reasons except:
   A. monitoring the patient's acid-base balance
   B. administering fluids and medications
   C. monitoring pressures
   D. drawing blood

3) A(n) _____ is inserted into a large vein such as the subclavian and advanced into the superior vena cava, proximal to the right atrium.
   A. PICC
   B. AV shunt
   C. CVC
   D. arterial line

4) A(n) _____ is a temporary connection between a vein and artery used for dialysis and for drawing blood.
   A. PICC
   B. external AV shunt
   C. arterial line
   D. CVC

5) The _____ are excellent sites for drawing labs on neonates and children under the age of 2.
   A. ankles
   B. antecubital veins
   C. wrists
   D. dorsal hand veins

6) _____ means that blood is supplied to an area by more than one artery.
   A. Collateral circulation
   B. Circulation stability
   C. Circumvented circulation
   D. Bilateral circulation

7) When performing an arterial blood gases collection, the site with the highest risk of infection is:
   A. radial
   B. brachial
   C. femoral
   D. umbilical

8) _____ should not be used for collection of ABGs because they alter the partial pressure of the gas in the blood sample.
   A. Syringes
   B. Butterfly infusion sets
   C. 22 gauge needles
   D. Evacuated tubes

9) A patient must be in a "steady state" for a minimum of _____ before collection of ABGs.
   A. 2 minutes
   B. 15 minutes
   C. 30 minutes
   D. 60 minutes

10) A blood culture bottle designed specifically for organisms that grow best when oxygen is not present is called a(n):
    A. aerobic bottle
    B. anaerobic bottle
    C. acid-base bottle
    D. broth media bottle

Critical Thinking

1) Your orders are to collect arterial blood gases from the patient in curtain three in the emergency room. The patient is comatose and collateral circulation cannot be determined in either wrist. Describe the collection process.

2) Nathan Taylor is an 8-week-old preemie in the NICU at the hospital where you are employed. Your orders are to collect a specimen for a CBC and urine culture. Nathan is critically ill and a PICC has been inserted. Although he is weak, he is also listless. Your hospital's protocol does not allow for a phlebotomist to draw from a PICC line. Describe the collection process.

Point-of-Care Testing and Other Laboratory Tests

OBJECTIVES

Upon completion of this chapter the student should be able to:

- Define and correctly spell each of the key terms.
- Define CLIA-waived laboratory tests.
- List primary regulatory agencies associated with waived laboratory tests.
- Describe the concepts of quality assurance, quality control, calibration, and range of values.
- Identify and describe the procedures, normal value ranges, and clinical indications for the following point-of-care testing procedures: hematocrit, hemoglobin, blood glucose, glucose tolerance test, cholesterol, activated coagulation time, prothrombin time, PTT, APPT, bleeding time, blood gases, electrolytes, BUN, fecal occult blood, pregnancy test, rapid strep test, and urinalysis.
- Describe the process employed for obtaining specimens for alcohol blood levels, forensic specimens, and drug testing.
- List and describe the procedure for following chain of custody.

OUTLINE

- History of Point-of-Care Testing
- Hematocrit
- Hemoglobin

(continues)

KEY TERMS
(continued)

hypokalemia
(**hi**-po-ka-**LEE**-me-ah)
intradermal
(**in**-tra-**DER**-mal)
ketonuria
(**kee**-to-**NUR**-ee-ah)
low-density lipoprotein
cholesterol (LDL)
occult (uh-**KULT**)
pCO$_2$
pH
point-of-care tests (POCT)
proteinuria
(**pro**-teen-**UR**-ee-ah)
prothrombin
renal calculi
sediment (**SED**-i-ment)
solute (**SOL**-yoot)
therapeutic (ther-a-**PU**-tik)
thromboplastin
(**throm**-boh-**PLAS**-tin)
transparency
turbidity (tur-**BID**-i-tee)

POINT-OF-CARE TESTS (POCTs)

Laboratory testing performed at the site of the patient, using portable or hand-held instruments.

- Blood Glucose
- Glucose Tolerance Test
- Cholesterol
- Coagulation Monitoring
- Bleeding Time
- Chemistry Panels
- Collection of Toxicology Specimens
- Therapeutic Drug Monitoring
- Paternity Testing
- Skin Tests
- Fecal Occult Blood Test
- Pregnancy Test
- Rapid Strep Test
- Urinalysis—Physical and Chemical Examination

HISTORY OF POINT-OF-CARE TESTING

With the creation in 1988 of the Clinical Laboratory Improvement Amendments (CLIA) and its implementation in 1993, the federal government exempted a group of clinical laboratory tests from the "universal" quality control requirements required by CLIA by establishing a category of tests called CLIA-waived tests. These tests were investigated by the Centers for Disease Control (CDC) and approved by the Health Care Financing Administration (HCFA) as procedures defined as "simple," requiring little laboratory expertise, involving no professional laboratory judgment, and that can be performed by a physician or health care professional under the supervision of a physician. These tests are then "waived" of the CLIA requirements in specific clinical settings. However, this does not mean that specific training is not required, and although the instruments are easy to use, manufacturer's guidelines and instructions must be explicitly followed. Quality control and quality assurance are just as essential for point-of-care tests as for any other laboratory procedure and are required of CLIA-certified laboratories. The phlebotomist has clearance by most hospital and laboratory standards to perform these CLIA-waived tests.

Because of the advances in technology that have made these tests portable, easy to operate, and accurate with reproducible results, the phlebotomist can perform these CLIA-waived tests at the patient's bedside, in the emergency room, or in ambulatory settings. These tests are referred to as **point-of-care tests (POCTs)**, as they are performed by the phlebotomist at the location of the patient. Point-of-care tests include: hematocrit, hemoglobin, blood glucose, blood gases, potassium, calcium, pH, sodium, blood urea nitrogen, prothrombin time, activated partial thromboplastin time, bleeding time, pregnancy tests, strep tests, and reagent strip urinalysis.

The phlebotomist may also collect specimens for various other tests that have been included in this chapter, such as drug testing, paternity testing, and therapeutic drug monitoring and toxicology studies.

It is important that the phlebotomist understands the quality control (QC) and quality assurance (QA) processes involved when performing point-of-care tests to ensure the accuracy of test results. Manufacturers of these portable, often hand-held devices include an instruction manual on how to operate the equipment as well as how to calibrate the instrument and how to perform QC procedures. The phlebotomist who performs POCT must comply exactly with the device's and QC requirements and maintain a log of when each procedure is performed and the test outcome.

Collecting a capillary specimen to perform a POCT is generally sufficient as the test requires only a minimal amount of blood. However, some of the special collections require that a venipuncture be performed. Remember to follow all Standard Precautions, patient identification, and documentation procedures.

Reference Value Range

Reference values are the normal values for laboratory tests, usually established using basal state specimens, and are determined for each POCT. These reference ranges have been established based on statistical findings of a representation of a population that has been tested. The statistic is based on a 95% finding; in other words, if 100 patients are tested 95 will have test values within the reference range. Tests with scores outside the reference range are abnormal. These range values allow for a physician to make a diagnosis with 95% accuracy.

Range values also affect quality control. Manufacturers of point-of-care instruments, knowing the reference ranges for each test, provide the laboratory a control specimen with known values. The phlebotomist performs a control "check" daily to ensure that when control specimens are analyzed they fall within the established range value. This control check is documented in a QC log book. If control specimens are not within the range, the equipment must be calibrated and/or recalibrated prior to testing of a patient specimen. Follow the manufacturer's guidelines to determine how often specific equipment must be calibrated.

Calibration of Equipment

Calibrating equipment is the process whereby the equipment is adjusted and realigned to operate within the normal value ranges. Calibration is accomplished by using a substance or device called a **calibrator**. The calibrator has a preloaded measurement or known concentration of the analyte being tested, which allows for the instrument to be adjusted to that value. The adjustment may be made by a manual operation, such as turning a dial or knob or tightening a screw. However, more modern POCT devices require the manufacturer or a specific repair facility to electronically or mechanically calibrate the equipment.

● HEMATOCRIT

The **hematocrit** (Hct) measures the volume of the patient's red blood cells as a percentage of whole blood in relationship to the plasma (Figures 13-1 through 13-4). The specimen is collected in a plastic microhematocrit tube. If the specimen is collected from a capillary puncture, the specimen is collected in a heparinized microhematocrit tube typically identified by a red band marked around the top of the tube. If the specimen is collected in an EDTA evacuated tube, a plain (containing no anticoagulant) microhematocrit tube, identified by a blue band marked on the tube, is used. The tube is filled a minimum of three-quarters full and must be free of air bubbles. One end of the tube is sealed with clay. Specially prepared clay trays are manufactured for this purpose. The microhematocrit tube is placed in the microhematocrit centrifuge with the clay end out (to the wall of the centrifuge). As the centrifuge must be balanced, two tubes are filled for each patient. The specimens are spun down for 5 minutes. Some microhematocrit centrifuges are equipped with built-in charts so the results can be read without removing the microhematocrit tubes. Separate laminated microhematocrit reader charts are also available to determine results if the centrifuge does not contain a chart. The top of the clay is lined up at the - 0 - line on the chart and the top of the plasma line is lined up with the top line of the chart. The result is determined by reading the line at which the red blood cells and buffy coat (white blood cells) separate. It is important to read and follow the instructions for whichever type of chart is used.

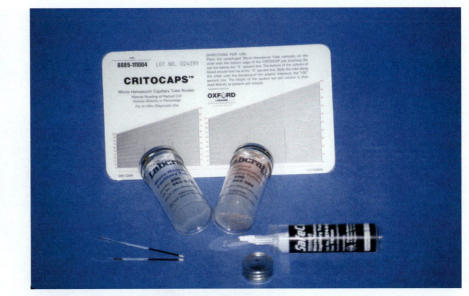

FIGURE 13-1: Microhematocrit tubes: heparinized and plain tubes (with hematocrit chart)

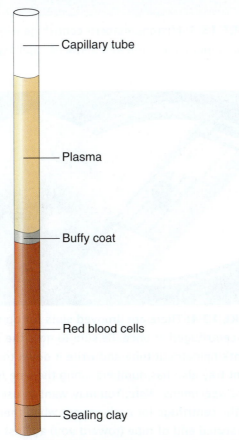

FIGURE 13-2: Diagram of packed cell column in the hematocrit showing separation of cellular components after centrifugation

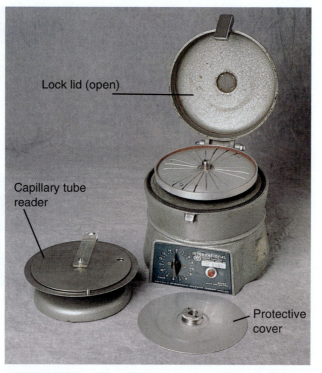

Lock lid (open)

Capillary tube reader

Protective cover

FIGURE 13-3: Microhematocrit centrifuge (right) with protective cover and lock lid (open) and a microhematocrit capillary tube reader (left)

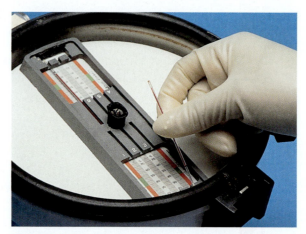

FIGURE 13-4: There are grooved slots for up to six microhematocrit tubes to be centrifuged at once. Be sure to note the space number for each patient's hematocrit tube and write it down to avoid confusion. The clay sealant tray also has numbers along the side to help you keep track of several specimens. *Note:* You may want to use the same number on the tray as in the centrifuge for each patient when there are two or more. Carefully place sealed end of tube (toward you) against the rubber padding in the microhematocrit centrifuge.

Hematocrits are ordered by the physician to aid in the diagnosis and monitoring of anemias and polycythemia.

Box 13-1: Reference Value Range—Hematocrit

Newborns	51–61%
1 Month	35–49%
6 Months	30–40%
1 Year	32–38%
6 Years	34–42%
Adult Males	42–52%
Adult Females	36–48%

HEMOGLOBIN

HEMOGLOBIN

The iron-containing protein pigment of the red blood cells, which carries oxygen from the lungs to the tissues.

Hemoglobin (Hgb) aids in the transportation of oxygen to all the cells of the body and the return of carbon dioxide to the lungs as a waste product to be expelled. Tests for hemoglobin levels are performed to aid in the diagnosis of anemias. Hemoglobin values vary with age, gender, and altitude. There are two basic devices used to measure hemoglobin. The Hb Meter Hemoglobinometer (Leica, Inc., Deerfield, IL) has been used for many years. This portable device consists of a base unit containing a light source and a graduated slide color scale and a special glass slide unit. The phlebotomist places a drop of blood on each side of the platformed slide. The drops of blood are then lysed by stirring vigorously with a hemolysis stick provided with the unit, thus releasing the hemoglobin contained within the red blood cells. The second slide is placed on top of the first slide and the unit is placed in the small metal clip. The clipped slides are then inserted into the slide chamber of the base unit. The light source button is depressed and the phlebotomist views the color scale by looking through the eyepiece. The slide knob on the side of the device is slowly adjusted until the two shades of green match. It is critical that the blood has been well mixed and that no air bubbles exist on the slide. The results are recorded by locating the number above the line on the slide knob. The second CLIA-waived procedure involves the use of a hand-held device called a HemoCue Hemoglobin System manufactured by HemoCue, Inc. (Figure 13-5). The test may be performed on venous, arterial, or capillary blood. The specimen is placed in a microcuvette specially designed for the system. The microcuvette is inserted into the machine and results are registered in the LED readout window of the machine. The results are recorded and the microcuvette is properly disposed of in a sharps container.

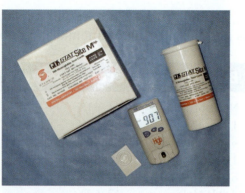

FIGURE 13-5: CLIA-waived hemoglobin testing equipment

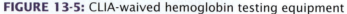

Box 13-2: Reference Value Range—Hemoglobin	
Adult Males	13.5–17.5 g/dL
Adult Females	12.5–15.5 g/dL
Early Childhood	10.0–14.0 g/dL
Newborn	16.0–23.0 g/dL

HYPERGLYCEMIC

Pertaining to the condition in which the blood sugar (glucose) is increased, as in diabetes mellitus.

HYPOGLYCEMIC

Pertaining to a condition in which the blood sugar (glucose) is abnormally low, as in hyperinsulinism.

FASTING BLOOD SUGAR (FBS)

The patient is required to restrict dietary intake for 12 hours prior to the collection of a specimen for testing for glucose levels in the blood.

2-HOUR POSTPRANDIAL (2-HOUR PP)

Collection of this specimen occurs 2 hours after the ingestion of the patient's last meal.

BLOOD GLUCOSE

Blood-glucose levels are most commonly performed to aid in diagnosis and management of diabetes mellitus in which patients are **hyperglycemic**. Blood-glucose testing also monitors **hypoglycemia**. It is one of the most frequently performed POCTs. Blood-glucose levels are routinely performed on whole blood from a capillary puncture, but some glucose monitor devices allow for anticoagulated venous blood specimens. Blood-glucose tests may be ordered stat or as a timed specimen. **Fasting blood sugar (FBS)** and **2-hour PP (postprandial)** are two types of timed requests. After a patient has ingested large amounts of carbohydrates it normally takes 2 hours for the patient's glucose levels to return to normal values. Glucose levels not performed at the designated times may lead to a misinterpretation of the results.

There are numerous manufacturers that produce glucose analyzers; they are relatively inexpensive and easy to use. The hand-held device is designed so patients may use the device at home. Most glucose analyzers require the use of a reagent strip, which must be kept in the airtight container in which they are packaged. The container may only be opened long enough to remove the reagent strip. Each reagent strip container is coded. The analyzer must be set to match the code of the container for all reagent strips in the container. This applies to the units that patients use at home, and must be part of the patient education process.

A capillary puncture is performed, the first drop of blood is wiped away, and the next drop of blood is placed on the reagent strip, which will either already have been inserted into the analyzer or which will now be inserted into the analyzer depending on the requirements of the analyzer used. The analyzer provides prompts through each step of the procedure. The analyzer determines the results and then displays them on the LCD readout screen. Some glucose analyzers use microcuvettes instead of reagent strips. The procedure is basically the same except that the microcuvette is filled with blood, rather than a drop of blood being placed on the reagent strip. The phlebotomist must perform the QC procedures prior to using the analyzer each day. A control reagent strip is provided by the manufacturer within each bottle of reagent strips. Follow the directions for performing the control procedure exactly. The procedure is the same as performing the test with the exception of adding a drop of blood to the reagent strip.

Some glucose analyzers have the capability to store multiple test results and compare one day's results with the previous day's results. Some devices are equipped with print capabilities.

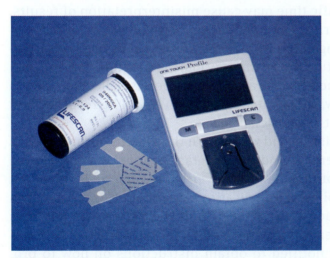 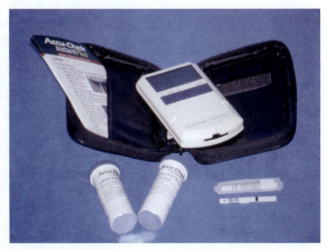

FIGURE 13-6: Blood glucose analyzers

Box 13-3: Reference Value Range—Blood Glucose	
Fasting glucose level	75–110 mg/dL

◗ GLUCOSE TOLERANCE TEST

GLUCOSE TOLERANCE TEST (GTT)

A test involving multiple collections of blood and urine over time to evaluate the metabolism of glucose. It is performed by giving the patient a measured amount of glucose either orally or intravenously.

The **glucose tolerance test (GTT)** is similar in nature to the 2-hour postprandial testing procedure. The major difference is that rather than ingesting a high-carbohydrate meal, the patient is given a commercially prepared glucose drink which consists of approximately 75 to 100 grams of glucose liquid for adults and about 1 gram per each kilogram of a child's weight. Occasionally a patient will not be able to tolerate this high concentration of glucose and may vomit. Contact the patient's nurse or physician for further instructions if this occurs. The test may need to be rescheduled for another time.

Glucose levels fluctuate normally throughout the day. A person with a healthy carbohydrate metabolism has blood glucose levels that return to the normal ranges of 65–110 mg/dL within 2 hours after ingesting high levels of carbohydrates or the glucose preparation. A diabetic patient, however, because of an inability to metabolize glucose, has glucose values that remain elevated over a longer period of time.

Timing of glucose tolerance testing is critical. Specimens not collected at a specific time may cause misinterpretation of results. Remember, it is normal for a patient's blood-glucose level to be elevated after the ingestion of a high-carbohydrate meal with glucose levels not returning to the normal parameters for approximately 2 hours. Therefore, if a GTT specimen is collected prior to this 2-hour window, an elevated glucose level will be recorded and misinterpreted by the physician.

The phlebotomist should verify with the patient or the patient's nurse that the patient has indeed been fasting for the required time period. The phlebotomist is also to verify that the patient has not taken any of the following medications or substances, as they can interfere with the accuracy of the GTT. If the patient has not been fasting or has taken any of the medications below, the patient's physician must be notified to obtain instructions on how to proceed. Typically the test is rescheduled for a time when the patient is in compliance.

- Salicylates
- Diuretics
- Alcohol
- Blood pressure medications
- Corticosteroids
- Anticonvulsive medications
- Estrogen or birth control pills

The exact procedure for glucose tolerance testing varies from institution to institution. However, each facility has specific procedures outlined in its procedure manual, so that testing is performed consistently within the same facility. The GTT procedure can vary in duration from 3 to 6 hours, with specimens being collected each half-hour or hour. Some facilities require a urine specimen to be collected at the same time as the blood specimen and a urine glucose reagent test performed.

Glucose tolerance testing can be performed on the same handheld devices as a fasting blood glucose or 2-hour postprandial test. More advanced devices can be used such as the ONE TOUCH® II Hospital Blood Glucose System (Lifespan, Inc., Milpitas, CA), which automatically stores QC data. The data are then linked via a laptop computer to the hospital's mainframe computer system, where the patient/client's permanent record is created and can be printed.

CHOLESTEROL

A recent importance has been placed on blood **cholesterol** levels. The medical community and the public have become increasingly concerned with HDL and LDL levels since the correlation between elevated cholesterol levels and heart disease was established. Cholesterol serves an important function as approximately 80% of cholesterol is used to manufacture bile acids that allow the body to digest lipids and fats. Cholesterol also functions in the production of hormones such as testosterone, progesterone, and estrogen and can be found in the skin in large amounts. Cholesterol located in the skin helps to keep the skin waterproof and aids in the prevention of evaporation of water from the body. Diet plays a very important part in cholesterol levels. Foods such as egg yolks, dairy products, and red meat are very high in cholesterol and, therefore, contribute to an increase in the cholesterol levels of individuals consuming large amounts of these foods. Increased cholesterol levels cause fats to deposit within the inner lining of the arteries, creating a condition known as **atherosclerosis**. As the fat is deposited, it narrows the lumen of the artery and causes the edges to be rough, which can result in blood clot formation. The artery may become so narrow that blood cannot circulate through, cutting off blood supply to vital organs. Blood clots may break off and cause a heart attack or stroke.

The overall cholesterol level has some diagnostic value. However, **high-density lipoprotein cholesterol (HDL)** and the **low-density lipoprotein cholesterol (LDL)** are much more diagnostic. HDL functions to transport the fat from the tissues to the

CHOLESTEROL
The most abundant steroid in animal tissues. It serves many functions in the body including manufacturing of bile acids that allows the body to digest lipids and fats. Some cholesterol is used to manufacture hormones such as testosterone, progesterone, and estrogen. Cholesterol is broken into two factions: high-density lipoprotein (HDL) and low-density lipoprotein (LDL). In most individuals, an elevated blood level of cholesterol constitutes an increased risk of developing coronary heart disease.

ATHEROSCLEROSIS
Pathologic condition in which fat deposits accumulate in the lining of the arteries.

HIGH-DENSITY LIPOPROTEIN CHOLESTEROL (HDL)
The "good" cholesterol.

LOW-DENSITY LIPOPROTEIN CHOLESTEROL (LDL)
The "bad" cholesterol.

liver to be metabolized into bile acids, and therefore is labeled the "good" cholesterol. LDL transports the cholesterol to the tissues, such as the lining of the arteries, where it is deposited as plaque, earning the term "bad" cholesterol.

There are a number of different waived cholesterol kits. The majority of these kits involve the use of a reagent strip imbedded with chemicals. The chemicals react similarly to the urine reagent strips in that the reaction to the chemicals involves the reagent strip changing colors, such as with the AccuChek™.

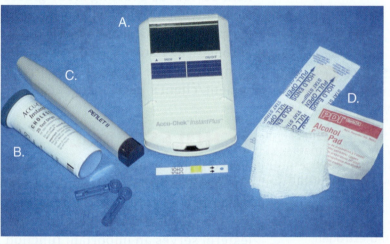

FIGURE 13-7: Supplies and equipment for cholesterol testing: (A) AccuChek™ Instant Plus; (B) Penlet lancet; (C) Cholesterol reagent strip; (D) Gauze, alcohol pad, and band aid

Another device that has gained in popularity because of its ability to not only determine blood cholesterol levels, but also HDL and LDL levels with a high degree of accuracy, is the Cholestech L.D.X.® Analyzer.

A cuvette or cassette is inserted into the analyzer in much the same way as glucose testing. The Cholestech L.D.X.® Analyzer is factory calibrated and the cassette is encoded with a magnetic strip, which is read by the analyzer, as each cassette is tested.

Quantitative controls are included in each type of cholesterol kit. Many of the kits must be stored in the refrigerator and warmed to room temperature before use. The following considerations must be observed to prevent possible errors in cholesterol testing:

● A fasting specimen is preferred.
● If using capillary blood, it must be free-flowing.
● If using venipuncture blood do not perform from tubes containing fluoride, oxalate, citrate, or EDTA as anticoagulants.

- Maximum and minimum values are determined for accuracy. For each type of cholesterol test, determine the limitations of the device used.
- Various substances can interfere with cholesterol testing. Read the accompanying literature of the test kit to determine what, if any, substance(s) interferes with the test results.
- Do not touch the reagent pads or pipette tips with fingers, gloved or ungloved.
- Quality Control measures must be performed with each run of client samples.
- Mix QC materials thoroughly by gentle inversion before testing.
- Do not use test kits or controls beyond the expiration dates.
- Capillary samples must be inserted into the cassette within 4 minutes of collection.

Box 13-4: Reference Value Ranges—Cholesterol

Desirable Cholesterol Level	<200 mg/dL
Borderline High Cholesterol	200–239 mg/dL
High Cholesterol Level	>200 mg/dL

COAGULATION MONITORING

HEMOSTASIS

An arrest of bleeding or of circulation. A stagnation of blood.

Coagulation tests provide information concerning the ability of the patient's blood to clot. **Hemostasis** is a critical factor when patients are being considered for surgical procedures or being treated for trauma, or for patient's with clotting disorders who are receiving coagulation therapy. The ability to provide coagulation results quickly is imperative in settings such as the emergency room, intensive care units, and operating rooms, and with dialysis patients. Coagulation testing is a convenient and reliable POCT, but the phlebotomist and laboratory personnel must take care during the processing of the specimen so as not to compromise the sample. Coagulation testing has a two-level quality control verification process in addition to a temperature control verification device. Coagulation studies must occur at 37.5° C to ensure accuracy of results.

There are several different types of hand-held instruments used for coagulation monitoring. Some devices use only a single drop of whole blood obtained from a capillary puncture while others use citrated blood obtained by venipuncture. Most of these devices provide results within 5 minutes. Coagulation monitoring includes ACT, PT, PTT, and APTT, which are addressed in the following sections.

Activated Coagulation Time (ACT)

ACT analyzes the activity of the intrinsic coagulation factors and is used to monitor heparin therapy. Heparin is an anticoagulant that is administered intravenously to minimize and control clotting. Heparin responds immediately but is difficult to control. Too much may cause uncontrollable bleeding and too little will not cause the desired response to prevent blood clots. Heparin therapy must be closely monitored and POCT provides the means to quickly and effectively do so. Once a patient's condition has stabilized, the patient may be placed on oral anticoagulant therapy such as warfarin (Coumadin), which is slower acting but easier to control. This can be monitored by the prothrombin test.

The ACT analysis is performed by collecting a small volume of blood in a prewarmed special gray top tube, containing a coagulation activator such as siliceous earth, silica, or celite. The phlebotomist assembles routine venipuncture equipment with the addition of a heat block or incubator, and a stopwatch or timer. A discard tube (red top) and a special gray top tube will be drawn.

To perform the ACT analysis:

- Perform a routine venipuncture and draw a 4 mL discard tube.
- Draw blood into the prewarmed tube containing the clot activator. Start the timer as soon as blood flows into the tube.
- When the vacuum in the tube is exhausted, mix the tube thoroughly and place in the heat block for 60 seconds. *Note:* Even though the gray top tube looks like all other evacuated tubes, it contains less vacuum. Draw only a small volume of blood, approximately 2 cc.
- After 60 seconds, rock the tube gently back and forth and visually inspect the blood for the first visible sign of a clot.
- If no clot is apparent, place the tube back into the heat block for 5 seconds. After 5 seconds remove from the block and inspect again.
- Repeat the procedure every 5 seconds until the first visible clot is observed. At the first sign of a clot, stop the timer and record the time.

There are a number of situations that can cause erroneous results. If the phlebotomist neglects to start the timer as soon as the blood enters the tube, values will be decreased. A traumatic draw or an inadequate sample will cause decreased values. If the tube is not mixed thoroughly the values will increase. Anticoagulant drugs, antibiotics, steroids, and barbiturates can also lead to erroneous results.

An automated version of the ACT test is available from the Hemochron system and is obtained from International Technidyne Corporation. With this system the machine does the mixing and timing automatically. A special tube with a black plastic cap provided by the manufacturer must be used.

Prothrombin Time (PT)

The PT procedure is often performed alone to monitor oral anticoagulation therapy (Coumadin) or is performed in conjunction with a PTT to give an accurate picture of the patient's total clotting abnormalities. Oral anticoagulants affect the synthesis of **prothrombin**, which is 1 of the 12 clotting factors produced by the liver. Clotting occurs naturally when trauma or injury to tissue releases tissue **thromboplastin**. Tissue thromboplastin, when combined with blood, activates the clotting mechanism. Prothrombin then converts to thrombin. Thrombin causes fibrinogen to form the fibrin matrix within the clot. Point-of-care testing with the Hemochron® Jr. device uses whole blood, and the PT normal values are 17 to 22 seconds. If PT is performed on plasma collected in sodium citrate tubes, the normal values are slightly less (11 to 13 seconds). It is important to read the manufacturer's literature for any POCT device as normal values may vary. Some devices compensate for using whole blood versus plasma. If using one of these devices, the normal value range for whole blood would be similar to plasma values.

Partial Thromboplastin Time (PTT) and Activated Partial Thromboplastin Time (APTT)

Either the PTT or the APTT is used to evaluate doses of heparin therapy. The procedure and results are similar; however, the "A" has been added to indicate that activation of a clotting factor has occurred to make the test more reproducible and sensitive. Values from whole blood differ from plasma values as with the PT procedure. Normal values for the PTT or APTT using plasma may be between 24 and 34 seconds, whereas whole blood values of 93 to 127 seconds are normal using the Hemochron® Jr. However, plasma-equivalent values are available based on statistical calculations. The CoaguChek™ is another POCT device that analyzes coagulation values.

Both devices are easy to operate and are portable. The Hemochron® Jr. requires approximately 50 units/L of whole blood be placed into a plastic cartridge. The CoaguChek™ requires less blood and uses programmed credit card–like cartridges that auto-

PROTHROMBIN

A plasma protein coagulation factor synthesized by the liver that is converted to thrombin in the presence of calcium ions.

THROMBOPLASTIN

The substance secreted by platelets when tissue is injured; necessary for blood clotting.

matically calibrate the device and correct for changes in the lot number of reagents. This technology uses a laser photometer to detect the formation of a clot.

BLEEDING TIME

The bleeding time test detects platelet function disorders by testing platelet plug formation in the capillaries. Bleeding times are sometimes performed prior to surgeries to determine any problems with hemostasis. Prolonged bleeding can occur because of abnormal platelet function. The ingestion of aspirin, other salicylate-containing medications, or a number of other medications within 2 weeks prior to the test may result in a prolonged bleeding time. A bleeding time test is performed using a standardized puncture performed in the earlobe, finger, or the inner surface of the forearm.

In 1910, bleeding times were routinely performed on the earlobe as described by Duke. However, with the exception of a few facial surgeons who feel that the circulation of the ear more closely resembles that of the face, physicians rarely request the use of the earlobe today. In 1941, Ivy modified the Duke bleeding time by requiring that the incision be performed on the volar surface of the forearm using a blood pressure cuff to maintain a constant pressure (Figure 13-8). A thin incision was made with a sterile lancet.

Today most laboratories use a modified version, controlling the width and depth of the incision by using an automated incision device such as the Surgicutt.

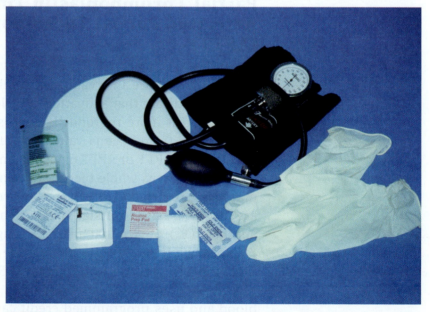

FIGURE 13-8: Supplies used for modified Ivy bleeding time procedure

Procedure 13-1

Modified Ivy Bleeding Time

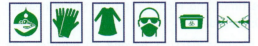

Equipment/Supplies

- Personal protective equipment
- 70% isopropyl alcohol pads
- Automated bleeding time device
- Sphygmomanometer (blood pressure cuff)
- Stopwatch, timer, or watch with sweep second hand
- Butterfly bandage or Steri-Strip

Method/*Rationale*

1. Gather equipment and supplies.

   Ensures everything is available to perform the procedure.

2. Wash hands/don personal protective equipment.

   Thorough handwashing aids in controlling the spread of infection. Remember, you must comply with Standard Precautions whenever you may come in contact with body fluids or blood.

3. Identify the patient.

   Ensures the procedure is performed on the correct patient.

4. Assemble equipment.

   Open the puncture device package. Open the alcohol wipe. Open the Steri-Strip package.

5. Explain the procedure.

   Helps ensure you will have the cooperation of the patient.

6. Position the patient. Seat the patient with the arm supported.

   The patient must be in a comfortable position with the arm securely supported.

7. Determine whether the patient has taken aspirin or any other salicylate-containing drug within the last 2 weeks. Advise the patient of the potential for scarring.

   Aspirin or other salicylate-containing drugs have the potential of thinning the patient's blood and rendering the test inaccurate. The blade of the bleeding time device has the potential to leave a small scar at the site of incision.

8. Select the site of incision.

   The lateral aspect of the inner surface (volar) of the forearm, distal to the antecubital area and devoid of bruises, hair, or surface veins, is the best site. The medial aspect of the forearm tends to cause the patient more discomfort and has a higher incidence of scarring. It may be necessary to shave the area if patients have excessive hair on the forearm.

9. Clean the site.

   Clean the site as if preparing for a venipuncture. Allow the site to air dry.

10. Place the blood pressure cuff around the arm.

    Inflate the cuff to 40 mm Hg. The time between inflation of the cuff and making the incision should be between 30 to 60 seconds. The pressure must be maintained throughout the entire procedure. Failure to maintain 40 mm Hg throughout the procedure will decrease bleeding time.

11. Remove the puncture device from its packaging.

    Do not allow the blade to touch any contaminated surface.

(continues)

Procedure 13-1 *(continued)*

12. Remove the safety clip and place the puncture device firmly on the forearm without pressing.

    A horizontal incision parallel to the antecubital crease is recommended.

13. Depress the trigger while simultaneously starting the timer.

    Failure to start the timing as soon as the incision is made will decrease the bleeding time.

14. Remove the device from the arm as soon as the blade has retracted.

    This is approximately 1 second.

15. Blot the blood flow at 30 seconds by bringing the filter paper close to the incision and absorbing or "wicking" the blood onto the filter paper.

    Do not touch the wound. Touching the wound will disturb platelet plug formation, thus increasing bleeding time.

16. Continue to blot every 30 seconds until blood no longer stains the filter paper. Stop the timer and record the time to the nearest 30 seconds.

    If bleeding persists beyond 30 minutes, the test is usually stopped and the time is recorded as 30 minutes or greater. Normal values are approximately 2 to 8 minutes.

17. Remove the blood pressure cuff, clean the arm, and apply a butterfly bandage or Steri-Strip. Cover with an adhesive bandage.

    Instruct the patient not to remove the bandage for 24 hours.

18. Dispose of puncture device in a puncture-resistant sharps container. Dispose of all contaminated articles in the appropriate biohazardous waste container.

19. Remove gloves and wash hands.

ELECTROLYTES

Substances that conduct electricity when dissolved in water. Acids, bases, and salts are common electrolytes, including potassium, sodium, and chlorine found in blood, tissue fluids, and cells.

PH

The degrees of acidity or alkalinity of a substance. The neutral point where a solution would be neither acid nor alkaline is a pH of 7. A number less than 7 would be acid and above 7 alkaline.

PCO$_2$

The symbol for partial pressure of carbon dioxide.

● CHEMISTRY PANELS

There are a variety of hand-held or portable devices available to perform POCT chemistry panels. These panels are groups of tests, such as blood gases and electrolytes, that are commonly ordered as stat tests by the physician. These analytes must be maintained in the body in very narrow ranges. When they are out of range they must be corrected quickly or the imbalance can lead to death. The test results must be supplied immediately and accurately and are often ordered in emergency and critical care situations.

The i-STAT (i-STAT Corp., Princeton, NJ), the IRMA (Diametrics Medical, Inc., St. Paul, MN), the AVL OPTI (AVL Scientific, Roswell, GA), the NOVA Stat Profile Analyzer (Nova Biomedical, Waltham, MA), and the Gem Premier (Instrumentation Laboratories, Lexington, MA) are all devices capable of measuring chemistry panels. These include values for a patient's **electrolytes**, blood gas values such as **pH**, **pCO$_2$**, and O$_2$ values, and **BUN**, glucose, and Hct values. The machines will initially calibrate, and once this is completed, a blood sample is injected into the device's sensors. The procedure takes less than 2 minutes. The cartridge is removed

BUN (BLOOD UREA NITROGEN)

Nitrogen in the blood in the form of urea, the metabolic product of the breakdown of amino acids used for energy production. BUN is a blood test that provides a rough estimate of kidney function.

ACIDOSIS

An actual or relative increase in the acidity of blood caused by an accumulation of acids or an excessive loss of bicarbonates.

ALKALOSIS

An actual or relative increase in blood alkalinity caused by an accumulation of alkalies or reduction of acids.

HYPOKALEMIA

Extreme potassium depletion in the blood.

HYPERKALEMIA

An excessive amount of potassium in the blood.

from the device and discarded in a biohazardous waste container. The results are displayed on the readout screen of the device and a printout can be generated.

Blood Gases

Arterial blood gases can now be measured by hand-held POCT instruments and include pH, partial pressure of carbon dioxide (pCO_2), and partial pressure of oxygen (PO_2). Analysis of the blood for these gases is important in helping to evaluate the extent of the deviation of acids and bases from the normal. Before appropriate therapy can be instituted, information obtained from those values is analyzed with respect to other laboratory results and clinical conditions.

pH is the measurement of the body's acid-base balance and indicates the patient's metabolic and respiratory status. The normal range for arterial blood pH is 7.35 to 7.45. Below 7.35 is referred to as **acidosis** and a pH level above 7.45 is considered to be **alkalosis**.

The pCO_2 levels measure the patient's ability to exchange air between the blood and lungs. pCO_2 measures the pressure exerted by dissolved CO_2 and is proportional with the pCO_2 in the alveoli. Rate and depth of respiration maintain CO_2 levels. An increase in pCO_2 is then associated with hypoventilation, while a decrease in levels is associated with hyperventilation.

The pO_2 levels measure the pressure exerted by dissolved O_2 in the plasma and indicate the lungs' ability to diffuse O_2 through the alveoli into the blood. pO_2 levels are used to determine the effectiveness of oxygen therapy.

Electrolytes

The most common electrolytes measured by POCT are sodium (Na^+), potassium (K^+), chloride (Cl^-), bicarbonate ion (HCO_3^-), and ionized calcium (Ca^{++}).

● Sodium functions in maintaining osmotic pressure and acid-base balance. It also aids in the transmission of nerve impulses. It is the most plentiful electrolyte in the serum or plasma.

● Potassium is primarily found within the cells of the tissue with very little found in the blood plasma or bones. It is only released into the blood plasma when cells are damaged and can be falsely increased if a blood specimen is hemolyzed. Potassium plays a major role in nerve conduction, muscle function, acid-base balance, and osmotic pressure. Potassium also influences cardiac output by helping to control the rate and force of heart contraction. Lack of potassium is called **hypokalemia**, and increased potassium is called **hyperkalemia**.

- Chloride resides in the extracellular spaces as sodium chloride (NaCl). Chloride is responsible for maintaining cellular integrity by affecting osmotic pressure and acid-base water balance. Chloride must be replaced along with potassium when treating a patient for hypokalemia.
- Bicarbonate ion helps transport carbon dioxide (CO_2) to the lungs and regulate blood pH. When hydrogen ions are released in the respiratory process it causes the blood to become more acidic. This, in turn, causes the bicarbonate ion to move from the cells to the plasma and is carried to the lungs where it re-enters the cell. This causes carbon dioxide to be released through the walls of the alveoli. The removal of carbon dioxide results in a decrease of hydrogen ions and an increase in the blood pH, which restarts the process. A decrease in ventilation (hypoventilation) causes an increase in CO_2 levels and production of more hydrogen ions, which can lead to acidosis. Hyperventilation decreases CO_2 levels and can lead to alkalosis.
- Ionized calcium is used by the body for critical functions such as muscular contraction, cardiac function, transmission of nerve impulses, and blood clotting. Approximately 45% of the blood's calcium is ionized calcium, and the remaining calcium is bound to proteins and other body substances. Only ionized calcium can aid in the above functions.

Blood Urea Nitrogen

A blood urea nitrogen (BUN) level is performed to provide a rough estimate of the patient's kidney function. Nitrogenous waste in the blood, in the form of urea, is the metabolic product of the breakdown of amino acids used for energy production. The normal concentration is 8 to 18 mg/dL. An increase in the blood urea nitrogen level usually indicates decreased renal function.

COLLECTION OF TOXICOLOGY SPECIMENS

Blood Alcohol Level and Forensic Specimens

Occasionally, law enforcement officials, for forensic or legal reasons, request a blood, urine, or other body fluid specimen. The most commonly requested tests are blood alcohol levels, drug levels, and specimens for DNA analysis.

A patient's blood alcohol (ethanol or ETOH) level may be ordered by the patient's physician to monitor alcohol intake, or, as mentioned above, the police department may request blood alco-

CHAIN OF CUSTODY

The procedure for ensuring that material obtained for diagnosis has been taken from the named patient, is properly labeled, and has not been tampered with en route to the laboratory.

hol levels be drawn for legal reasons. If this is the case, the phlebotomist must follow a special protocol as with all other forensic specimens, referred to as a **chain of custody** (Figure 13-9). Chain of custody requires detailed documentation to track the specimen from the time it is collected until the results are reported. The specimen must be accounted for at all times. If the documentation is incomplete or inaccurate, legal action may be impaired.

A special form is used to identify the specimen and the person or persons who obtained the specimen. Particular attention must be paid to the date, time, and place of the collection. The person from whom the specimen was obtained and the signature of the person obtaining the collection must both be on the form in the appropriate place. Identification of the person and the collection of the specimen must both be performed in the presence of a witness; frequently this witness is a police officer. Special seals and containers are required for the specimen. A phlebotomist who performs the collection of a specimen may be summoned to appear and testify in court.

When collecting a specimen for blood alcohol levels, the typical 70% isopropyl alcohol wipes are not used in skin preparation, as they may affect the results of the alcohol content determination. Iodine preparations also contain alcohol and likewise are not used. A non-alcohol-containing alternative such as green soap and water are used instead. A gray top, sodium fluoride evacuated tube is required for specimen collection. This tube may or may not have an anticoagulant depending on whether there is a need for serum or plasma. Red top and green top evacuated tubes may also be used. Alcohol is volatile and easily evaporates, so care should be taken to completely fill the tube until the vacuum is depleted. The stopper should not be removed until absolutely necessary for testing.

Collection of Drug Testing Specimens

Drug testing is required by many organizations, including major corporations, athletic organizations, airlines, and government agencies. Drug testing can be part of pre-employment requirements, random testing, or for cause testing. As with forensic and blood alcohol testing, drug testing requires the special protocols of chain of custody. Whether or not it is being performed for legal reasons, drug testing always has legal implications. Drug testing procedures require that the special donor preparation and collection procedures defined by the National Institute on Drug Abuse (NIDA) be followed exactly. Table 13-1 describes the drugs most commonly tested for as part of the drug screening process and how long they are detectable in the body, depending on frequency and amount of usage.

USA LABS
ID#

Referred by

Health Care Provider
Address
Phone

DO NOT WRITE
IN THIS AREA

CHAIN OF CUSTODY

STEP 1 — TO BE COMPLETED BY EMPLOYER/COLLECTOR.
DONOR IDENTIFICATION—PLEASE PRINT

LAST NAME _____

FIRST NAME _____ M.I. ____

SOC. SEC. NO. _____ — _____ — _____

EMPLOYEE NO. _____

DONOR I.D. VERIFIED ☐ PHOTO I.D.

☐ EMPLOYER REPRESENTATIVE

_____
SIGNATURE OF EMPLOYER REP.

REASON FOR TEST (CHECK ONE)
☐ (1) PRE-EMPLOYMENT ☐ (2) POST ACCIDENT ☐ (3) RANDOM
☐ (4) PERIODIC ☐ (5) REASONABLE SUSPICION/CAUSE
☐ (6) RETURN TO DUTY
☐ (99) OTHER (SPECIFY)

TESTS REQUESTED:

TOTAL TESTS ORDERED ☐

SPECIMEN ☐ Urine ☐ Blood (SUBMIT ONLY ONE SPECIMEN WITH EACH REQUISITION)

STEP 2—COLLECTOR, FOR URINE SPECIMENS, READ TEMPERATURE WITHIN FOUR MINUTES OF COLLECTION.
CHECK THE BOX IF TEMPERATURE IS WITHIN THE SPECIFIED RANGE ☐90°–100°F / 32°–38°C

OR RECORD ACTUAL TEMPERATURE HERE: _____

STEP 3—TO BE COMPLETED BY COLLECTOR.

COLLECTION SITE

COLLECTION DATE _____ TIME _____ ☐ AM PM _____
ADDRESS

REMARKS _____
CITY _____ STATE _____ ZIP _____
( )
PHONE

I certify that the specimen identified on this form is the specimen presented to me by the employee identified in Step 1 above, and was collected, labeled and sealed in the donor's presence.

COLLECTOR'S NAME PRINT (FIRST, M.I., LAST)   SIGNATUE OF COLLECTOR

STEP 4—TO BE INITIATED BY THE DONOR AND COMPLETED AS NECESSARY THEREAFTER.

PURPOSE OF CHANGE	RELEASED BY SIGNATURE	RECEIVED BY SIGNATURE	DATE
A. PROVIDE SPECIMEN FOR TESTING			
B. SHIPMENT TO LABORATORY			
C.			

COMMENTS:

Self-stick   identification
Labels for sealing specimen:
(123) (123) (123) (123)

SPECIMEN PACKAGE INTEGRITY WAS ☐ACCEPTABLE ☐UNACCEPTABLE WHEN RECEIVED IN LAB.

RECEIVER'S INITIALS

FOR OFFICE USE

FIGURE 13-9: Sample chain of custody form

Table 13-1: Drugs Most Commonly Detected in Drug Screens

Drug or Drug Family	Common Names	Detectable (Time)	Comment
Alcohol		2–12 hours	
Amphetamines	Methamphetamine, speed, crystal, crank, ice	1–3 days 2–7 day	Single/light use Frequent/chronic use
Barbiturates	Downers, Seconal, Fiorinal, Tuinal, Phenobarbital	2 days to 4 weeks	Varies considerably with drugs in this class
Benzodiazepines	Valium, Librium, Xanax, Dalmane, Serax	1 week to >30 days	Varies considerably with drugs in this class
Cocaine (as metabolite)	Crack	1–3 days 3–14 days	Single/light use Frequent/chronic use
Cannabinoids	Marijuana, grass, hash	1–7 days >30 days	Single/light use Frequent/chronic use
Methadone	Dolophine	1–4 days	Single/light use
Opiates	Heroin, morphine, codeine, Dilaudid, hydrocodone	2–4 days >7 days	Single/light use Frequent/chronic use
Phencyclidine	PCP, angle dust	2–7 days >30 days	Single/light use Frequent/chronic use
Propoxyphene	Darvon, Darvocet	1–2 days >7 days	Single/light use Frequent/chronic use

(Courtesy Tox Talk, Sonora Laboratory Sciences, Phoenix, AZ, 1996)

Donor preparation requirements include the following:
- Positive identification of the donor via picture identification, such as a driver's license.
- Explain the test purpose and procedure.
- Advise the donor of his or her legal rights. The donor has the right to refuse the test if it is a requirement for pre-employment. The company requesting the test is advised of the donor's refusal. If the test is random or for cause, the donor will have previously signed a consent form with the company requesting the test.
- Each organization requesting drug testing will have outlined the exact procedures to follow in its Policy and Procedure Employment Manual, although all companies requesting drug screening must follow NIDA's general guidelines. For example, an athletic organization may require that a visual collection be performed, whereas a delivery company might not require a visual collection.

- A special collection area must be prepared or maintained for urine collections. If the donor is being tested at the health care facility, the facility may have a special lavatory set aside only for drug testing. If the phlebotomist is performing a collection off-site, or at the facility of the company requesting the drug test, the bathroom must be prepared. Both facilities must initially be prepared and maintained to NIDA's standards throughout the collection process.

- To prepare the lavatory, access to water must be eliminated. Faucets must be taped off. (A special tape is used that tears easily, but cannot be pulled free from the surface once applied. If removed or torn it will leave a telltale sign that it has been tampered with.) Toilet tank lids must be taped shut. A blue dye is placed in the toilet water, and must be replaced for subsequent collections. The lavatory must be inspected for hidden urine samples or other substances that could affect the test. If there are cabinets under the sink, inspect the cabinets and tape them shut. Investigate waste receptacles, paper towel dispensers, and under the toilet bowl.

- Once the facility is prepared and the correct donor is identified, open the drug testing collection kit in front of the patient. Ask the donor to fill in the required areas on the chain of custody form. Some forms provide space for the donor to list any prescribed medications he or she is taking. The donor may be asked to provide proof that the medication was prescribed, if part of the company's protocol.

- A witness must be present in the lavatory during the collection of the specimen to ensure that the required patient provides the sample. Drug testing collection kits provide a collection container with a temperature strip attached, to ensure the specimen is freshly voided. The temperature of the specimen is written on the chain of custody form.

- A split sample may be requested for confirmation or parallel testing. In this case the sample that is collected in the collection cup is poured into two separate containers.

- The specimen from the collection cup is poured into the container(s) with the patient witnessing the procedure. Evidence seals are attached to the chain of custody form, and the specimen ID number from the chain of custody form is stamped on the evidence seal as well. Once the specimen is in the transportation container, remove the evidence seal from the form and place it over the lid so that it covers both sides of the container. The donor and the collector both initial the seal and the collector writes the date and time of collection in the appropriate space.

- The specimen is then placed in a tamper-proof bag and sealed in the presence of the donor.
- The form is completed and signed by the donor.
- The collector signs the form and indicates the date, time, and collection site.
- The specimen is then delivered to the laboratory for testing.
- All laboratory personnel and anyone else (including delivery personnel) who handle the specimen will document their involvement by signing the chain of custody form until the results are reported.

THERAPEUTIC DRUG MONITORING

THERAPEUTIC

Pertaining to results obtained from treatment.

Many prescribed drugs have varying effects dependent on the dosage of the drug. Because exact dosages are required to produce the desired effect of the medication, physicians order **therapeutic** drug monitoring (TDM) to manage individual patient drug treatment. Ordering TDM allows the physician to establish drug dosages, maintain dosages at beneficial levels, and avoid drug toxicity. Timing of urine and blood collections during specific drug administration is critical for safe and beneficial treatment and must be consistent. This is a team effort between the patient's physician, nursing staff, and pharmacy. The phlebotomist is critical in this team approach, as the timing of collection is critical. Therapeutic drugs require monitoring and evaluation at peak and trough drug levels in order for the physician to determine a safe and effective dose. Peak levels are collected when the highest serum concentration of the drug is anticipated, which is typically 30 to 60 minutes after administration. Peak levels screen for drug intoxication and/or monitor if the blood level is within the therapeutic range for that day. Trough levels are collected when the serum concentration of the drug is at its lowest point, usually just prior to administration of the next scheduled dose. Trough levels are monitored to ensure that levels of the drug stay within the range of therapeutic effectiveness.

PATERNITY TESTING

Paternity testing is performed to determine the probability that a specific individual fathered a child. Typically paternity testing eliminates the possibility of paternity, rather than proving paternity. Paternity testing can be requested by physicians, lawyers, child support enforcement bureaus, or by individuals. The tests performed are based on ABO and Rh typing as well as testing for other proteins on the surface of red blood cells. Paternity testing also requires chain of custody procedures, and it may require fingerprinting of the individual. The mother, child, and alleged father are all tested. This procedure is rapidly being replaced by DNA testing.

SKIN TESTS

The nursing staff of inpatients typically performs skin tests. However, some independent laboratories offer skin testing, especially tuberculosis testing, as part of their services for outpatients. It is therefore important that the phlebotomist be familiar with this procedure. Skin testing involves the injection of minute amounts of allergens or disease-producing microorganisms that stimulate an antibody reaction. These injections are given **intradermally**. The TB test, also called a PPD test, is the test for tuberculosis and is the most common type of skin test. Other skin tests include the Schick test for diphtheria, the Dick test for susceptibility to scarlet fever, Coccidioidomycosis (Cocci) test for an infectious fungus disease, and the Histoplasmosis (Histo) test for past or present infection by the fungus *Histoplasma capsulatum.*

INTRADERMAL

Within the substance of the skin.

FECAL OCCULT BLOOD TEST

The detection of **occult** blood in a patient's stool (feces) is an important diagnostic tool in the early detection of colorectal cancer and other digestive disorders including gastric ulcers and colitis. The test is performed using a specially designed kit containing a small cardboard card that feces are smeared onto. The specimen can be collected and tested on-site or the kit can be sent home with the patient to collect the specimen and then returned to the laboratory. There are many CLIA-waived fecal blood test products available. HemaCheck and Hemoccult® Sensa Test are two examples. The primary reaction is caused by a color reaction which occurs as a result of the mixture of hemoglobin and gum guaiac. Some of the kits use a filter paper that has been impregnated with gum guaiac; other kits add it as a reagent. All kits use visual color comparison to determine results. The two parts to this procedure are equally important. The first part is patient prep and collection of the specimen. The patient is instructed about the appropriate dietary requirements. For example, the patient must not eat red meat, turnips, or horseradish for at least 2 days prior to testing and throughout the duration of the test. They must discontinue the use of aspirin and iron intake for at least 1 week prior to the test. They must discontinue taking vitamin C and anti-inflammatory drugs. The patient is

OCCULT

Obscure; concealed, hidden.

Procedure 13-2

Skin Test

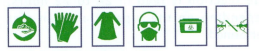

Equipment/Supplies

● PPE
● Tuberculin syringe with a ¹/₂-inch, 26 to 27-gauge needle
● 70% isopropyl alcohol wipe
● Diluted antigen
● 2 × 2 gauze pads
● Sharps container
● Biohazardous waste container

Method/*Rationale*

1. Gather equipment and supplies.

   Ensures all equipment is available to perform the procedure.

2. Wash hands/don personal protective equipment.

   Thorough handwashing aids in controlling the spread of infection. Remember, you must comply with Standard Precautions whenever you may come in contact with body fluids or blood.

3. Identify the patient.

   Ensures the procedure is performed on the correct patient.

4. Assemble equipment.

   Attach the needle to the syringe as needed. Open the alcohol wipe.

5. Explain the procedure.

   Helps ensure you will have the cooperation of the patient.

6. Position the patient. Seat the patient with the arm supported.

   The patient must be in a comfortable position with the arm securely supported.

7. Draw 0.1 mL of diluted antigen into the tuberculin syringe.

   If a single dose vial is used, remove the protective plastic cap covering the vial, uncap the needle, insert the needle into the vial, withdraw the required dose, and resheath the needle. If a multidose vial is used, wipe the rubber stopper of the vial with an alcohol wipe. Then draw 0.1 mL of air into the syringe, inject the air into the vial, withdraw the required dose into the syringe, and resheath the needle. Do not allow the needle to touch any contaminated surface.

8. Select the site—the volar surface of the forearm below the antecubital crease.

   Areas with scars, burns, rashes, bruises, excessive hair, or superficial veins should be avoided.

9. Clean the site with a 70% isopropyl alcohol wipe and allow to air dry.

   Using a 70% isopropyl alcohol, wipe clean the site in a circular motion from point of insertion outward. Allowing the site to dry lessens the stinging sensation felt by the patient. The evaporation and drying process helps to destroy microbes.

10. Hold the arm in the same manner as for a venipuncture with the skin pulled taut with the thumb.

    Pulling the skin taut allows for a smoother insertion of the needle, causing the patient less discomfort.

11. Insert the needle.

    The syringe is held at a 15 to 20-degree angle and the needle is inserted just under the skin, just past the bevel.

(continues)

Procedure 13-2 *(continued)*

12. The syringe plunger is pulled back slightly to make certain a vein has not been entered.

    Blood will pull into the hub of the needle if a vein has been entered. If a vein has been entered, remove the needle from the patient's arm. Prepare a new syringe and select a new site. Begin the procedure again. A diluted antigen must never be injected into a vein.

13. Slowly inject the diluted antigen into the patient's skin, creating a distinct, pale elevation of the skin approximately 6 to 10 mm in diameter. This is commonly called a wheal or bleb (Figure 13-10).

    The needle must be inserted barely under the skin. If the needle is too deep a wheal will not form.

14. Remove the needle; do *not* apply pressure or a bandage to the site.

    Maintain the arm in position until the site has closed. Applying a bandage may cause irritation or absorb the antigen and distort the test results.

15. Dispose of equipment and supplies.

    Place the needle in a puncture-resistant sharps container. Soiled supplies, if any, are disposed of in a biohazardous waste container. All other waste is disposed of in a waste receptacle.

16. Remove gloves and wash hands.

17. The reaction is read in 24 to 72 hours, depending on the type of antigen test performed.

    Interpretation of the test is based upon the presence or absence of erythema (redness) or induration (hardness). A negative test will produce erythema and induration of 5 mm or less. A doubtful test result will demonstrate erythema and induration between 5 and 9 mm in diameter. If this result occurs the test is repeated. A positive test will produce erythema and induration of 10 mm or greater in diameter.

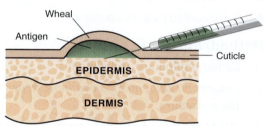

FIGURE 13-10: A raised wheal will form when the antigen is properly administered with an intradermal injection.

only allowed to eat small amounts of chicken, tuna fish, peanuts, popcorn, or bran cereal. A high-bulk diet of breads and cereals, and plenty of vegetables, such as lettuce, spinach, and corn and plenty of fruits such as prunes, grapes, plums, and apples, should be eaten for a minimum of 1 week prior to the collection. The patient must be instructed in the appropriate collection techniques, especially if the collection is to take place at home. The patient is provided with three collection kits, each containing a wooden applicator stick and a cardboard test apparatus. The patient should fill out completely the required information on the cover of the cardboard kit, especially the date and time of collection.

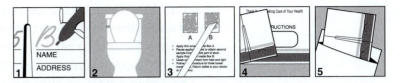

1. Remove slide from paper dispensing envelope. Using a ball-point pen, write your name, age, and address on the front of the slide. **Do not tear the sections apart.**
2. Fill in sample collection date on section 1 before a bowel movement. Flush toilet and allow to refill. You may use any clean, dry container to collect your sample. Collect sample before it contacts the toilet bowl water. Let stool fall into collection container.
3. Open front of section 1. Use one stick to collect a small sample. Apply a thin smear covering Box A. Collect second sample from different part of stool with same stick. Apply a thin smear covering Box B. Discard stick in a waste container. **DO NOT FLUSH STICK.**
4. Close and secure front flap of section 1 by inserting it under tab. Store slide in any paper envelope until the next day. **Important: This allows the sample to "air dry."**
5. Repeat steps 2-4 for the next two days, using sections 2 and 3. After completing the last section, store the slide overnight in any paper envelope to air dry.
   The next day, remove slide from the paper envelope and place in the Mailing Pouch, if provided. Seal pouch carefully and **immediately return to your doctor or laboratory.**
   Note: Current U.S. Postal Regulations prohibit mailing completed slides in any standard paper envelope.

IMPORTANT NOTE: Follow the procedure exactly as outlined above. Always develop the test, read the results, interpret them and make a decision as to whether the fecal specimen is positive or negative for occult blood BEFORE you develop the Performance Monitors®. Do not apply Developer to Performance Monitors® before interpreting test results. Any blue originating from the Performance Monitors® should be ignored in the reading of the specimen test results.

READING AND INTERPRETATION OF THE HEMOCCULT® TEST
the world's leading test for fecal occult blood

Negative Smears*

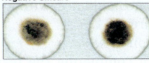

Sample report: negative
No detectable blue on or at the edge of the smears indicates the test is negative for occult blood.
(See **LIMITATIONS OF PROCEDURE.**)

Negative and Positive Smears*   **Positive Smears***

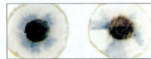

Sample report: positive
Any trace of blue on or at the edge of one or more of the smears indicates the test is positive for occult blood.

FIGURE 13-11: Hemoccult® Sensa test (Courtesy of Beckman Coulter, Inc.)

Instruct the patient to flush the toilet before beginning and to collect the specimen in a clean container. Care should be taken so that water from the toilet is not collected with the specimen. There are a variety of methods that may be employed to accomplish this: 1) Specially designed toilet "hats" can be fit over the toilet bowl under the seat; 2) Saran wrap can be fit over the bowl in much the same manner as the toilet "hat"; 3) a paper plate may also be used to collect the stool specimen. Once the specimen is collected, the patient is instructed to smear the specimen on the paper side of one cardboard kit. The patient must take a sample from a completely different part of the specimen and smear the second sample on the other test area. The wooden stick is then discarded. If collected in a medical facility, the wooden stick must be discarded in a biohazardous waste container. The cardboard slide pack is sealed and either mailed or delivered to the lab. If mailed, all postal regulations for biohazardous substances must be followed. This procedure is commonly repeated for 3 consecutive days.

The second part of this procedure is the testing of the specimen. When the specimen arrives in the laboratory, the appropriate barrier precautions are used. Open the back of the slide pack and apply the color developer supplied in the kit. Handle the reagents with care; some are flammable and poisonous. Any blue color change is a positive reaction. Always compare the reaction to the picture of positive and negative reactions that accompanies the kit. As with all other point-of-care testing, it is imperative that quality control measures be taken. A control area is provided on each cardboard slide. Follow the manufacturer's guidelines in quality control testing. Document results and dispose of cardboard kits in a biohazardous waste container.

Possible sources of error when performing a fecal occult blood test include:

● Noncompliance with dietary restriction or collection procedures.
● Expired kits.
● Not completing the test within 2 days of collection of specimen. Patients who mail the hemoccult kit to the laboratory must be reasonably sure that the test will reach the laboratory within the 2-day window.
● Reading results within the required time of 30 to 60 seconds (or manufacturer's requirements).

PREGNANCY TEST

There are a wide variety of test kits available to perform pregnancy testing. However, only the simplest tests, with the minimum of steps using color comparisons, are CLIA-approved for waived testing.

Pregnancy tests determine the levels of **human chorionic gonadotrophin (hCG or HCG).** HCG is present in increasingly higher levels during pregnancy, in both urine and blood, and peaks between the 50th and 80th day of gestation. Then the levels start to decrease. HCG disappears shortly after delivery. HCG may not be present in sufficient amounts for the first 1 to 2 weeks after conception, so it is possible to have false-negative test results during this time period. If test results are negative in this time frame, it is best to wait a few days and repeat the test. It is also possible to have false positive results as HCG has been found to increase in conditions such as choriocarcinoma or malignant tumors of the

HUMAN CHORIONIC GONADOTROPHIN (HCG)

A hormone produced by the placenta that appears in both urine and serum, beginning approximately 10 days after conception, the presence of which is an indication of pregnancy.

ovaries or testes. Various medications may also interfere with the test by producing false positive or negative results.

CLIA-waived pregnancy tests are typically one-step tests (Figure 13-12), such as the QuickVue® One-Step HCG-Urine test or the CARDS® QS®.

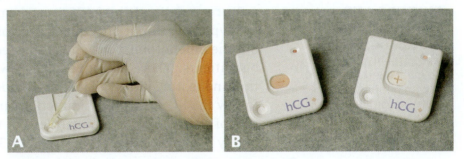

FIGURE 13-12: (A) A drop of urine is placed in the urine test unit. (B) The package instructions will specify how the test is to be interpreted. The most common interpretation is with a negative sign (left) and positive sign (right).

With all one-step tests it is important that the urine be fresh and free of detergents, protein, hematuria, and excessive bacterial contamination, as these may invalidate test results. The first morning specimen has the highest concentration of HCG and is thus the most optimum specimen to test. If the sample cannot be tested immediately, the specimen should be refrigerated, as HCG deteriorates over time at room temperature.

Quality Control is as important in HCG testing as it is with all laboratory procedures. A positive and negative control test should be performed with each patient's specimen, making sure to accurately document each control result. Most pregnancy tests must be kept refrigerated and warmed to room temperature before performing the test. Make sure to check the kit's expiration date before using.

RAPID STREP TEST

A rapid strep test is performed to determine the presence of a Group A beta-streptococcal infection. It is typically performed when a patient has a sore throat or tonsillitis and strep is suspected as the causative agent. It is especially important to determine if strep is the causative agent in children and young adults. Strep A can reside and thrive in the kidneys, causing chronic kidney infections, and lead to permanent kidney damage, scarlet fever, rheumatic fever, endocarditis, or glomerulonephritis. Strep A can be detected by bacterial culture or by a rapid slide or tube test.

CULTURE AND SENSITIVITY (C&S)

The process by which bacterial organisms are grown on media and identified, and an antibiotic susceptibility (sensitivity) test is performed to determine which antibiotics will be effective against the organism.

There are definite advantages to performing a rapid strep test versus performing a bacterial culture. Time is the number one advantage. If the test results from a rapid strep test are positive, then antibiotic therapy can be started right away. If a bacterial culture is performed, the results will not be available for 24 to 48 hours. If the results are questionable from a rapid strep test, a bacterial **culture and sensitivity (C&S)** can be performed to confirm results.

Typically, throat specimens are collected by the nursing staff, but the phlebotomist may be requested to collect the specimen on outpatients. There are several CLIA-waived throat culture collection and testing kits available. It is important that the phlebotomist follow the manufacturer's directions included with the kit. Collection of a throat culture, regardless of the brand of the kit, is commonly performed as in Procedure 13-3.

URINALYSIS—PHYSICAL AND CHEMICAL EXAMINATION

The physical and chemical analysis of urine involves simple observation and color comparisons, which can be accomplished with reasonable accuracy and very little training. However, their value in clinical diagnosis can be immeasurable. The trained phlebotomist can perform these tasks with ease and accuracy and provide the physician with helpful diagnostic information.

The description of urine's physical characteristics includes color, appearance, clarity or transparency, odor, and foam. Urine color can vary from almost completely colorless to black and a variety of colors in between. The procedure for observing a urine specimen's color should be consistent within the laboratory. For example, if the urine specimen's color is routinely observed while in a urine collection cup, all urine specimens are to be observed the same way. If the color is observed after the urine has been poured into a urine centrifuge tube, then all urine specimens are observed in this manner, as the color may vary by degrees from one to the other. The institution sets a policy for this procedure to ensure consistency. If only the physical and chemical properties of the urine specimen are to be observed, it is much more economic to keep the specimen in the original collection cup rather than pouring it into a centrifuge tube. If a microscopic urine test is to be performed by laboratory personnel, the specimen will be poured into a centrifuge tube.

Normal urine color is described as yellow, gold, amber, or straw, and may be further clarified by pale, light, or dark (i.e., pale yellow or dark amber). The color of a normal urine specimen is directly

Procedure 13-3

Rapid Strep Test

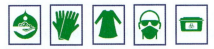

Equipment/Supplies

- PPE
- Culturette system
- Tongue depressor
- Strep A one-step kit (should include reagents, cartridges, cuvettes, tubes or slides, dropper, mixing sticks, as needed)
- Biohazardous waste container

Method/*Rationale*

1. Gather equipment and supplies.

   Ensures all equipment is available to perform the procedure.

2. Identify the patient.

   Ensures the procedure is performed on the correct patient.

3. Explain the procedure.

   Helps ensure you will have the cooperation of the patient.

4. Assemble equipment.

   Open the culturette wrapper and remove the culturette. Twist the cap to break the seal.

5. Wash hands/don personal protective equipment.

   Thorough handwashing aids in controlling the spread of infection. Remember, you must comply with Standard Precautions whenever you may come in contact with body fluids or blood.

6. Position the patient. The patient's mouth should be at the phlebotomist's eye level. Ask the patient to tilt the head back and open the mouth. Hold the culturette securely and carefully remove the cotton-tipped applicator. Place the tongue depressor on the tongue and ask the patient to say "ahhh."

   This allows the phlebotomist to clearly see to the back of the patient's throat.

7. Collect a sample by moving the cotton tip to the back of the mouth and tonsils, sweeping the cotton tip from side to side.

   Do not allow the cotton-tipped to touch the tongue, sides of the mouth, or uvula.

8. Remove the cotton tip without touching any parts of the mouth. Remove the tongue depressor and discard into a biohazardous waste container.

9. Carefully replace the applicator into the culturette tube without touching the sides of the tube. Insert the applicator as far as possible and twist the cap to secure.

   This ensures that the specimen is not contaminated.

10. Once the applicator is secured, invert the tube and break the preservative capsule so that the cotton tip is completely covered.

    If the specimen is being transported to the laboratory prior to testing, the specimen will be preserved.

(continues)

Procedure 13-3 *(continued)*

11. Label the tube and attach a completed requisition.

12. Disinfect areas. Remove gloves and PPE and discard appropriately in biohazardous waste container. Wash hands.

13. Transport specimen to laboratory and perform rapid strep test, or prepare specimen for shipment to outside lab if required.

14. To perform rapid strep test, wash hands and apply gloves.

15. Bring all specimens and reagents to room temperature before performing test.

16. Remove a test well, cuvette, or cartridge from the foil pouch.

17. Use a new disposable pipette included in test kit, and place the number of drops of solution recommended by the manufacturer in the test well, cuvette, or slide.

    Do not touch the specimen test site.

18. Wait for the specified time suggested by the manufacturer. Read the reaction at the precise time.

19. Always compare the unknown color reaction to a test well, cuvette, or slide prepared from a positive control and a negative control to determine validity and accurate interpretation of the results.

    Some kits have built-in controls. A colored line must develop in the positive control area or the patient's test results are invalid.

20. Record patient's results and the results of the positive and negative controls.

21. Discard all disposable material into a biohazardous waste container. Disinfect the work area and dispose of specimens according to institutional policy.

22. Remove gloves and wash hands.

SOLUTE

A dissolved substance in a solution.

TRANSPARENCY

In reference to urine, the ability or difficulty to see through a specimen.

TURBIDITY

Opacity caused by the suspension of flaky or granular particles in a normally clear liquid.

SEDIMENT

The substance settling at the bottom of a liquid.

CLARITY

The range of clearness to turbidity of a specimen.

related to the concentration of the specimen's **solutes**. The higher the concentration, the darker the urine. Concentration may vary depending on the time of day the specimen is collected. First morning specimens will often have a darker color. The urine has a higher concentration of solutes because it has been collecting overnight in the bladder, while a random mid-day specimen may appear lighter in color because it has been diluted by fluid intake. The normal colors of urine are caused by three urinary pigments: urochrome (yellow), uroerythrin (red), and urobilin (orange/yellow).

Abnormal urine colors come in a wide variety. Some are clinically significant while others are simply caused by ingestion of certain foods or medications. It is important that the phlebotomist recognize the difference between pathologic and nonpathologic colors (Table 13-2).

Transparency of a urine specimen appearance includes **turbidity**, **sediment**, and **clarity**. The specimen must be well mixed prior to examination so that any sediment that has settled in the bottom of the container is evenly distributed throughout the specimen. The specimen must be observed in a clear container so there is no distortion.

Table 13-2: Urine Colors—Causes or Clinical Significance

Color	Cause Or Clinical Significance
Colorless, pale yellow, light straw	Excessive fluid intake, diabetes mellitus
Dark yellow, amber	Concentrated specimen, excessive fluid loss caused by vomiting, dehydration, fever, excessive exercise
Orange, Red-orange	Carrots, vitamin A or beta-carotene, antibiotics to treat UTI
Red	Blood, food dye
Deep yellow-brown	Bilirubin (look for bright yellow foam)
Yellow-green	Biliverdin (bilirubin converting to biliverdin), old specimen
Green, blue-green	Pseudomonas infection (UTI) Interfering substances include Clorets, Indican, Methocarbamol, Amitriptyline
Blue	Food dye
Dark brown, black	Melanoma

Terms used to describe the transparency of the urine specimen include clear, hazy, cloudy, turbid, and milky. The transparency can be further clarified if a microscopic examination is performed.

A normal, freshly voided specimen will appear clear. Substances found in the urine that will impair its clarity and cause the specimen to appear hazy, cloudy, turbid, or milky include epithelial cells, white blood cells, red blood cells, crystals, fats, protein, bacteria, or a variety of other contaminates including toilet tissue, medications such as antibiotics, talcum powder, or radiographic material. A urine specimen may be cloudy because of crystals and cells that will centrifuge out; bacteria will not. It is also important to take into consideration whether or not the specimen has been refrigerated. Even a clear specimen will become cloudy upon refrigeration because of the precipitation of amorphous urates or phosphates. A specimen that has been left standing at room temperature for any length of time will also become hazy to cloudy as bacteria will multiply at room temperature. Some of the above substances are normal constituents of urine in small amounts. Bacteria and epithelial cells are only pathologic in larger quantities. Chemically testing specimens (reagent strips) may help to differentiate an increase in some of these substances; however, for a definitive clarification, a microscopic examination must be performed. It is not the phlebotomist's responsibility to make these differentiations but to simply report all observations and allow the physician to interpret or order further testing. Microscopic urinalysis not a CLIA-waived test.

Other characteristics of the urine specimen are odor and foam. Although urine specimens are no longer wafted to determine odor, as it presents a health risk to the health professional, strong urine odors are hard to avoid. A freshly voided specimen should have an aromatic odor. Urine may have a strong fruity or sweet smell from acetone caused by diabetic acidosis, starvation, or dieting. A foul or putrid odor suggests that the urine is not freshly voided, or may be associated with the growth of bacteria; decomposition of urine containing cystine or pus will have the odor of rotten eggs. A strong ammonia odor occurs especially during decomposition of urine on standing (alkaline fermentation) or retention within the urinary bladder and may be related to some bacterial infections. Another important diagnostic element is the presence of foam, especially the appearance of "lasting" white foam, which may suggest the presence of increased protein and perhaps renal disease. The presence of deeply pigmented yellow foam on yellow-brown or yellow-green urine may indicate the presence of bilirubin or biliverdin. The phlebotomist should proceed with caution as this may indicate hepatitis.

Remember to wear the appropriate PPE when handling urine specimens.

The chemical analysis of a urine specimen by using the reagent strip, sometimes called the dipstick method, may include the evaluation of glucose, protein, bilirubin, urobilinogen, pH, blood, ketones, nitrite, leukocytes, and specific gravity. The Multistix® (Miles Diagnostics, Elkhart, IN) and the Chemstrip® (Boehringer Mannheim, Indianapolis, IN) are two brands of reagent strips that are very similar and dominate the medical market. The reagent strips are thin white plastic strips with a number of absorbent pads attached, one for each analysis. Each pad is impregnated with all necessary reagents for a color change to occur. After the strip has been dipped into the urine, the color is then compared at a specific time to a color chart on the product bottle. The number of tests on the strip can vary. Some tests are available individually. Every facility determines how many tests are to be included to screen for urine chemistries.

To perform a reagent strip test, guidelines and procedures must be followed exactly to obtain accurate and reliable results (Figures 13-13 and 13-14). Remove the strip(s) from the manufacturer's bottle, which must be stored in a cool, dry, and dark place.

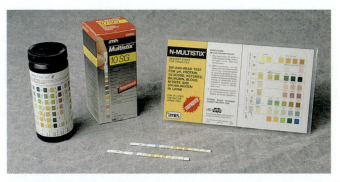

FIGURE 13-13: Multistix reagent strips with color-coded chart are used for chemical analysis of urine.

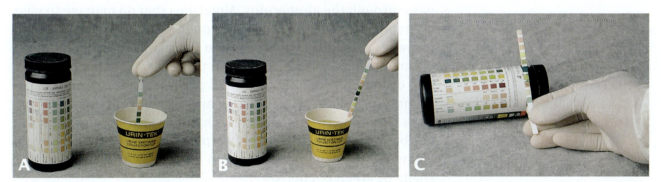

FIGURE 13-14: (A) Immerse the reagent strip in the urine sample. (B) After immersing the reagent strip, tap it lightly to remove excess urine. (C) Read the reagent strip by matching the color on the strip to a color on the container.

Never refrigerate the bottle. Never remove more than the number of strips that are to be used immediately. Once the strip(s) is removed, replace the lid and keep it tightly closed. Discard any bottles and strips that are out-of-date, even if the bottle has never been opened. Do not remove the desiccant from the bottle. Make sure the urine specimen has been well mixed. Completely immerse the strip into the urine specimen and wipe the excess specimen off the strip against the rim of the tube or specimen container. The strip may also be blotted with an absorbent paper. Keep the strip in a horizontal position to prevent the mixing of reagents from one pad to another. Following the manufacturer's recommendations, begin timing at the start of immersion. Each pad's timing requirements are listed on the color-comparison chart on the side of the bottle. Note the results of each reagent pad at the exact time indicated. For some tests, the reaction continues to change after the designated time. Therefore, accurate timing is critical.

Reagent Pads

- pH: Urinary pH is the measure of the acidity or alkalinity of the specimen. The measurement of the urine pH may identify a respiratory, metabolic acid-base balance disorder, a urinary tract infection, or **renal calculi** formation. Urinary pH varies from 5 to 9, with 7 being considered neutral. Acidity is less than 7 and alkaline is greater than 7. If urine from the protein pad is allowed to run over the pH reagent pad, an alkaline specimen can produce an acid result.

- Protein: In normal urine there is no (or very little) protein. The normal range is reported as negative to trace amounts. This is because protein is a rather large molecule and normally will not pass through the glomerulus. Molecules that do manage to pass are typically reabsorbed back through the glomerular tubules. However, if there is damage to the Bowman's capsule, as might occur in renal disease, the large protein molecules may pass into excreted urine. This is called **proteinuria**. Albumin is the primary protein found in urine, and the reagent strip test detects only the presence of albumin; other types of proteins will not be detected. The reagent strip changes through shades of green; as the amount of protein in the urine increases, the shade of green deepens.

- Glucose: The value of determining the presence of glucose in the urine, **glucosuria**, is for the diagnosis and management of diabetes mellitus. Glucose is a metabolic threshold substance that spills over into the urine when the blood concentration surpasses approximately 170 mg/dL (the amount required for body function). The reagent strip for glucosuria is enzymatic and a specific test; in other words, it is only positive if glucose is present. The color changes vary based on the concentration of glucose. The color chart ranges from negative to 2,000 mg/dL or 0.1 to 2.0%. The reagent strip manufacturers suggest that if the test pad is positive the dipstick process be repeated with strict adherence to the timing of the test.

- Ketones or ketone bodies are normal end-products of fat metabolism. The detection of their presence in urine is important because their presence may be toxic to the brain. Ketones are most often elevated in patients with diabetes. However, ketones may be present in patients with severe vomiting, dieting, and starvation. The muscles of the body normally utilize ketones, but when the supply of carbohydrates is jeopardized or depleted as in extreme dieting, the body increases the metabolism of fat for energy and **ketonuria** is the result.

RENAL CALCULI

Kidney stones.

PROTEINURIA

Protein, usually albumin, in the urine.

GLUCOSURIA

Sugar (glucose) in the urine.

KETONURIA

The formation or excretion of ketones in the urine.

HEMATURIA

Blood in the urine.

HEMOGLOBINURIA

The presence in urine of hemoglobin free from red blood cells.

The interpretation of a positive reaction is sometimes difficult. One reason for this is that the ketone pad is located next to the bilirubin pad and may be confused with the color of the positive ketone reaction.

● Blood is detected in the urine as either intact red blood cells **hematuria**, or as hemoglobin from lysed cells, **hemoglobinuria**. Blood can be present as part of a pathologic process or it can be nonpathologic. Nonpathologic blood could be caused by contamination of the specimen from menstrual blood. If blood is present because of kidney damage, it suggests damage of the glomerular membrane or bleeding along the urinary tract. Myoglobin, a muscle form of hemoglobin, will also give a positive reaction.

The reaction on the reagent pad may vary from speckled to full color change. The speckled color is associated with the presence of intact red blood cells, while the uniform color change corresponds to free hemoglobin.

● Bilirubin in the urine is a significant indicator of liver disease, such as hepatitis and cirrhosis, disease of the gallbladder, and cancer. Bilirubin is a normal end-product of the breakdown of hemoglobin, as a part of red blood cell destruction. It is normally present in the blood but not in the urine. A positive reaction produces a color change from tan to pink. It is easy to confuse the bilirubin color pad with a ketone reaction.

● Urobilinogen is a product of further disintegration of bilirubin after it passes from the bile ducts into the intestines. The bilirubin reaction and the urobilinogen reaction give the physician valuable diagnostic information when studied together. Urobilinogen then continues to be transformed by bacteria into urobilin. Urobilin is one of the normal urinary chromogens, a strong urinary pigment. Urobilin is also responsible for the normal color of feces, but it is not detectable by the reagent strip test. It is possible, however, to have an increased urobilinogen and normal-colored urine. It is also possible to have abnormal-colored urine and a normal urobilinogen result. It is abnormal to have a negative urinary urobilinogen value unless the bile duct is obstructed.

● A nitrite test and the leukocyte test are both performed to screen for urinary tract infections (UTIs). The nitrite test is an indirect method to detect significant bacteria in the urine—it detects the presence of nitrites rather than bacteria. The test is based on the assumption that the organism causing the UTI can convert nitrates (normally present in urine) to nitrites (normally absent in urine). In order for this test to be somewhat accurate, the urine must have been in the bladder for at least 4 hours; if present, the bacteria must have time to convert the nitrates to nitrites. The patient may have a UTI that is caused by other organisms giving a negative test result. The leukocyte test helps to further determine the presence of a UTI.

● Leukocytes (white blood cells) are often present in bacterial urinary tract infections. A positive nitrite test, in conjunction with a positive leukocyte test, is often indicative of a urinary tract infection. The reagent pad changes to shades of purple in direct relationship with the numbers of leukocytes present. Besides the nitrite and leukocyte tests, other chemical results that clinically support the UTI findings may include a urinary pH that is alkaline, positive blood, and positive protein reactions.

● Specific gravity: The specific gravity of urine evaluates the kidneys' ability to concentrate and dilute. Until recently, specific gravity was only performed with the use of a refractometer or urinometer. These two methods, however, are not CLIA-waived and the reagent strip method for determining specific gravity has gained a wider acceptance. Although not as accurate as the refractometer and urinometer, in many situations the specific gravity reagent strip is adequate, and it is an easier and faster procedure. The reagent pad color changes are easy to interpret.

SUMMARY

The phlebotomist can perform a wide variety of CLIA-waived tests at the patient's bedside, in the emergency room, or in ambulatory settings, because of the advances in technology that have made these tests portable, easy to operate, and accurate with reproducible results. Technology is ever changing and as advancements are made, the well-trained phlebotomist is in an excellent position to continue to develop as well. Maintaining the integrity and quality control of point-of-care testing is an integral part of this advanced technology. Waived point-of-care testing has become a valuable component of today's health care.

❚ COMPETENCY CHECK-OFF SHEETS
Modified Ivy Bleeding Time Competency Check

Given all the equipment and supplies, the student will be required to perform, within 10 minutes, a bleeding time test. A "0" in more than two areas or an overall score of less than 80% will require the procedure to be repeated for competency.

Points to Be Awarded:	5 pts	2.5 pts	1 pt	0 pts	total pts
1 Assemble equipment and supplies					
2 Verify physician's orders					
3 Wash hands/don PPE					
4 Identify patient					
5 Explain procedure					
6 Position the patient					
7 Determine adherence to medication restrictions (aspirin)					
8 Select incision site					
9 Clean site					
10 Apply blood pressure cuff/inflate to 40 mm Hg					
11 Perform incision/start timer					
12 Blot blood at 30-second intervals until bleeding stops					
13 Remove blood pressure cuff/clean arm					
14 Apply Steri-Strip or butterfly bandage					
15 Instruct patient in wound care					
16 Dispose of sharps and contaminated supplies					
17 Wash hands					
18 Record results in patient chart					

Total Points Possible: _____ Total Points Earned: _____

Start Time: _____ End Time: _____

Instructor Signature: _____ Date: _____

Student Signature: _____ Date: _____

Cholesterol Test Competency Check

Given all the equipment and supplies, the student will be required to perform, within 10 minutes, a cholesterol test. A " 0" in more than two areas or an overall score of less than 80% will require the procedure to be repeated for competency.

Points to Be Awarded:	5 pts	2.5 pts	1 pt	0 pts	total pts
1 Assemble equipment and supplies					
2 Verify physician's orders					
3 Wash hands/don PPE					
4 Identify patient					
5 Explain procedure					
6 Ask patient about adherence to dietary restrictions					
7 Remove reagent strip from container					
8 Replace lid on container					
9 Correctly perform capillary puncture					
10 Wipe away first drop of blood					
11 Place drop of blood on reagent strip/insert reagent strip into analyzer					
12 Read result					
13 Clean and disinfect device					
14 Dispose of sharps and contaminated supplies					
15 Wash hands					
16 Record results in patient chart					

Total Points Possible: _____ Total Points Earned: _____

Start Time: _____ End Time: _____

Instructor Signature: _____ Date: _____

Student Signature: _____ Date: _____

HCG Urine Test Competency Check

Given all the equipment and supplies, the student will be required to perform, within 10 minutes, a HCG urine test. A "0" in more than two areas or an overall score of less than 80% will require the procedure to be repeated for competency.

Points to Be Awarded:	5 pts	2.5 pts	1 pt	0 pts	total pts
1 Assemble equipment and supplies					
2 Verify physician's orders					
3 Wash hands/don PPE					
4 Identify patient					
5 Explain procedure					
6 Instruct patient in collection of specimen					
7 Perform test following manufacturer's guidelines					
8 Dispose of contaminated supplies					
9 Wash hands					
10 Record results in patient chart					

Total Points Possible: _____ Total Points Earned: _____

Start Time: _____ End Time: _____

Instructor Signature: _____ Date: _____

Student Signature: _____ Date: _____

Microhematocrit Competency Check

Given all the equipment and supplies, the student will be required to perform, within 10 minutes, a microhematocrit. A "0" in more than two areas or an overall score of less than 80% will require the procedure to be repeated for competency.

Points to Be Awarded:	5 pts	2.5 pts	1 pts	0 pt	total pts
1 Assemble equipment and supplies					
2 Verify physician's orders					
3 Wash hands/don PPE					
4 Identify patient					
5 Explain procedure					
6 Position patient					
7 Correctly perform capillary puncture					
8 Fill two microhematocrit tubes— 3/4 full with no air bubbles					
9 Seal one end of each tube with clay sealer					
10 Centrifuge microhematocrit tubes— 3 min.					
11 Read percentage					
12 Dispose of sharps and contaminated supplies					
13 Wash hands					
14 Record results in patient chart					

Total Points Possible: _____ Total Points Earned: _____

Start Time: _____ End Time: _____

Instructor Signature: _____ Date: _____

Student Signature: _____ Date: _____

Physical and Chemical Urinalysis Competency Check

Given all the equipment and supplies, the student will be required to perform, within 10 minutes, a physical and chemical urinalysis. A "0" in more than two areas or an overall score of less than 80% will require the procedure to be repeated for competency.

Points to Be Awarded:	5 pts	2.5 pts	1 pt	0 pts	total pts
1 Assemble equipment and supplies					
2 Verify physician's orders					
3 Wash hands/PPE					
4 Identify patient					
5 Explain procedure					
6 Instruct patient in specimen collection					
7 Perform physical UA					
8 Perform chemical UA					
9 Dispose of contaminated supplies					
10 Wash hands					
11 Record results in patient chart					

Total Points Possible _____ Total Points Earned: _____

Start Time: _____ End Time: _____

Instructor Signature: _____ Date: _____

Student Signature: _____ Date: _____

Collection of Throat Culture and Rapid Strep Test Competency Check

Given all the equipment and supplies, the student will be required to perform, within 10 minutes, a throat culture and rapid strep test. A "0" in more than two areas or an overall score of less than 80% will require the procedure to be repeated for competency.

Points to Be Awarded:	5 pts	2.5 pts	1 pt	0 pts	total pts
1 Assemble equipment and supplies					
2 Verify physician's orders					
3 Identify patient					
4 Explain procedure					
5 Wash hands/don PPE					
6 Position the patient					
7 Collect specimen					
8 Select site					
9 Invert tube to activate preservative					
10 Label tube—complete requisition					
11 Bring reagents to room temperature					
12 Remove test well, or cuvette from pouch					
13 Place recommended solution in well or cuvette					
14 Wait specified time					
15 Compare color reaction—patient and controls					
16 Disinfect work area/dispose of contaminated supplies					
17 Wash hands					
18 Record results in patient chart					

Total Points Possible: _____   Total Points Earned: _____

Start Time: _____   End Time: _____

Instructor Signature: _____   Date: _____

Student Signature: _____   Date: _____

Skin Test Competency Check

Given all the equipment and supplies, the student will be required to perform, within 10 minutes, a skin test. A "0" in more than two areas or an overall score of less than 80% will require the procedure to be repeated for competency.

Points to Be Awarded:	5 pts	2.5 pts	1 pt	0 pts	total pts
1 Assemble equipment and supplies					
2 Verify physician's orders					
3 Wash hands/don PPE					
4 Identify patient					
5 Explain procedure					
6 Position the patient					
7 Draw 0.1 mL of NaCl (sterile water) (*This would be diluted antigen if not practicing*)					
8 Select site					
9 Clean site					
10 Insert needle					
11 Aspirate to check for blood					
12 Inject NaCl—creating a 6 to 10 mm wheal					
13 Withdraw needle					
14 Do not apply pressure or bandage					
15 Dispose of sharps and contaminated supplies					
16 Wash hands					
17 Record results in patient chart					

Total Points Possible: _____ Total Points Earned: _____

Start Time: _____ End Time: _____

Instructor Signature: _____ Date: _____

Student Signature: _____ Date: _____

STUDY AND REVIEW EXERCISES

Defining Key Terms

Write the definition for each of the following key terms.

1) 2-hour postprandial (2-hour pp) _____

2) acidosis _____

3) alkalosis _____

4) atherosclerosis _____

5) BUN _____

6) calibrator _____

7) chain of custody _____

8) cholesterol _____

9) clarity _____

10) culture and sensitivity (C&S) _____

11) electrolytes _____

12) fasting blood sugar (FBS) _____

13) glucose tolerance test (GTT) _____

14) glucosuria _____

15) hematocrit _____

16) hematuria _____

17) hemoglobin _____

18) hemoglobinuria _____

19) hemostasis _____

20) high-density lipoprotein cholesterol (HDL) _____

21) hyperglycemic _____

22) hyperkalemia _____

23) hypoglycemic _____

24) hypokalemia _____

25) human chorionic gonadotrophin (HCG) _____

26) intradermal _____

27) ketonuria _____

28) low-density lipoprotein cholesterol (LDL)_____

_____

29) occult _____

30) pCO$_2$ _____

31) pH _____

32) point-of-care tests (POCT) _____

33) proteinuria_____

34) prothrombin _____

35) renal calculi_____

36) sediment_____

37) therapeutic_____

38) thromboplastin _____

39) transparency_____

40) turbidity _____

Reviewing Key Points

1) List the primary regulatory agencies associated with waived laboratory tests.

2) Describe the procedure to perform a microhematocrit.

3) Describe the chain of custody process when collecting a forensic specimen.

4) Define CLIA-waived laboratory tests.

5) What are the reference value ranges for a fasting blood glucose level?

Sentence Completion

1) The _____ were created in 1988 and implemented in 1993.

2) _____ of equipment is the process whereby the equipment is adjusted and realigned to operate within the normal value ranges.

3) A _____ is inserted into the cholesterol analyzer in much the same way as a test strip is inserted into the glucose analyzer.

4) The _____ test is performed to monitor oral anticoagulation therapy.

5) A _____ measures the volume of a patient's red blood cells as a percentage in relationship to the plasma in a predetermined amount of whole blood.

6) _____ are the measurement of a patient's pH, pCO_2, and PO_2 levels.

7) When performing a skin test 0.1 mL of a diluted antigen is injected _____. The most common skin test is called a PPD and is test for tuberculosis.

8) Physical characteristics of a urine specimen include _____, appearance, clarity, odor, and foam.

9) The most common electrolytes measured by POCT are sodium, potassium, _____, bicarbonate ion, and ionized calcium.

10) Blood-glucose levels are most commonly performed to aid in diagnosis and management of diabetes mellitus in which patients are _____.

Multiple Choice

1) Freshly voided urine will have a distinctive _____ odor.
   A. putrid
   B. aromatic
   C. fruity
   D. ammonia

2) Albumin detected in the urine is found in a condition called:
   A. hyperkalemia
   B. glucosuria
   C. proteinuria
   D. ketonuria

3) Drug testing procedures require that the special donor preparation and collection procedures defined by _____ be followed exactly.
   A. CLIA
   B. CDC
   C. NCCLS
   D. NIDA

4) The ACT analysis is performed by collecting what color top tube, which contains a clot-enhancing substance such as silica?
   A. Gray
   B. Red
   C. Lavender
   D. Green

5) When performing a _____ a small incision is made in the patient's forearm and the blood is blotted at 30 second intervals.
   A. PTT
   B. pro time test
   C. GTT
   D. bleeding time test

6) _____ levels are performed to aid in the diagnosis and treatment of anemias.
   A. HGB
   B. HCT
   C. PTT
   D. ACT

7) A _____ test is performed after the patient has fasted for 12 hours and then given a commercially prepared drink.
   A. PTT
   B. GTT
   C. ACT
   D. HCT

8) _____ functions in the manufacturing of bile acids and the production of hormones and helps to keep the skin waterproof.
   A. Keratin
   B. Ketone
   C. Cholesterol
   D. Bilirubin

9) _____ is primarily found within the cells of the tissue; it is only released into the blood when cells are damaged. It plays a major role in nerve conduction, muscle contraction, and acid-base balance.
   A. Sodium
   B. Bicarbonate ion
   C. Ionized calcium
   D. Potassium

10) A(n) _____ requires that detailed documentation tracks a forensic specimen from the time of collection until the results are reported.
   A. itinerary
   B. bill of lading
   C. chain of custody
   D. writ of transportation

Critical Thinking

1) The laboratory that you work for has requested that you perform an off-site drug collection for cause (an accident has occurred). You arrive at the company and are shown to the lavatory that you are to use for the collection. Describe the process of preparing the lavatory before you can begin the collection.

2) The physician has ordered that a modified Ivy bleeding time be performed on Mrs. King prior to surgery. You identify the patient and gather the supplies. What questions will you ask Mrs. King before beginning the procedure? What, if any, information will you tell her about the test?

Professional Communication Skills

CHAPTER
14

KEY TERMS

articulate
code-blue
communication
cultural diversity
customer
distress
empathy
ethics
eustress
integrity
kinesics (kih-**NEE**-six)
professionalism
standards

OBJECTIVES

Upon completion of this chapter the student should be able to:

- Define and correctly spell each of the key terms.
- Identify and demonstrate the correct techniques for verbal and nonverbal communication.
- Demonstrate and explain the criteria for being a "good listener."
- Describe the appropriate methods for answering the telephone.
- Demonstrate the ability to accurately record a telephone message.
- Define cultural diversity and identify the phlebotomist's role in communicating across cultures.
- List and describe the five stages of grief, providing examples of each stage.
- Describe the procedures for do-not-resuscitate orders and a code-blue.
- Identify methods for keeping healthy as a health care provider.
- Describe techniques to manage time and stress.
- Outline the procedures for problem solving and conflict resolution.
- Describe the phlebotomist's role in providing client/patient customer service.

● INTRODUCTION

The most important skill that a successful health care provider can possess is the ability to interact compassionately with patients, clients, and their families. This is often not an inherent trait, but a skill that is developed. A well-trained phlebotomist will not only be able to perform required technical procedures, but also be able to perform them while demonstrating professionalism, compassion, and empathy. The phlebotomist interacts with numerous people every day: patients, coworkers, supervisors, family members, and friends of the patient. Interactive communication skills are as important to the phlebotomist as venipuncture skills. In addition, bedside manner reflects directly on the facility employing the phlebotomist. The phlebotomist is a customer service agent for the laboratory and, as such, must always demonstrate a professional demeanor.

PROFESSIONALISM

The conduct, behavior, and qualities that characterize a professional person.

INTEGRITY

To adhere to a strict ethical code. To be in an undiminished or unimpaired state.

ETHICS

A system of principles governing medical conduct. It deals with the relationship of the health care professional to the patient, the patient's family, associates, and society at large.

STANDARDS

That which is established by custom or authority as a mode or rule for comparison of measurement.

● PROFESSIONALISM

Professionalism is the ability to perform work-related duties and responsibilities with a high degree of respect for the profession itself and for the client/customer. A professional phlebotomist exudes confidence, is appropriately attired, and demonstrates the ability to perform required tasks in a positive and caring manner. Personal **integrity**, the ability to do what is right even when no one is watching, and a positive attitude are integral components of professionalism. The phlebotomist must be caring and cheerful, dependable, even-tempered, polite, tactful, efficient, and calm while complying with the ethical standards set by society, the medical profession, and the employer.

Ethics are the **standards** that have been established to address the basic principles of right and wrong conduct. Hospitals and laboratories have established codes of ethics. The following list of principles are common to all medical codes of ethics:

- Do not intentionally harm anyone.
- Work within your scope of practice, using sound judgment, and act as any reasonable professional would act.
- Respect the rights of the patient (i.e., confidentiality, privacy, informed consent, and the right to refuse treatment).

VERBAL AND NONVERBAL COMMUNICATION

COMMUNICATION

Transmission of a message from a sender to a receiver.

Communication skills require two active participants: the person sending the message and the person receiving it. In the communication process, the sender communicates to the listener by symbol. The listener receives the symbols and interprets the sender's message. The messages can be sent either verbally or nonverbally. With today's technology both verbal and nonverbal communication can be transmitted in a variety of media. For example, the spoken word, music, facial expressions, touch, gestures, posture, appearance, and tone of voice can all be transmitted by direct physical contact or by high-tech media such as computers. Regardless of the mechanism of communication, for it to be effective, the listener must receive and understand it. We can send a message, but if the message is not understood in the manner in which it was meant, we have failed to communicate.

Verbal Communication

ARTICULATE

Distinct and clear enunciation of words, phrases, and sentences.

For effective verbal communication to take place, the sender of the message must be **articulate**. In other words, the sender must choose language that is appropriate and easily understood, use good diction, and enunciate each word, paying attention to tone and quality of voice. As a medical professional, the phlebotomist must remember that it is not necessary to impress the patient by using medical terms that may not be understood. Industry terminology used with coworkers, such as antecubital, hemostasis, hematoma, or even venipuncture, may not be understood by the patient and may be interpreted as something very frightening. *Use words to express, not impress.* Use terms that are appropriate for the age of your patient. For example, current trendy slang terms and language should never be used when communicating with an 82-year-old patient. In fact, slang terms and abbreviations should be avoided altogether. Be brief, concise, and accurate when presenting information and answering questions. For example, if a patient asks why you need to draw blood and the reason for the test, the best response is to tell the patient that the doctor has ordered laboratory tests to monitor and/or aid in the diagnosis of the patient's current condition. If the patient continues questioning, encourage the patient to discuss questions with the physician.

Another area to consider when communicating is how the message is presented. Use a strong clear voice and exude confidence. The tone of the phlebotomist's voice plays an important role as well. For example, the statement, "Ask your doctor," can be delivered and received in a variety of ways. If the phlebotomist's demeanor is friendly and helpful, the patient will perceive this communication in a positive manner. If the phlebotomist is grumpy or seemingly put out, the patient will receive this communication very differently. The phlebotomist's nonverbal communication contributes to the overall message and often has more effect than the words that are spoken.

Nonverbal Communication

If phlebotomists do not take pride in themselves, how is it possible to take pride in the profession, or to expect respect from others? How the phlebotomist physically presents herself is the first nonverbal communication. Most facilities require a certain dress code because they know that the physical impression their employees give establishes how future interactions with other health care providers will proceed. The phlebotomist is to be neat, clean, well-groomed, and have good posture. This communicates to the patient that the phlebotomist is confident and capable. Uniforms and/or lab coats must be clean and pressed and in good repair. Never wear anything that would distract or offend a patient. Duty shoes are to be clean and well-kept. Jewelry should be kept to a minimum. Use of perfume and cologne is discouraged. Hair should be neat and clean, with no extreme hairstyles or colors. It should be worn off the collar or pulled into a clip, ponytail, or braid. Nails must always be clean and well groomed. Particular attention is always paid to personal hygiene. Clean teeth, fresh breath, and use of antiperspirant/deodorant must be part of the phlebotomist's daily routine.

It has been stated that approximately 80% of all communication is nonverbal. Nonverbal communication is multidimensional and involves body movement, gestures, facial expression, eye contact, touch, use of space, and appearance. The most lasting nonverbal communication from the phlebotomist is a warm smile. Smiling sincerely conveys to the patient that you care.

The next important step in developing patient rapport is the nonverbal communication of establishing and maintaining eye contact. It tells the patient that the phlebotomist cares enough to recognize the patient as an individual and not just another case. Making eye contact with a patient should be done on eye level. It is unprofessional and intimidating to patients to have the health care provider looking down on them. When explaining procedures or giving a patient instruction, sit down, especially if the patient is in a hospital bed or wheelchair.

Be sure that gestures match the spoken word. People trust nonverbal communication messages over the spoken word, especially when the two conflict. If the phlebotomist walks into a patient's room smiling and with a sweet disposition, but continuously looks at his or her watch and looks around the room while the patient is speaking, the patient will receive the message that the phlebotomist does not truly care about his or her feelings and only wants to be done with the chore of caring for the patient.

Not only does the phlebotomist communicate with the patient nonverbally, but she can also learn a great deal about the patient by watching for nonverbal communication clues. Often the patient's expression will describe how he or she is feeling even when the patient says he feels fine. The study of body language is called **kinesics**.

KINESICS

Systematic study of the body and the use of its static and dynamic position as a means of communication.

Medicine is a contact profession. Generally, patients appreciate being touched in a thoughtful and caring manner by a medical professional. Touching can be a comforting means of nonverbal communication (e.g., holding a patient's hand through a particularly painful procedure). However, not all patients are comfortable with being touched. The phlebotomist must be sensitive to the patient's needs. It is impossible to perform a venipuncture without touching the patient. Establishing a favorable rapport in the beginning will lessen the patient's apprehension about being touched with a needle. Communicating effectively will comfort the patient. Verbally communicate to the patient what is to be expected at each step of the procedure, and ask for permission before touching.

Learning to Be a Good Listener

As a phlebotomist you must be ready to actively listen. There is a big difference between hearing and listening. Hearing is the result of sound waves hitting the eardrums and the brain processing the sound into language. Listening is the result of understanding the words and taking action or responding appropriately. Everyone has at one time or another pretended to listen. Do not make this mistake with patients. Valuable information will be missed, and a lack of interest and caring will be the message communicated.

The average person can absorb approximately 500 to 600 words per minute. The average speaking rate is 120 to 150 words per minute. Therefore, the average person has time to "wander off" when someone is speaking. Studies have shown that the average listener retains and comprehends only about 25% of what has been said. Active listening requires concentration and skill, and when these skills are applied, the phlebotomist can increase comprehension and retention of information. To actively listen, the phlebotomist gives the patient his undivided attention, acknowledges the message sent, and offers an appropriate response or takes the appropriate action. This is accomplished by first staying focused on the patient and not allowing distractions to interrupt. Acknowledgement of the message can occur by a simple nod of the head, direct eye contact, or a verbal response that the message was heard. The phlebotomist should summarize in his own words, what the patient has said, asking the patient questions for further clarification as needed.

Other Considerations in Health Care Communication

Communication between a health care provider and a patient is often more complicated than in other situations. The patient may be frightened, ill, or suffering. Patients commonly reach out for comfort and reassurance through conversation. The phlebotomist must respond to patients in a calm and respectful manner, using a communication style that includes trust, empowerment, and empathy.

When a person is ill, several emotional responses may occur. The patient may feel a loss of control and this feeling may permeate the individual's sense of well-being. The human psyche needs to feel some control over the decisions that are made. Illness may take away the ability to perform "normal" daily functions. The patient's physician may order frightening tests or procedures, or the patient may hear she is to be admitted to the hospital, where complete care will be transferred to the health care system. The patient may begin to feel helpless and that all control has been taken away, and may act in anger or respond by refusing a procedure or test. The phlebotomist who is patient, takes time to allow the patient to assimilate information, and gives the patient the opportunity to participate in decisions, will gain the patient's cooperation. If a patient can participate in decision making, she may feel enough gain of control to agree to necessary tests and procedures. Empowering a patient to make the right decisions about health care is a responsibility that belongs as much to the phlebotomist as to the patient's other health care providers. Allowing a patient to participate in health care decisions aids the healing process.

Patients do best when they believe that their health care providers are giving the best possible care. This trust must be established early in the health care provider/patient relationship. It is more difficult for the phlebotomist who spends only a minimal amount of time with a patient to establish a trusting relationship. However, it must be done. When the phlebotomist acts in a professional, confident manner, great strides are made in establishing this trust level.

Empathy is defined as an objective awareness of and insight into the feelings, emotions, and behaviors of another person. Empathy is not the same as sympathy. With empathy, one substitutes oneself for the other person. By putting himself in the patient's shoes and trying to understand how difficult it is to be ill, the phlebotomist may be able to provide the necessary support. A patient needs a supportive health care provider who will listen with an empathetic ear. Patients do not want, nor do they need, someone to feel sorry for them or to react out of sympathy. Allow the patient to express concerns and fears. Talking helps to validate the patient's feelings, and gives the patient a sense of control.

Never label your patients with their conditions, such as "the gallbladder in room 203" or "the diabetic in room 112." Labeling belittles the patient and hinders the healing process. Patients need to feel that their health care providers acknowledge them as unique individuals. Each patient has special requirements, wants, and needs, and these cannot be addressed if the patient is a nonperson, or "the case in room 203." It is the phlebotomist's responsibility to assure the patient that his or her personal desires are met.

Barriers to Effective Communication

One of the most frequent barriers to effective communication is the terminology of medicine itself. It is best to speak in terms that the patient will understand, but without talking down to the patient. Explain procedures thoroughly in lay terms.

A patient with a hearing impairment requires a different style of communication. Enunciate terms loudly and clearly. Depending on the degree of the impairment, a sign language translator may be necessary. The phlebotomist should write down all instructions and procedural directions for the hearing-impaired patient. Ensure that the patient understands the procedure thoroughly before beginning it. Allow the patient to ask questions, and confirm that he or she understands. If there is a concern about whether the patient understands a procedure, a patient advocate can be requested, or a family member or friend can be invited to be present.

Every patient has the right to informed consent. Non-English speaking patients and those for whom English is their second language have special concerns. Several geographic locations in the

EMPATHY

Objective awareness of and insight into the feelings, emotions, and behavior of another person.

CULTURAL DIVERSITY

The cultural identity of groups of people, their environments, ideas, values, traditions, institutions, and technologies.

United States are predominantly non-English speaking. For example, in rural Alaska, where Yupik is the predominant language of elder Alaskan natives, or in the southwestern United States, where Spanish is the predominant language spoken, it is beneficial to health care providers to learn the basics of the local language. Larger facilities that are located in these regions typically employ interpreters to assist non-English speaking patients. Some institutions provide basic requests and/or instructions printed in the predominant languages of the area. Often non-English speaking patients understand basic directions through the use of hand signals or sign language. Always treat the patient with respect, and honor the dignity of the patient. Practice principles of **cultural diversity**. Be certain that the patient understands the procedure completely before beginning. If learning the predominant, non-English language of the area, practice basic requests with a native speaker, as mispronunciation of terms may only further confuse patients.

A patient's state of health and level of consciousness play an important role in the communication process. Often, patients are heavily medicated or have altered levels of consciousness. These situations pose a special communication challenge. Explain instructions and procedures carefully, even if the patient appears unresponsive. Ask the patient's nurse or physician for clarification of status prior to invasive procedures.

The patient's comfort zone must also be taken into consideration. Each of us has an area or space around the body that we want others to respect. Invading a patient's comfort zone, or "space," may put the patient on the defensive and shut down communication by being too close. Some patients have a wide comfort zone, while others' are very limited. Comfort zones are also culturally based. Some cultures encourage speakers to stay very close to each other, while others require that a greater distance be maintained. Comfort zones are also related to gender. For example, negative past experiences may cause a female patient to feel uncomfortable with a male phlebotomist who she feels is invading her comfort zone.

Telephone and Computer Communication

The telephone is an essential communication tool and requires special communication consideration. The basic tenets of communication still apply; there is a message sender and a receiver. Of course, most nonverbal communication is unavailable. Only the sender's voice can communicate; personal emphasis cannot be added by a facial expression or the shrug of a shoulder. Enunciation of words, pitch, and voice quality become even more important than they are in face-to-face encounters. The phlebotomist should speak clearly, in a conversational tone of voice, neither too loudly nor too quietly, and convey confidence and warmth.

Even though most people have been using the telephone to communicate since childhood, there is a need to review the professional use of the telephone for the phlebotomist. Proper telephone etiquette is essential. Remember that the phlebotomist represents the employer's business; a client/patient may be gained or lost by your telephone manners. Telephone etiquette can be summed up in one phrase: *Be courteous*. Following these basic guidelines will lead to excellent telephone skills.

● Answering the telephone:

Answer the phone within a maximum of three rings. Before speaking—*smile*. Then keep the smile in your voice throughout the conversation. Treat the person on the other end of the line as you would treat a person standing in front of you. Be expressive; do not speak in a monotone. Be alert, attentive, and discreet. Use good listening skills and avoid slang.

Box 14-1: Avoid the Use of Slang

AVOID:	SAY INSTEAD:
"Huh?"	"I beg your pardon. I did not understand you" *or* "Would you repeat that please?"
"OK"	"Yes"
"Un-uh"	"Of course"
"Bye-bye"	"Goodbye"
"Yeah"	"Yes" *or* "Certainly"
"Nah"	"No"
"Watcha doin?"	"What are you doing?"
"Ya"	"You"

Greet the caller by acknowledging the time of day: "Good morning," "Good afternoon." Identify the employer: "County Hospital—Laboratory." Identify yourself: "Lori Parker." Ask what you can do for the caller: "How may I help you?"

● The conversation:

Obtain the caller's name early in the conversation. Write it down and use it at least three times during your conversation. If you cannot help the caller you must redirect the call.

● Answering multiple phone lines:

Answer all incoming calls in a timely manner by the third ring. Do not wait until you have finished with the first call to answer a second. Put the first caller on hold (using the guidelines below), answer the second call, and after you ask if you may put the caller on hold, return to the first call. If you suspect the first call may be lengthy, return to the additional callers and ask if you may take a message and return their calls. Give the callers an idea of how long it will be before the call is returned.

● Putting a caller on hold:

There are occasions when the caller must be put on hold. This is handled as follows:

1. Ask the caller if you may put him or her on hold.

2. Wait for a response.

3. Explain to the caller why you must put him or her on hold.

4. Thank the caller for holding when you return to the call.

● Taking a message:

There are occasions when the phlebotomist is required to take a phone message, for example, if the call is not for you and the person the call is intended for is unavailable. The following information is critical and must be recorded accurately when taking a message:

• The caller's name (spelled correctly). Ask the caller to spell his or her name if you cannot understand it or are uncertain of the spelling.

• Company name (as applicable).

• Telephone number (including area code if it is a long distance call).

• Time of call.

• Message (recorded exactly).

• Repeat all information back to the caller before hanging up.

Most facilities provide telephone message pads (Figure 14-1). Keep a pen or pencil and paper or phone message pad close to the telephone. Do not make a caller wait for you to find these supplies.

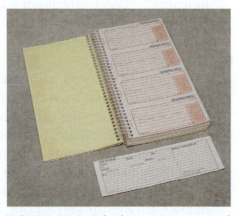

FIGURE 14-1: Telephone message pad

● End of call:

Always end the call on a positive note. Repeat any actions that you and the caller agreed to during the conversation. Ask the caller if you can do anything else for him or her. Tie up any loose ends. Thank the caller for calling. Let the caller hang up first, so that the caller is not accidentally hung up on mid-sentence. Write down important information immediately after ending the call.

● Phlebotomist telephone considerations:

Most facilities do not allow employees to make or receive personal telephone calls while they are on duty. Become familiar with your facility's policy regarding telephone usage immediately upon employment. Depending on the facility's protocols, the phlebotomist may or may not be allowed to give test results over the telephone. It is never appropriate to give patient information to anyone other than the patient, and for this reason, test results are typically not given to anyone over the phone. Some test results require interpretation and explanation, which is another reason why test results are not given over the phone. The phlebotomist is not usually allowed nor trained to give detailed explanations of test results. Giving a patient test results borders on diagnosing, which the phlebotomist is not legally allowed to do.

Computers have become an essential communication tool in the medical laboratory. Most medical facilities, including hospitals and smaller independently owned laboratories, use the computer to communicate with other medical facilities or to communicate with other departments within the facility. The rules of communication and etiquette apply to all computer use, whether within the facility or for outside communication. Computer skills are discussed in Chapter 5.

CULTURAL DIVERSITY

The world's population is incredibly diverse. Patients come from all walks of life and every background. How does cultural diversity affect the phlebotomist and the delivery of health care? The phlebotomist must understand that cultural differences exist, and must strive to respond appropriately to all patients. More than 100 languages are spoken in the school systems in New York, Chicago, and Los Angeles. Over 30 million people in the United States speak English as their second language. The point is not that we must learn to speak multiple languages, but that we must realize just how diverse our world is, and treat all people (regardless of their language or ethnicity) with consideration and respect.

Even though the world is diverse, we usually respond to individuals (regardless of their culture) as if we are all from the same culture. We often assume that everyone thinks and behaves in the same manner as we do. We are conditioned to do this from childhood, and most of our conditioning or learned behavior exists on a subconscious level. We are not even aware that we have expectations about how people should behave, but they are there. On an intellectual level we may recognize this, but often intellect is no match for a lifetime of conditioning. To break this conditioning, we must first develop an understanding of cultural differences and then understand how our individual beliefs relate. The phlebotomist must be sensitive to the cultural needs of patients. These may be tied to religious beliefs as well. For example, the patient who does not wish to have medical intervention of any kind because of religious beliefs will experience having blood drawn as a violation. Or perhaps the patient's culture uses Eastern medicine, and the patient would rather have acupuncture than pain medication. In such situations, the patient's wishes must be honored. Many large medical facilities have bioethics committees that make decisions about when Western medical intervention should occur or be withheld. These are not decisions that can be made by the phlebotomist. When in doubt about your role, defer to the patient's nurse or physician. The most important point to remember is that all patients deserve to be treated with the utmost respect.

DEATH AND DYING

The phlebotomist will very likely establish professional relationships with and provide services to patients who are terminally ill or near death. Death, however, is a part of life and an experience we all face. Accepting the fact that death is a natural result of the life process and does not necessarily reflect failure of the health care delivery system may help the phlebotomist to respond to patients' needs in a more caring manner. Elderly patients with significant health problems may be expecting death and look forward to the release from pain, loneliness, and suffering. The death of a younger patient may be more difficult for health care providers and the patient's family to accept. Each person deals with dying differently and does not follow the same steps in grieving. The phlebotomist will not only interact with the patient, but also with the patient's family and friends who may be visiting the patient.

If the phlebotomist finds a patient who is unconscious and unresponsive, she is to first notify the nurse, who will call a **code-blue**. Unless the phlebotomist is assigned specific duties in the resuscitation effort, she should remain calm and stay out of the way. The phlebotomist should be prepared to assist, if asked, and/or help other patients in the room.

Some patients will have do-not-resuscitate (DNR) orders, requesting that they do not receive any heroic measures if they need to be resuscitated. However, unless a DNR order is in the patient's chart, every effort must be made to resuscitate the patient. A phlebotomist who is trained in Basic Life Support—cardiopulmonary resuscitation (BLS-CPR)—may be called on to assist with resuscitation.

Stages of Grieving

Patients who are aware that they are dying will progress through a series of steps called the stages of grief. Their families will progress through these stages as well. These stages of grief are outlined by Elizabeth Kubler-Ross, a psychiatrist who has done extensive work on the grieving process. The stages of grief are set forth in her book, *On Death and Dying,* published by Macmillan. The stages include:

● Denial
● Anger
● Bargaining
● Depression
● Acceptance

CODE-BLUE

A coded message broadcast over a hospital's public address system. Code-blue indicates the need for an emergency team to respond to a patient in cardiac or respiratory arrest.

Box 14-2: Stages of Grief

● Denial	Person refuses to accept the truth. The patient may say, "I'm too young to die" or "I'm sure that they will find a cure."
● Anger	Patient may act out feelings, directing anger to caregivers and family. The patient may say, "I don't deserve this. How could God [or nature, or my doctor] do this to me?"
● Bargaining	The patient attempts to "make deals" for remission or for more time to live. The patient may pray and say, "If you will only let me live, I promise to be a better person, give to charity, or stop drinking."

(continues)

Box 14-2: Stages of Grief *(continued)*

● Depression   The patient comes to the realization that the situation cannot change and feels saddened over things that will be left unfinished. When bargaining fails, depression sets in. The patient reviews his or her life and may feel sad about all the things that were done or not done. The patient mourns losses and begins to move into the last phase, acceptance.

● Acceptance   The patient recognizes that death is part of life. The patient is calmer and more in control. The patient may start to put his or her affairs in order. The patient may begin to make funeral arrangements and give away personal belongings.

Some patients will progress through these stages in an orderly fashion and reach the acceptance stage as a natural part of life. Others will never reach the acceptance level, but will stop at another stage. Some patients will jump around and may go back and forth through the phases before experiencing acceptance. Remember, this experience is not the same for everyone.

As a health care provider, it is critical that feelings about death and the phlebotomist's own mortality be examined. When the phlebotomist first encounters patients who are dying, the experience can be frightening and stressful. This is especially true if the phlebotomist has worked with the patient over a long period of time, or if the patient is a young person. With time, experience, and personal growth, it becomes easier to be supportive and caring.

There is no way for the phlebotomist to completely prepare for the first experience of a patient's death. The following are suggestions that may help:

● Talk with friends, family, and other medical professionals about your feelings about life and death.
● Discuss your feelings about death with a member of your spiritual affiliation.
● Give yourself permission to grieve, to feel sad, and to express those feelings.
● Understand that over the course of time and with experience, the task becomes easier.
● Offer physical support to the patient's visitors. Become familiar with community resources so that you can provide directions to meetings, or the names and telephone numbers of support groups.

KEEPING THE HEALTH CARE PROVIDER HEALTHY

The phlebotomist working in medical facilities will be exposed to a variety of conditions that may pose health risks to him. It is important that the phlebotomist maintain a healthy lifestyle. Get plenty of sleep (8 hours per night), eat balanced, nutritious meals, drink plenty of water (8 glasses per day), and exercise. Having a healthy lifestyle boosts the immune system and lessens the risk of contracting illnesses. Managing time effectively, managing stress, and learning effective ways to solve problems all contribute to maintaining health and strengthening job performance.

Time Management

Life is hectic. We rarely take time to do such things as sit back and enjoy a sunny afternoon with a good book and a cool glass of lemonade. Work schedules, family responsibilities, and household chores keep us busy. How do we balance all these responsibilities? The answer is time management. The phlebotomist can start by investing in a daily planner. Planners come in a variety of shapes and sizes and can be as simple as a monthly wall calendar, or considerably more complex such as a hand-held computer. It is helpful before making a purchase to make a list of your needs. Do you need to keep track of your work schedule and your personal address book, or will you also need to keep track of your children's or supervisor's schedules? Does your address book need to include work contacts as well as personal contacts? Do you need a "Things to Do" section, or a means to track work priorities? All of these, and possibly other needs, must be addressed.

Once you have selected a planner that will accommodate your particular needs, matrix it. In other words, fill in all the addresses and telephone numbers you want to have handy. Fill in commitments that do not change throughout the year, such as birthdays and anniversaries. Then fill in your work schedule and regularly scheduled events that your children or others in your life may have. For example, you may have regularly scheduled staff in-service training the second Wednesday of every month or your child's hockey practice every Monday night. Once these are entered, make a list of all the tasks that must be accomplished every month, every week, and every day, and allot the same time each week to accomplish these tasks. For example, do your laundry every Saturday afternoon from 1:00 to 4:00. Walk your dog from 6:00 to 6:30 every morning. Now that you have accounted for all your "Must Do's," schedule in recreational time, time for friends and family, and schedule time just for you. You will be surprised at just how much "extra" time you do have.

Stress Management

Stress is a constant element in our day-to-day lives, both at work and at home. **Eustress** is healthy or manageable stress and is considered good stress. **Distress** is abnormal, unhealthy, or extreme stress and is considered to not be good. Eustress consists of happy events that still cause us stress, such as a wedding, the birth of a child, or a promotion at work. This type of stress can help motivate us to achieve, to win, and to succeed. However, even eustress can become distress if not managed effectively.

All stress can cause physiologic changes in the human body, such as elevated blood pressure, increased heart rate, increased respiration rate, increased body metabolism, and increased blood flow to the muscles. This is the "fight or flight" response discussed in Chapter 3—Anatomy and Physiology. If we are unable to cope with stress, it can literally incapacitate us and make us ill. Rest usually helps us to return to a normal state, but even rest will not completely restore an individual who has been stressed at high levels for long periods of time. Like a rubber band that has been stretched too tight for too long, that individual may never completely return to normal. In addition to the health care professional's personal stress, he or she also works with patients who are stressed. This can add to the health care professional's stress, creating a vicious cycle. The health care professional must be able to recognize his or her own stress and effectively manage it, before being able to help patients manage their stress. The following are suggestions for lowering stress levels:

● Manage time efficiently.
● Learn and practice relaxation techniques, such as deep breathing exercises or "minivacations."

EUSTRESS

A term used to describe normal, healthy, or manageable stress.

DISTRESS

Physical or mental pain or suffering. A term used to describe abnormal, unhealthy, or extreme stress.

Box 14-3: Minivacation

An excellent way to relieve stress and tension is to take minivacations throughout the day. Find a quiet place where you can take a 10-minute break without being interrupted or disturbed. If possible, dim the lights. Sit in a comfortable chair with both feet on the ground in front of you. Rest your hands on the arms of the chair or on your lap. Close your eyes, take three deep breaths from your belly up, inhaling through your nose and exhaling through your mouth to the count of six. Visualize your favorite vacation spot; it could be a sandy beach, with the sound of the water lapping at the shore, the sun warming your barefoot toes; or it could be a mountain stream surrounded by pine trees and wildflowers; or perhaps you could imagine yourself riding a camel through the Sahara desert. Pick whatever spot holds a happy and relaxing memory for you. You can also borrow the memory of a favorite vacation spot or make one up. See yourself relaxing and enjoying the scenery. Try to incorporate as many of your senses as possible. Be aware of the sounds surrounding you, the smells, the tastes, and what you see. Feel yourself relax; allow all the tension of the day to be released, perhaps through your barefoot toes out into the warm sand. Once you have established your spot, you will be able to return as frequently as you like. If you are nervous about falling asleep and not getting back to work on time, set a timer.

- Eat nutritious foods and exercise regularly. Talking a 10-minute walk greatly reduces stress.
- Give yourself permission to have "alone" time.
- Read interesting books or articles just for fun.

Take time every day to concentrate on reducing your stress levels. Take your stress "temperature." Depending on where the level is, take appropriate steps to lower the level.

Problem Solving

Conflicts occasionally arise in any work situation. The professional phlebotomist understands this and is able to utilize problem-solving techniques to resolve conflicts smoothly and quickly. The steps of problem solving include:

- Defining the problem in a nonthreatening way. Never place blame.
- Identifying all possible solutions—"brainstorming." Do not evaluate possible solutions at this point, just explore as many options as you can.
- Evaluating options that are satisfactory to both parties involved in the conflict.
- Deciding on an acceptable solution.
- Implementing the solution.
- Evaluating the effectiveness of the solution after it has been implemented for a time.

When the conflict involves another party, which most conflicts do, take the following steps:

- Listen without judgment to the other party's position. Use all the listening skills previously covered in this chapter.
- Sincerely try to understand the other party's position.
- Summarize to the other party what you have heard.
- Clearly state your position, and explain why you feel the way you do.
- Ask the other person to explain why he or she feels the way he does.
- Summarize and come to an agreement on what your differences really are. You many only agree to disagree.

Part of your responsibility as a health care provider is to keep the lines of communication open and to provide patients with a safe and comfortable environment to facilitate healing. Resolve conflict quickly and move on to more positive, uplifting endeavors.

) CLIENT/PATIENT CUSTOMER SERVICE

CUSTOMER

A person, patient, or client to whom goods are delivered or services are rendered.

Customer service is an integral part of every profession, and phlebotomy is no exception. The dictionary definition of a **customer** denotes a person with whom one has dealings. The phlebotomist interacts with customers daily: patients, patients' families and friends, physicians, and coworkers. Customer service is an art and is essential to every successful business, including health care. In providing excellent customer service, attitude is everything. It is not just giving the customer what he or she wants, but giving the customer more than is expected. For example, you may be the most efficient phlebotomist on staff, able to collect blood every time; there has not been a vein you could not hit. However, if in addition to this exceptional service you perform your task with a smile and an empathetic ear, then you have offered exceptional customer service.

) SUMMARY

The ability to communicate effectively begins with a few easy steps. Learn to be a good listener. Speak on a level that your patient will understand. Be empathetic, respect your patient's needs, allow for the grieving process, and take steps to keep yourself healthy.

STUDY AND REVIEW EXERCISES
Defining Key Terms
Write the definition for each of the following key terms.

1) articulate_____

2) code-blue _____

3) cultural diversity_____

4) communication _____

5) customer_____

6) distress _____

7) empathy _____

8) ethics _____

9) eustress_____

10) integrity _____

11) kinesics _____

12) professionalism_____

13) standards _____

Reviewing Key Points

1) Identify methods for keeping healthy as a phlebotomist.

2) List the criteria for being a good listener.

3) Describe the procedure for responding to an unresponsive patient with a "DNR" order in the chart.

4) Identify three key points relating to client/patient customer service.

5) List the information that must be included in an accurate telephone message.

Sentence Completion

1) _____ involves the transmission of a message from a sender to a receiver.

2) _____ is a term used to describe abnormal, unhealthy, or extreme stress.

3) If the phlebotomist finds a patient who is unresponsive, not breathing, and without a pulse, a _____ will be broadcast over the hospital public address system, indicating an emergency response team should respond to the patient's room.

4) The phlebotomist should display _____ towards a patient.

5) _____ is the ability to perform work-related duties and responsibilities with a high degree of respect for the profession itself and for the client/customer.

Multiple Choice

1) Facial expressions are a method of _____ communication.
   A. long-distance
   B. verbal
   C. nonverbal
   D. expressive

2) Which of the following should *not* be part of the phlebotomist's daily routine?
   A. Bathing
   B. Use of perfume or cologne
   C. Use of deodorant
   D. Brushing teeth

3) The average person can absorb approximately _____ words per minute, but can speak at a rate of _____ words per minute.
   A. 500 to 600, 120 to 150
   B. 300 to 400, 120 to 150
   C. 500 to 600, 100 to 120
   D. 300 to 400, 100 to 120

4) What type of listening means that we are not only listening but are responding to the speaker's communication by letting the speaker know that we have understood?
   A. Passive
   B. Active
   C. Aggressive
   D. Interactive

5) Which one of the following is a barrier to effective communication?
   A. English as a second language
   B. Hearing impairments
   C. Patient's level of consciousness
   D. All the above

6) Which element of communication is absent when communicating via the telephone?
   A. Sender
   B. Receiver
   C. Verbal
   D. Nonverbal

7) The telephone must be answered in a minimum of _____ rings.
   A. 1
   B. 2
   C. 3
   D. 4

8) Of the following, which is not a vital piece of information to obtain when taking a phone message?
   A. Name
   B. DOB
   C. Phone number
   D. Date

9) Which one of the following does not usually enter into the stages of grief?
   A. Denial
   B. Anger
   C. Depression
   D. Joy

10) An event such as the birth of a child, a wedding, or a promotion at work causes what type of stress?
   A. Eustress
   B. Distress
   C. Emstress
   D. Astress

Critical Thinking

1) Mrs. Killian is a 45-year-old mother of three. She has just been diagnosed with terminal cancer. She has been hospitalized and you are to "draw" labs from her this morning. When you arrive she is crying hysterically, with her 8-year-old daughter wrapped in her arms. The child looks at you with obvious confusion and fear in her wide-eyed stare. Describe the stages of grief the mother and daughter are in and what you as the phlebotomist can do.

2) You have orders to draw labs on the patient in room 313. Mr. Hiljardo speaks no English and you do not speak Spanish. Describe how you will gain informed consent to draw his blood.

Employment Skills

OBJECTIVES

Upon completion of this chapter the student should be able to:

- Define and correctly spell each of the key terms.
- Create a career marketing plan.
- Identify the three main steps in outlining a career marketing plan.
- Identify your skills or market value.
- Define the three different types of skills and give examples of each.
- Identify your potential employment obstacles and describe methods to overcome them.
- Describe the steps of organizing your job search.
- Identify methods used to research potential companies/organizations.
- Define and describe networking.
- List common networking errors.
- Demonstrate the ability to present a professional image.
- Demonstrate the ability to write a resume and cover letter.
- Correctly complete a job application.
- Demonstrate the ability to interview for employment.
- Describe the actions of follow-up after an interview.

OUTLINE

- Introduction
- Marketing Plan
- Product Analysis
- Market Analysis
- Product Presentation

❶ INTRODUCTION

You have now finished studying all the specific technical skills involved in becoming a phlebotomy technician. You have had an opportunity to practice blood draws and become proficient at point-of-care testing. You have learned medical terminology, how hospitals and laboratories are set up, medicolegal issues, OSHA standards, emergency procedures, and everything in between. Now it is time for the most important step: finding employment.

Marketing Plan

The first step in finding a job is setting a goal to get a job. This may seem obvious. Of course you want a job; you just went through months of training to achieve just that. However, you might be surprised at how many graduates complete training programs and never work in their profession. Finding the perfect job does not happen by chance, it takes dedication and hard work on your part. You might say that finding that perfect job is a job by itself. Start by taking a 3×5 card like those you have been diligently using as study cards, and write in large letters across the top, *"I have the perfect job for me."* Underneath this statement make a list of all the conditions that make the job perfect for you. Keep this card with you throughout your job search. Read it every day. Picture yourself working at your perfect job. Imagine what your coworkers and supervisor(s) will be like, what you will wear, how much money you will make, what benefits you will have, and so forth. The more details you can imagine, the better. Now that you can really see yourself working at your perfect job, it is time to put your career-marketing plan together.

Career marketing is what you do to provide prospective employers a positive presentation (sales) of your strengths (skills), using verbal and nonverbal communication skills to generate interest and motivate an employer to offer you a position.

Because finding a job is a job, it is important to have a career-marketing plan, which is an outline of what steps to take to become employed. There are three main steps:

1. Product Analysis
   - Identifying your skills or **market value**.
   - Identifying your potential employment obstacles.
2. Market Analysis
   - Researching the company/organization.
   - **Networking**.
   - Generating job leads.
   - Scanning the classified and job ads.

MARKET VALUE

What a product (you) is worth to the consumer (employer); characteristics and skills that are valuable in the employment market.

NETWORKING

Meeting with people you know, or have just met, to discuss your career plans.

3. Product Presentation
   - Presenting a professional image.
   - Writing the perfect resume and cover letter.
   - Completing the application.
   - Interviewing.
   - Follow-up.
   - Staying employed.

Let's examine each of these in detail.

● PRODUCT ANALYSIS

Society teaches us not to speak highly of ourselves in public. If you do, you are labeled a braggart or egotistical, two traits not often admired. However, when you are in the job market you must exhibit confidence and communicate a high level of self-esteem. You must tell the possible future employer why you are the best person for the job. You must "sell" your skills and knowledge. This might be a little easier if you think of yourself as a product. Do you believe in what you are saying about the strengths of that product? If you do, you will present the product with a natural ease and enthusiasm and the end result will be a win/win situation. Learn to be flexible, take risks, and to not be afraid of the word "no." Do not take a "no" as a personal rejection. The best person is not always hired. Buyers do not always purchase the right or best product. Learn something from the experience that you can use. Keep trying despite any temporary setbacks.

Identifying Your Skills or Market Value

The first step in preparing to sell any product is to know the product's strengths and weaknesses. You need to examine your personal work, life, and educational experiences to identify your strengths (skills) and weaknesses (employment obstacles). Remember that employers only want to hire self-assured applicants who can talk about their skills and what they can offer a company. What are the positive qualities (skills) you have to offer a prospective employer? These skills should include past work experiences, education, training, or attitude-related characteristics. Always be honest with yourself in order to be honest with the employer.

3-T'S

Training—Transferable skills—Traits

TRAITS

Personal attributes, characteristics, and/or behavior that you consistently demonstrate and that describe you (e.g., cheerful, outgoing, hard working).

Three Types of Skills—3-T's (see Box 15-5)

1. Training/Education—(I learned how to do it):

    Knowledge that you acquire as a result of formal education and on-the-job training and formal education. Program diplomas and certification validate a proven level of knowledge and skill to a future employer. Examples of knowledge and skills include drawing blood, point-of-care testing, and medical terminology. Other examples could include first aid and basic life support for health care provider certification.

2. Transferable—(I have done it):

    General work-related skills that do not change from one job to another job; these skills transfer with you from job to job (Boxes 15-1 and 15-2). Use story examples to illustrate these skills. Examples include typing, account receivable/account payable skills, customer service, office skills, and management skills. The transferability of these skills includes the ability to work in an office with patients in stressful situations.

3. Traits—(I will fit in or adapt):

    ● Positive Personality **Traits**—Your attitude as determined through nonverbal communication. Examples of these are friendly, outgoing, cheerful, enthusiastic, thoughtful, methodical, slow to anger, patient, kind, and sincere (Boxes 15-3 and 15-4).

    ● How you do things—Examples of these qualities include hardworking, dependable, flexible, organized, and detail-oriented.

Identifying Your Potential Employment Obstacles

In almost every sales situation, customers will raise objections to the product. Customers want to buy the best product possible and be sure it will do what it says and will benefit them. If not addressed properly, these concerns about the product become reasons for not buying (hiring) the product (you).

Similarly, employers want to hire the most qualified and personable candidate who will "fit in" their office, department, or company. Employers will raise objections that are employment obstacles which you must prepare to overcome. Perhaps your grades were less than perfect while in school, or your attendance record has not been the best, and once, 10 years ago, you were fired from your job. Does this mean you are unemployable? Definitely not.

When you start the job-searching process it is just as important to make a list of your weaknesses as your strengths. Employers may ask some difficult questions during the interview process; it is best if you have verbally rehearsed your responses beforehand.

Box 15-1: Transferable Skills Assessment

Following is a list of transferable work skills. Indicate all the skills you have from the list by placing a Y (yes) or N (no) by each item.

Skills	Yes/No	Skills	Yes/No
Accounting	_____	Leadership	_____
Administrative	_____	Maintenance	_____
Analysis	_____	Management	_____
Artistic	_____	Marketing	_____
Audio-Visual	_____	Mechanical	_____
Budgeting	_____	Meeting Deadlines	_____
Cash Handling	_____	Meeting the Public	_____
Computer Skills	_____	Merchandising	_____
Consulting	_____	Negotiating	_____
Coordinating	_____	Operating Office Equip.	_____
Cost Analysis	_____	Organizing Projects	_____
Counseling	_____	Personnel	_____
Creating Displays	_____	Planning	_____
Customer Service	_____	Policy Writing	_____
Data Processing	_____	Public Speaking	_____
Designing	_____	Purchasing	_____
Equipment Maintenance	_____	Record Keeping	_____
Financial Planning	_____	Recruiting	_____
Food Preparation	_____	Research	_____
Fundraising	_____	Sales	_____
Inspecting	_____	Telephone Skills	_____
Instructing	_____	Written Communication	_____
Language Interpreting	_____		

Box 15-2: Transferable Skills Assessment—The Final Five

Now look at your list from Box 15-1 and the skills you marked with a Y. From all the transferable skills you marked with a Y, select a total of five that are the most accurate description of you and list them below. Next to each, write one example of when you used that skill.

1. _____
   _____

2. _____
   _____

3. _____
   _____

4. _____
   _____

5. _____
   _____

Box 15-3: Personal Traits Skills Assessment

Following is a list of traits. Determine if you have each trait. Place a Y by those you have and an N by those you lack.

Skills	Yes/No	Skills	Yes/No
Able to make a decision	_____	Imaginative	_____
Accepts supervision	_____	Intelligent	_____
Alert	_____	Learns quickly	_____
Assertive	_____	Loyal	_____
Attentive to details	_____	Mature	_____
Authentic	_____	Methodical	_____
Calm	_____	Modest	_____
Cheerful	_____	Motivated	_____
Committed to growth	_____	Open-minded	_____
Concentrates	_____	Optimistic	_____
Conscientious	_____	Orderly	_____
Cooperative	_____	Patient	_____
Courageous, risk-taker	_____	Persistent	_____
Curious	_____	Performs under stress	_____
Dependable	_____	Playful	_____
Diplomatic	_____	Poised	_____
Discreet	_____	Polite	_____
Dynamic	_____	Punctual	_____
Eager	_____	Reliable	_____
Efficient	_____	Resourceful	_____
Emotionally stable	_____	Responsible	_____
Energetic	_____	Self-confident	_____
Enthusiastic	_____	Self-controlled	_____
Expressive	_____	Self-respectful	_____
Flexible	_____	Sense of humor	_____
Friendly	_____	Sincere	_____
Generous	_____	Spontaneous	_____
Good judgment	_____	Tactful	_____
Hard worker	_____	Tidy	_____
Helpful	_____	Tolerant	_____
Honest	_____	Trustworthy	_____
Initiative	_____	Versatile	_____

Everyone has employment obstacles, and identifying yours is half the battle to win a job.

During a job search, you should first reduce the possibility of objections by creating the best image and impression possible. Second, during the interview, you must listen for and be prepared to respond quickly, positively, and briefly to employer concerns. Let us look at one example.

Box 15-4: Personal Traits Skills Assessment—The Final Five

Now look at your list from Box 15-3 and the traits you marked with a Y. From all the traits you marked with a Y, select a total of five that are the most accurate description of you and list them below. Next to each, write one example of when you used that trait.

1. _____
   _____

2. _____
   _____

3. _____
   _____

4. _____
   _____

5. _____
   _____

Box 15-5: Assessment Summary—Three T's

ASSESSMENT SUMMARY

Review the different types of skills (training, transferable, traits) that you acquired through working through Box 15-1 to 15-4. List these skills in the corresponding section of the triangle below.

THREE T'S

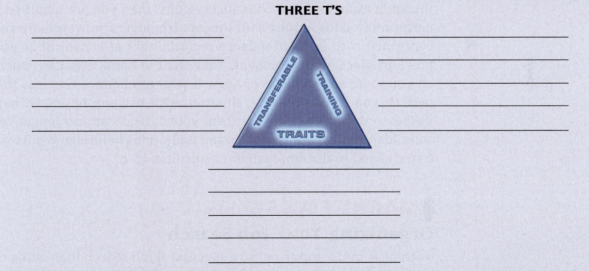

Using your skills triangle as an outline, develop a paragraph describing ". . .you should hire me for the position of phlebotomy technician because . . ."

Remember to include:

● Where you acquired these skills; prepare vivid, but brief, "success stories."
● Descriptions of how you acquired these skills.
● Qualities that make you different from other applicants.
● Why you want this position.
● What you will do for the company.

An employer may state, "You seem qualified, but you also seem a little too young for this position." The objection really is not your age, but whether or not you are mature and responsible enough to handle the job responsibilities. The best way to overcome this objection is to convince the interviewer that you are mature; support your claim by giving specific examples. You might say, "I am very mature for my age. Since the time I turned 14, I started to babysit. I have been responsible for children as young as 2 years old and handled one serious emergency situation. During this time, I received only praise concerning my performance. I will bring this same attitude of responsibility to this job."

Other obstacles to employment might be transportation, wardrobe, daycare, or illness. After you have made your personal list, eliminate all the obstacles you can; for example, how you will get to work if you do not have a car (will you take the bus or carpool). Perhaps you have daycare but they will not take your child if he or she is sick. You must have backup daycare with a provider who will care for your sick child. Your sister, mother, aunt, or close friend will usually help out in a pinch. Start planning your interviewing wardrobe before it is time to interview—not the day of the interview. As far as your grades are concerned, most employers expect that if you have graduated from an accredited program and have taken a national certification exam and passed it successfully, then you are qualified to perform the skills required for the job. Employers, however, are very concerned with your attendance record either at school or at your previous place of employment. They want to know they can depend on you to be on the job every day. If your attendance was less than perfect, you can correct the situation with makeup hours. Perhaps the reasons you were absent from your last job are no longer reasons. Identifying your obstacles and limitations beforehand puts you a step ahead in the employment game (Box 15-6).

● MARKET ANALYSIS
Organizing Your Job Search

Nothing is more important to a successful job search than being organized. First, you need to develop a daily and weekly job search schedule to stay on task. Second, you need to have a job search organizer to track the status of all your employer contacts.

● How much time should you spend looking for a job?

You need to spend as much time as necessary to get the job. Your goal should be between 25 and 40 hours a week. Remember that looking for a job is a job in and of itself.

Box 15-6: Obstacle Inventory

Obstacle Inventory Worksheet

In the column on the left-hand side, list all the potential objections you can think of that might come up during an interview. In the column to the right, write how you would overcome this objection. Examples are: age, gender, physical ailments, experience level, termination, job hopping, financial issues, relationship status, young children, no daycare, undependable transportation, arrests, and so forth.

(*Note:* Remember, these are not items you should bring up. They are things you should be aware of and ready to respond to in case they do come up during an interview.)

OBSTACLES   RESPONSE TO OVERCOME

_____   _____

_____   _____

_____   _____

_____   _____

_____   _____

_____   _____

_____   _____

_____   _____

_____   _____

_____   _____

_____   _____

_____   _____

_____   _____

_____   _____

_____   _____

_____   _____

_____   _____

- When is the best time to contact employers?

  The best days and times, from best to least effective, are listed in order below:
  - Tuesday through Friday mornings, 8:00–11:30 AM
  - Monday through Thursday afternoons, 1:00–4:30 PM
  - Monday morning, 8:00–11:30 AM, and Friday afternoon, 1:00–4:30 PM
  - Saturday morning and afternoons
- How should I organize my time?
  - Step 1—Purchase a daily planning calendar.
  - Step 2—Use the calendar to create a daily/weekly job search schedule.

    Mark out times during each day you will be spending on job search activities.
  - Step 3—Use a career search organizer.

    Create a form to write down and keep track of your entire employer contact list and the status of each contact.

Personal Marketing Card

One handy job-search tool you can create inexpensively for yourself is a personal marketing card (PMC) or mini-resume. The PMC is a 3 × 5 card with concise information typed on it relating to you and the position you desire. This card can be used in a variety of ways, such as a business card to introduce yourself to prospective employers. You can leave them with friends, post them on bulletin boards, leave them at businesses, attach them to applications, or leave them with an interviewer. This is a very inexpensive way to advertise your desires, skills, and contact information.

The following are guidelines for creating a personal marketing card:

- Type all information.
- Be concise—use short sentences.
- Be honest.
- Make everything relate to your job objective.
- Be positive.
- Write at length and then edit.
- Include your relevant education, training, transferable skills, and traits.

Example:

Percy Tonsil   Home: (555) 257-1643

                          Message: (555) 361-1754

Position: Phlebotomy Technician

Skills: *(These are job-related skills showing performance/results)

      *6 years experience customer service

      *1 year volunteer community hospital

      *Nationally Certified Phlebotomy Technician

      *Competent with Point-of-Care Testing

      *CPR Certified

      *Proficient at all methods of blood collection

      **(These are special conditions)

      **Will work any shifts

      ***(These are desirable work traits)

      ***Honest

      ***Reliable

      ***Well-organized

      ***Hardworking

Researching the Company/Organization

As you are developing your career-marketing plan, one of the first responsibilities is to do investigative work. Make a list of all the laboratories, hospitals, health care facilities and clinics in your area, check out the Internet, and use library resources. Contact local employers and personnel offices. Gather pertinent information about each company, such as how long it has been in business, size of the company/organization, salary ranges, days and hours of operation, different shifts, and so forth. When communicating with prospective employers, project an informed interest. The more information you have about the company, the easier it will be for you to make informed decisions. Another method is to visit the independent laboratory or hospital. Some laboratories and hospitals have brochures that will provide information about the company. If you are able to visit and tour the laboratory/hospital, observe personnel interacting with each other and with their clients. Ask yourself if the surroundings appear pleasant, clean, and safe. Is this a place you would like to work?

Networking

To access the job market, practice networking. This has proven to be a very successful career marketing tool. Networking is talking with people you know about your career plans. Ask them to help by referring you to people they know and to other professionals. You then follow up on all referrals that come your way. As a member of today's professional workforce, making and keeping contacts is essential to your career. Networking often influences employment and promotion.

Getting Started

To get your network started, list the names of everyone you know. They do not necessarily need to be just close friends or relatives. List everyone you have met in the last year. List all the groups you can think of and then list individual names of people in each group. Examples of networking groups:

- Friends
- Relatives
- Former employers
- Former coworkers
- Classmates from grade school through high school, vocational school, and so forth
- Members of your church
- Members of your social clubs
- Members of your athletic club
- Members of your professional organizations
- People who sell you things (at the store, insurance, etc.)
- People who provide you with services (hairdresser, gardener, etc.)
- People who you play sports with
- Neighbors

Once you have determined the groups of people you know, begin to list everyone you know within each group. Then begin to contact each person on your network list.

Present Yourself Well

- Always be neat, friendly, polite, and well-organized.
- Show interest in what the other person has to say.
- Start with people you know best.
- Unless you know the person well, make an appointment for a meeting.

REFERRAL

A name of a person or company given to you to contact as part of your career-marketing plan.

Get Two Referrals

One of the primary objectives of networking is to get the names of other people whom you can contact. Get two **referrals** from everyone you talk to and then follow up by contacting those people.

Follow Up on Referrals

Contact the people whose names you receive as referrals and make an appointment with them.

● Keep the meeting brief.
● If the person cannot help you with employment information, ask for two more referrals from them.
● This process will continue to perpetuate and expand your networking groups.

Send Thank-You Notes

It is very important that you immediately send thank-you notes to all the people you contact. Send them on the same day that you speak with them. Sending thank-you cards is a simple act of appreciation, and it reinforces the one-to-one relationship you are working to develop.

Common Networking Errors

Problems will occur when you only go through the motions of contacting others. It is not enough to just meet someone and conduct a 15-minute interview, or to ask others for leads, or to pass along your resume. Whether you are approaching a colleague, a friend, a family member, or a stranger, your presentation will make the difference. Be prepared.

Make sure to offer any information, help, or insight you have in return. Networking should be mutually beneficial. Thank the contact and make plans to meet again. Keep the contact aware of your future career moves and ask about his or her plans. Perhaps you know someone he or she would like to meet.

Generating Job Leads

Locating Prospective Employers

● Look in the Yellow Pages and make a list of all prospective employers.
● Use your research techniques to obtain the name of the hiring authority and other information.
● Rank each employer from 1 to 3, based on your ideal job.
● Practice your contacting techniques until you are comfortable.
● Start with the #3's and call them first, then #2's, then #1's.

Visit Without an Appointment

● Dress professionally.
● Bring current portfolio. (Resume—References—Certificates, etc.)
● Ask to see the hiring authority (manager).

- If unavailable, make an appointment to see the manager.
- When you are able to see the manager, sell yourself.

Call Prospective Employers for an Appointment

- Call the hiring authority and follow the four-part telephone contact dialogue (Box 15-7).

Box 15-7: The Four-Part Phone Contact Dialogue

Introduction:
Hello Mr./Ms. Future Employer, my name is _____.
Is now a good time for you to take a few minutes to talk to me?
Thank you.

Position:
I'm interested in a position as a phlebotomy technician with your laboratory.

Hook:
State your qualifications as listed on your personal marketing card.
I have over two years of customer service experience plus one year of volunteer work at the local hospital. I've just graduated from a phlebotomy technician program with a 95% GPA and have taken a national certification exam. I have good written and verbal communication skills, can handle pressure well, and meet deadlines. I am organized, get along well with others, and have good telephone skills. I am hardworking, reliable, and a problem-solver.

Close:
If you have an opening, when is the best time for me to come in to further discuss my skills and qualifications?

- Learn to get past guardians of the organizations (e.g., receptionists).
- Be polite, friendly, and nonpushy but confident.
- Do not appear pushy.
- Be brave; ask yourself, "What is the worse thing that can happen?"
- Present yourself and your qualifications in 30 seconds or less and ask for an appointment.
- Write out exactly what you want to say and practice out loud until you are comfortable.

Responding to Advertised Positions

Only about 20% of available jobs are advertised and 80% to 90% of available job hunters see these advertisements. This means that the competition for these jobs is very high. The key to getting an advertised job is to respond quickly, work to separate yourself from the competition, and be persistent. Jobs are advertised in several publications: Classified Want Ads, Federal/State Employment Service (Job Service), Employment Agencies, Temporary Employment Agencies (Job Pools), and the Internet.

Follow the same procedures with advertised positions as you would for a referral: make contact, set an appointment, interview, and follow through.

The Internet poses a unique method of job hunting. There are a variety of Web sites that post job listings. The general method for pursuing this type of job search requires that you connect to the Internet. Most search engines allow you to put in key words, such as "Phlebotomy Technician Job Listings" or "Allied Health Job Listings." The search will display a variety of organizations that post jobs on the Web. Some Web sites list current employment opportunities that you can apply for specifically. Other Web sites will ask you to submit your resume via E-mail and they will contact you as positions become available. Internet job searching is an excellent method for locating potential positions if you plan on relocating to another area, state, or country. Follow the same procedures as advertising and one-on-one contacting. Follow through with thank-you notes and so forth.

PRODUCT PRESENTATION
Presenting a Professional Image

Dressing for success is key during the interview process. Even though you may be wearing a uniform once hired, you must present a professional image to be hired. The interviewer will make a first impression about you in the first 30 seconds of meeting you. Make this impression count. The progression of the interview will be determined by this first impression. We are a visual society. If you are sloppily dressed, all the skills and experience in the world will not overcome your appearance. The following are guidelines regarding professional appearance during the interviewing process:

1. Always appear neat and clean.
   - Fingernails—trimmed neatly; no garish colors.
   - Make-up—Subdued; no harsh eye-shadow colors.
   - Shoes—polished, with modest heel.
2. Be aware of odors
   - Avoid all scents except breath mints or sprays (no gum).
   - No perfume, after-shave, or hand cream.
   - Clean clothes. No perspiration stains or stale cigarette odor.

3. De-accessorize
   - Less is better with jewelry size, amount, and color.
   - Avoid pins reflecting religious or organizational affiliation.
   - Cover tattoos if possible.
   - Remove any jewelry from visible pierced body parts (other than ears).
   - Do not carry a large purse or backpack.
   - Do not wear sunglasses, hats, or ball caps.
4. Accessorize
   - Wear a watch; choose a conservative style.
   - Carry a portfolio with the following inside:
     - 3 copies of your resume
     - 3 copies of your reference list
     - Sample application (completed)
     - Copy of any applicable certifications, diplomas, or awards
     - Copy of any letters of recommendation
     - Two forms of identification (one picture I.D.)
     - Pen and paper
5. Prepare for the unexpected. Bring:
   - Spot remover
   - Extra pair of earrings
   - Two safety pins
   - Extra tie
   - Static guard
   - Extra pair of panty hose
   - Scotch tape or sewing kit
   - Extra pair of shoes
   - Fingernail file
   - Dental floss
   - Comb/brush
   - Raincoat
6. Always dress conservatively to moderately
   - The goal is to project a business-like appearance.
   - If in doubt, dress more conservatively.
   - Tight-fitting clothing flatters no one.
   - Use conservative colors, necklines, hemlines, and tie patterns.
   - Unless research says otherwise, it is best to wear a jacket or blazer.
   - Consider the season; be aware of color and weight of fabric.

The following guidelines reflect the most professional and appropriate business attire recommended for interviewing.

Women's Dress Guidelines:

1. Best styles
   - Good quality, conservative cut.
   - Calf-length skirt or dress is okay but not ankle length.
   - Blue, black, gray, beige, or tan are the preferred primary colors.
   - Best combinations (ranked in order of preference):
     - A structured jacket, blouse, and knee-length straight skirt.
     - An unstructured jacket and dress.
     - Pant suit, blouse with skirt or slacks.
2. Blouses:
   - Good quality, simple style.
   - Long sleeves.
   - Moderate neckline that shows no cleavage.
   - No gaps between buttons.
3. Stockings:
   - Beige, tan, or neutral hose are best.
   - Match hem of skirt and shoes or darker.
   - No bold, black, white, or pastel colors.
   - Avoid glitzy look, patterns, or lines.
4. Shoes:
   - Classic, medium-heeled, enclosed toe pumps.
   - Wear flats or heels up to 2 inches.
   - Wear same color as hemline of dress or darker.
   - No sandals. Avoid overly dressy shoes.
5. Accessories:
   - Printed silk scarves, high quality jewelry, pearls, or necklace.
   - Keep accessories to a minimum.

Men's Dress Guidelines:

1. Best styles:
   - Tailored, good quality suit of solid color or muted pinstripe.
   - Dark blue or gray suit.
   - No casual cut of sport coat (i.e., patched elbows or pockets).
   - Jacket sleeve to cover wrist bone.
   - Jacket length to cover buttocks.
   - Lapels should be 3 to $3\frac{1}{2}$ inches in width.
   - Trouser waistband never to be lower than the navel.
   - Trouser length to break slightly in front.

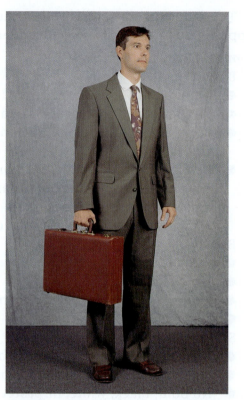

FIGURE 15-1: Phlebotomist appropriately dressed and prepared for the interview

- Best Combinations (ranked in order of preference):
  - Matched two-piece suit.
  - Sports coat and trousers.
  - Shirt and tie with trousers and vest.
2. Shirt:
   - Good quality solid white or pale blue shirt.
   - Subdued and color coordinating pattern or stripe.
   - Cuffs to show no more than ½ inch beyond jacket sleeve.
   - Shirt to fit well, clean, and pressed.
3. Tie:
   - Conservative, good quality tie that complements outfit.
   - Avoid faddish prints, loud colors, bold patterns, clip-on or bow ties.
   - Tie to reach to middle of belt buckle.
   - Tie width at largest point not to exceed 3 inches.
4. Socks:
   - Match color of pants or darker.
   - Match color of shoes or darker.
   - Calf-length sock with good elastic.

5. Shoes:
   ● Match color of pants or darker.
   ● Oxford or slip on.
   ● Black or brown.
   ● Clean, polished, and in good condition.

Writing the Perfect Resume

Nothing is more important to your total professional image than a well-written and complete **resume**. Whatever design or content you choose for a resume, it must emphasize your strong points and accomplishments as well as a detailed work history.

Think of your resume as a sales brochure. Your resume must be persuasive. It must excite the reader, arouse interest, and stimulate a desire to meet you in person.

Your resume is not your biography or your memoirs, but rather a summary of your skills and qualifications that apply to the position you are seeking. A good resume is a well-structured, easy-to-read presentation of your capabilities and accomplishments.

Resumes are usually one page in length and should never be more than two pages. Most professionals agree that a one-page resume is best. Identify only your most pertinent information and organize the details in the most concise way possible. Your resume should include the following information:

1. Contact information: Your complete name, permanent address, and local telephone number with area code at the top of the page. If you have more than one phone number (i.e., message number, cell phone number, pager), list in priority.

2. Objective (optional): Keep your career objective general in nature. If you do not include your objective on your resume you must include it in your cover letter (i.e., a career in the allied health field as a Phlebotomy Technician).

3. Education: List the school, including city and state, from which you have or will graduate. Include your date of graduation, certification, and academic honors. GPA is optional.

4. Experience/employment history: Present paid and volunteer experience in reverse chronologic order. Include job titles, dates of employment, and duties/responsibilities for each position. If you participated in a sponsored externship, describe here. Include location, city, and state.

5. References: State that references are available on request.

RESUME

A typed document describing your employment history, education, and objectives, given to prospective employers as a means of providing background information prior to or during an employment interview.

When writing your resume:

Do:

- Be specific.
- Use action verbs.
- Laser print on quality paper.
- Proofread carefully.
- Re-read it as if you are the prospective employer.

Don't:

- Misspell anything.
- Include personal information (hair color, height, number of children, religious affiliations, etc.).
- Forget to include your telephone number.
- Type it on a typewriter.
- Forget to highlight your selling points.

Keep in mind the following suggestions as you begin developing your resume:

- Sell yourself: Create a good first impression.
- Use action words (Box 15-8).
- Be consistent: Choose a pattern of spacing and order of information. Be consistent throughout.
- Present information in reverse chronological order: List education and work experiences with the most recent first.
- Check for grammar: Misspellings and poorly constructed sentences communicate negative impressions about a candidate.
- Ensure your resume is neat and visually appealing: Select high quality paper in white, off-white, or gray. Reproduce the final version professionally.

There are many styles of resumes. Two of the most current trends in resume writing are included in Box 15-9. To keep current with resume trends, do research on the Internet or at the library every time you update your resume. There are several Web sites dedicated specifically to resume writing.

Cover Letter

COVER LETTER

A letter of introduction accompanying your resume to prospective employers.

Providing a prospective employer a well-written **cover letter** is essential to presenting and introducing your resume. The cover letter and resume complete your professional image. It is one of the most important letters you will write. It introduces you and your qualifications and is one of the key steps leading to the interview (Box 15-10).

Box 15-8: Resume Action Words

administered	counseled	impressed	referred
advanced	created	increased	refined
advised	decreased	influenced	regulated
alerted	delegated	initiated	reinforced
amplified	designed	innovated	reorganized
analyzed	determined	inspected	represented
arranged	developed	inspired	reproduced
assessed	devised	interviewed	researched
assisted	devoted	introduced	reshaped
broadened	diagrammed	invented	restored
budgeted	dignified	investigated	revamped
calculated	directed	managed	reviewed
catalogued	displayed	measured	revised
chaired	distributed	observed	scheduled
coached	drafted	operated	secured
collected	edited	ordered	selected
combined	embraced	performed	solved
comforted	encouraged	planned	supervised
complied	enlightened	predicted	supported
composed	enthused	prepared	sustained
computed	established	programmed	taught
condensed	excelled	promoted	trained
conducted	exhibited	provided	translated
constructed	experimented	raised	updated
contacted	explained	recommended	visualized
coordinated	idealized	recorded	wrote
corresponded	implemented	recruited	

A cover letter has several purposes:

● The business letter format introduces your resume to a prospective employer.

● Generates interest in your resume by highlighting your strongest qualifications.

● Demonstrates your writing and thinking skills.

● Requests an interview and thanks the interviewer for his or her time and effort.

Guidelines of Cover Letters

Do:

● Type a cover letter on standard $8 \times 11\frac{1}{2}$ inch paper that matches the resume paper in color and weight.

● Prepare an original letter for every resume delivered or mailed.

Box 15-9: Resumes Examples

MADELINE A. WILSON

1967 EAST 176TH AVENUE

CITY, STATE ZIP

Telephone: (555) 834-9458

JOB OBJECTIVE: To obtain a career position in the Allied Health field as a Phlebotomy Technician.

HIGHLIGHTS OF QUALIFICATIONS

➤ 10 years of sales and customer service
➤ Fluent in English and moderate Spanish
➤ Confident—compassionate—responsible
➤ Quick learner—dependable—hard working
➤ Earned Phlebotomy Technician diploma in 1999 with practical experience

PROFESSIONAL EXPERIENCE

Phlebotomy Skills:

➤ Proficient in the collection of blood specimens by means of capillary puncture and venipuncture by evacuated tube, syringe, and butterfly draws.
➤ Practiced point-of-care tests to include: cholesterol, blood glucose, pregnancy, bleeding time, prothrombin time, hematocrit, hemoglobin, urine dipstick, and strep testing.
➤ Trained in patient instruction in the collection of: skin tests, amniotic and cerebrospinal fluids, gastric secretions, semen, stool, and tissue specimens.
➤ Applied procedures for collection of tolerance tests, forensic specimens, drug screening, postprandial glucose test, and cold agglutinin.
➤ Received instruction in various specialty collections such as: pediatric, arterial blood gases, procedures for fistulas, indwelling catheters, and inpatient and ambulatory care procedures.

Office Skills:

➤ Accounts payable/accounts receivable.
➤ Maintained inventory and stock.
➤ Operate MS Word, MS Publisher 2000, MS Office, Adobe Photoshop 5.0.
➤ Type 40 WPM.

Patient Care Skills:

➤ Provided point-of-care testing for homebound patients, pre-employment, random, probable cause, and accident, and drug and alcohol screening.
➤ Collected blood and other specimens; prepared and packaged specimens for transportation.
➤ Performance of accurate vital signs.
➤ Obtained electrocardiogram for physician interpretation.

WORK HISTORY

    1999–1999 **AXTLM**, City, State—Phlebotomist
    1998–1999 **Safeway**, City, State—Shift Manager

EDUCATION AND TRAINING

School, City, State

Nationally Accredited

Phlebotomy Technician Specialist Diploma—1999

National Basic Life Support CPR Certification—Current

REFERENCES AVAILABLE UPON REQUEST

DANIELLE FRANKLIN
123 Green Mountain, Apt. #12
Anchorage, Alaska 99512

Home: (555) 243-9876

HIGHLIGHTS OF QUALIFICATIONS:
- Four years of clerical experience
- Seven years of public relation skills
- Motivated, problem-solver
- Cheerful, dependable, and hard working

PROFESSIONAL EXPERIENCE:

Medical Skills
- Proficient in the collection of blood specimens; over 200 capillary punctures and 200 venipunctures by evacuated tube, syringe, and butterfly draws.
- Practiced point-of-care tests to include: cholesterol, blood glucose, pregnancy testing, bleeding time, prothrombin time, hematocrit, hemoglobin, urine dipstick, and strep testing.
- Trained in patient instruction in the collection of: skin tests, amniotic and cerebrospinal fluids, gastric secretions, semen, stool, and tissue specimens.
- Applied procedures for collection of tolerance tests, forensic specimens, drug screening, postprandial glucose test, and cold agglutinin.
- Received instruction in various specialty collections such as: pediatric collections, arterial blood gases, procedures for fistulas and indwelling catheters, and inpatient and ambulatory care procedures.
- Learned and practiced blood-banking procedures and therapeutic phlebotomy.
- Mastered understanding and implementation of OSHA and CLIA regulations.

Customer Service Skills
- Made reservations for clientele and wrote tickets
- Telephone sales and marketing
- Prepared meeting packets for employees and pay roll

WORK HISTORY
08/98–08/99	**Ouzinkie Tribal Council**, Ouzinkie, Alaska—*Laborer*	
1996–1998	**Ouzinkie School**, Ouzinkie, Alaska—*Substitute Teacher*	
06/97–08/98	**Kodiak Housing Authority**, Ouzinkie, Alaska—*Carpenter*	
07/95–08/97	**Ouzinkie Tribal Council**, Ouzinkie, Alaska—*Office Clerk*	
06/94–10/94	**Markair**, Kodiak, Alaska—*Ticket Agent*	
09/93–04/94	**Ouzinkie City Office**, Ouzinkie, Alaska—*Office Clerk*	
06/93–05/94	**Ouzinkie Tribal Council**, Ouzinkie, Alaska—*Gym Director*	

EDUCATION AND TRAINING
Career Academy, Anchorage, Alaska
Nationally Accredited—ACCSCT
Phlebotomy Specialist Diploma—April 2000
National Certification—Phlebotomist, April 2000

REFERENCES AVAILABLE UPON REQUEST

- Write in a positive tone and generate interest by being employer-focused (written to meet the needs of the employer).
- Proofread it and ask at least one other person to proofread it.
- Date and sign the cover letter using blue or black ink.
- Use an appropriate business letter format.
- Personalize each letter by addressing it to a specific individual, using his or her correct title, business name, and address.
- Be positive, honest, and sincere and give an impression of modest confidence.

Don't:
- Mail a resume without a cover letter.
- Use trite phrases or trendy slang.
- Use the first name of the employer.
- Use business stationery.
- Exceed one page.
- Overuse the personal pronoun "I."
- Address the letter "To Whom It May Concern" or use unusual greetings such as "Dear Friend."
- Handwrite your cover letter.
- Use a reproduced form letter or preprinted letter.
- Cover all the same material included in your resume.
- Mention salary, fringe benefits, vacation time, and so forth.

Parts of a Cover Letter
- Return address: Use the address that you want return correspondence directed to. Your return address is always listed first.
- Date: Position on the first line to the left side of the page.
- Inside Address: Include correctly spelled name of the person you want to receive the letter, his or her title, company name, and full address. Skip one line after the date and type flush with the left margin of the letter. Use either the title Mr. or Ms. Use Mrs. only if you know for certain that the person wishes to be addressed by Mrs.
- Salutation: Used to greet the person to whom you are writing. Skip one line after the address and type flush with left margin of letter. Use Dear, Mr. or Ms., the last name, and a colon.
- Body: Contains the message for the addressee and is normally three paragraphs long with a double space between each paragraph. Type flush with the left margin of the letter.

- Paragraph one (statement of interest): Introduces resume, states the position you are seeking, states how you heard about the position.
- Paragraph two (value selling statement): Briefly summarize your 3-T's (Training, Transferable, Traits) (Box 15-5).
- Paragraph three (action/appreciation): Ask for an interview, the job, or consideration. Thank the employer.
- Complimentary closing: Word grouping used to bring the message or text to a close. Skip one line after the last paragraph and type flush with the left margin of the letter; use the word "sincerely."

Box 15-10: Cover Letter Examples

Patty Belle
Third Avenue South
City, State Zip
(555) 123-4567

Today's Date

Mr./Ms. Future Employer:

Please accept the enclosed resume outlining my qualifications for the phlebotomy technician position that was advertised in the Sunday edition of the *Anchorage Daily News*.

My successful professional experiences include two years of retail sales and customer service and one year of professional office management. I led my region three times in total sales volume. I have recently graduated from Career Academy with a 100% attendance rate, and honors, in the top 10% of my class. This training resulted in my certification as a phlebotomy technician specialist, and provided hands-on experience in nearly every facet of this industry. My strong interpersonal and communicative skills and the ability to work well with other people will help your company succeed.

I would like to schedule an interview, at your convenience, to further discuss my skills and qualifications for your position. You may reach me at (555) 123-4567. If I am not available, my answering machine will take your message. If I have not heard from you by Tuesday, March 28, I will call to determine your interest.

Thank you in advance for your time and consideration.

Sincerely,

Patty Belle

Enclosure

(continues)

Box 15-10: Cover Letter Examples *(continued)*

KATHLEEN N. BROOKS
8885 Blackberry Drive
City, State Zip
(555) 243-9876

September 23, 20—

Southcentral Foundation
Mr. Kaiser Epstein
Staffing Services/HR Department
670 W. Fireweed Lane
Anchorage, Alaska 99503

Re: Phlebotomy Technician Position

This letter is in response to your advertisement for a Phlebotomy Technician. This position is of great interest to me. I am ready to transition my qualifications into a challenging Phlebotomy Technician position with a respected institution like Southcentral Foundation.

In addition to my background as a Nationally Certified Phlebotomy Technician, my experience and training has expanded to include ECG Technician as well. I am very active in the local chapter of the Phlebotomy Technician Association. I also possess experience and education in point-of-care testing and I am BLS-CPR certified.

I earned praise from my externship coordinator while fulfilling practical work experience requirements. I passed the National Phlebotomy Technician Certification Examination with a 93%. My overall GPA in school was 96.8%.

Along with an excellent ability to problem solve and make sound decisions, I am highly organized and computer proficient. I am confident in my skills and feel I am a viable candidate for your position. Please review the attached resume for additional information regarding my training and experience.

Thank you for your consideration. I appreciate your time in reviewing my qualifications and look forward to speaking with you in person at your earliest convenience.

Sincerely,

Kathleen N. Brooks, NCPT

Enclosure

- Signature line: Your full formal name. Skip four lines after the complimentary close and type your name flush with the left margin of the letter. Sign your name in blue or black ink above the signature line.
- Enclosure line: Indicates if there is an enclosure. Type the word "enclosure" two lines after the signature line and flush with left margin.

Completing the Employment Application

Box 15-11: Employment Application

APPLICATION FOR EMPLOYMENT

IDENTIFICATION

AN EQUAL OPPORTUNITY EMPLOYER. This organization does not discriminate in hiring for employment because of race, color, religious creed, national origin, sex, age or marital status. No questions on this application are intended to secure information to be used for such dicrimination.

PLEASE PRINT OR TYPE

NAME (Last) (First) (Middle) (Nickname)	SOCIAL SECURITY NUMBER

PRESENT ADDRESS (No. and Street) (City) (State) (Zip)	TELEPHONE NUMBER

POSITION DESIRED	SALARY REQUIRED	DO YOU HAVE A VALID DRIVERS LICENSE? If yes provide DL#

DATE AVAILABLE	LOCATION RESTRICTIONS	ARE YOU AT LEAST 21 YEARS OF AGE? ( ) YES ( ) NO

WILLING TO WORK SHIFTS, NIGHTS, WEEKENDS, HOLIDAYS OR OVERTIME IF NECESSARY? Specify any limitations

U.S. CITIZEN? ( ) YES ( ) NO	IF NO, VISA TYPE	DO YOU HAVE A CURRENT PASSPORT? ( ) YES ( ) NO	REFERRED BY:

RELATIVES EMPLOYED BY:

HAVE YOU EVER BEEN REFUSED A BOND? ( ) YES ( ) NO
(IF YES, PROVIDE THE NAME AND ADDRESS OF EMPLOYER):

HAVE YOU EVER BEEN CONVICTED OR PLEAD "NO CONTENDERE" TO ANY CRIME OTHER THAN A MINOR TRAFFIC VIOLATION IN THE LAST FIVE YEARS? ( ) YES ( ) NO
(If Yes, Explain):

PERSONAL

DO YOU HAVE ANY PHYSICAL HANDICAPS AND/OR LIMITATIONS WHICH MAY AFFECT YOUR ABILITY TO PERFORM THE JOB FOR WHICH YOU HAVE APPLIED? ( ) YES ( ) NO
(If Yes, Explain):

HAVE YOU EVER FAILED A PHYSICAL EXAMINATION?

LIST DATES AND REASONS FOR HOSPITALIZATIONS AND/OR WORKERS COMPENSATION CLAIMS IN PAST FIVE YEARS.

ESTIMATE NUMBER OF WORK DAYS MISSED DUE TO ILLNESS IN PAST TWO YEARS _____

EMERGENCY CONTACTS

NAME	PHONE	ADDRESS	RELATIONSHIP

MILITARY

SERVICE STATUS
( ) VETERAN ( ) ACTIVE ( ) INACTIVE ( ) ADVANCED ROTC ( ) NATIONAL GUARD ( ) RESERVE

BRANCH OF SERVICE	SPECIALTY TRAINING	DATES OF SERVICE	HIGHEST RANK ATTAINED

PRINCIPAL DUTIES

(continues)

Box 15-11: Employment Application *(continued)*

REFERENCES

LIST THREE PERSONAL REFERENCES THAT HAVE KNOWN YOU FOR AT LEAST FIVE YEARS.
(NOT RELATIVES)

NAME	PHONE	ADDRESS	RELATIONSHIP

EDUCATION

SCHOOLS	NAME/CITY/STATE	FROM/TO	GRADUATED	TYPE OF DEGREE LICENSE OR CERTIFICATE	MAJOR/MINOR TYPE OF TRAINING
HIGH SCHOOL					
COLLEGE					
GRADUATE SCHOOL					
VOCATIONAL/TECHNICAL					

COURSES, WORKSHOPS, SEMINARS AND OTHER SPECIALIZED OR ADVANCED TRAINING:

TECHNICAL LICENSES HELD/EXPIRATION DATES:

INDICATE THE AREAS IN WHICH YOU ARE PROFICIENT

TYPING (WPM)____ TELEX____ DATA ENTRY____ COMPUTER OPERATIONS____ PAYROLL____
WORD PROCESSING____ ACCOUNTING____ DRAFTING____ DICTATION EQUIPMENT____
ENGINEERING____ AUDIO-VISUAL EQUIPMENT____ PBX EQUPMENT____ 10-KEY ADDING____

ADDITIONAL INFORMATION

INDICATE THE IMPORTANCE OF THE FOLLOWING REASONS FOR WANTING TO JOIN ORGANIZATION
PLACE (1) BESIDE THE REASON WHICH IS MOST IMPORTANT TO YOU (2) BESIDE THE SECOND MOST IMPORTANT
REASON, UNTIL YOU HAVE RANKED THEM ALL

USING TECHNICAL SKILLS____ PAY____ BENEFITS____ PROVIDING A SERVICE TO OTHERS____
OPPORTUNITY FOR ADVANCEMENT____ DEALING WITH THE PUBLIC____ VARIED DUTIES____
INDEPENDENCE ON THE JOB____ USE OF MANAGERIAL SKILLS____
OTHER (SPECIFY)_____

WHAT ARE YOU OFFERING THAT DISTINGUISHES YOU FROM OTHER CANDIDATES?

STATE YOUR LONG-TERM GOALS AND PROFESSIONAL EXPECTATIONS.

EMPLOYMENT

EMPLOYMENT RECORD: List your employment history for the past five years beginning with the most recent or present employer. Indicate name under which employed if different than this application. Complete application fully, do not indicate "see resume".

IMPORTANT: State full particulars of all employment covering full disposition of your time whether employed or not. If employing company is out of business, so state. If you have been conducting your own business, give names, phone numbers, and addresses of at least two clients whom we can contact. If time between employers exceeds 60 days, explain what you were doing during the period

MAY WE CONTACT YOUR PRESENT EMPLOYER? { } YES { } NO (Yes after interview)	
FROM MO/YR	TO MO/YR	NAME OF BUSINESS
ADDRESS	NATURE OF BUSINESS: Nature of business (e.g., retail, health care)
POSITION HELD (Your duty title)	NAME OF SUPERVISOR:
DUTIES (Be very specific)	SALARY: (Hourly Rate)

REASON FOR LEAVING (Be positive. If it can't be positive, then leave it blank or write, "Would prefer to explain at interview"; e.g., pursue education, career change, personal leave, family management).

FROM	TO	NAME OF BUSINESS
ADDRESS		NATURE OF BUSINESS:
POSITION HELD		NAME OF SUPERVISOR:
DUTIES		SALARY:

REASON FOR LEAVING

FROM	TO	NAME OF BUSINESS
ADDRESS		NATURE OF BUSINESS:
POSITION HELD		NAME OF SUPERVISOR:
DUTIES		SALARY:

REASON FOR LEAVING

AGREEMENT

I UNDERSTAND THAT SUBMISSION OF THIS APPLICATION, AND ITS ACCEPTANCE BY ANY EMPLOYEE OF _____, DOES NOT OBLIGATE_____ TO INTERVIEW ME, OR OFFER EMPLOYMENT OF ANY FASHION.

I FURTHER UNDERSTAND THAT IF EMPLOYMENT IS OFFERED, IT IS OFFERED "AT WILL". THEREFORE, I MAY TERMINATE MY EMPLOYMENT WITH _____ AT ANY TIME, WITH OR WITHOUT NOTICE, AND _____MAY TERMINATE MY EMPLOYMENT AT ANY TIME, WITH OR WITHOUT NOTICE. I CERTIFY THE INFORMATION PROVIDED HEREON IS ACCURATE AND COMPLETE AND UNDERSTAND THAT OMISSIONS OR FALSE STATEMENTS ARE SUFFICIENT GROUNDS FOR _____ TO REFUSE TO HIRE ME OR, IF HIRED, TO DISMISS ME.

I AUTHORIZE _____ TO CONTACT EMPLOYERS, SCHOOLS, AND REFERENCES CONCERNING MY WORK ETHICS, ATTENDANCE, TIMELINESS, SALARY, PERFORMANCE, AND CHARACTER. FURTHER, I AUTHORIZE SAID EMPLOYERS, SCHOOLS, AND REFERENCES TO RELEASE SAID INFORMATION ABOUT ME TO_____.

I UNDERSTAND TO QUALIFY FOR SOME POSITIONS I MUST SUCCESSFULLY COMPLETE A REQUIRED TRAINING PROGRAM AND MAINTAIN QUALIFICATIONS DURING THE COURSE OF MY EMPLOYMENT.

I UNDERSTAND ANY OFFER OF EMPLOYMENT IS CONDITIONAL UPON MY SUCCESSFULLY PASSING THE REQUIRED DRUG TEST, A FIVE-YEAR BACKGROUND CHECK, AND PROVIDING ADDITIONAL PERSONAL DATA REQUIRED BY STATE AND FEDERAL REGULATIONS AND STATUTES, AND FOR BENEFIT ADMINISTRATION.

I UNDERSTAND _____ HAS A DRUG-FREE PHILOSOPHY AND I MAY BE TERMINATED ANY TIME UNAUTHORIZED DRUGS ARE DETECTED ON MY PERSON OR IN MY SYSTEM.

NOTE: Always read the agreement. Then date and sign the application. This is a legal document and must be signed to be valid.

SIGNATURE   DATE

The application is the first formal "test" a potential employer will give, and it often occurs before he or she meets you in person. Applications are designed for you to provide information. The employer may use the application process to screen out applicants. Information received on an application must be accurate.

You are evaluated and screened based on neatness and accuracy of the information. Submitting a neat and complete application will make a positive impression. Your opportunity to secure an interview will be increased. Employers assume that if you cannot fill out an application properly then you will not be able to follow other directions. If the application is sloppy, they will assume your work will be sloppy.

Remember: An overwhelming percentage of the applications received by most companies are:

- Not typed
- Messy
- Incomplete
- Completed incorrectly (directions are not followed)
- All the above

Box 15-12: Ten Unbreakable Rules for Filling Out Applications

1) Read and follow all written directions.
2) Type or neatly print (block letters) your application.
3) No incomplete or missing information.
4) Keep original application neat and clean.
5) All information must be positive.
6) Write N/A if the item does not apply to you.
7) Match your strengths (skills) to job-needed skills.
8) Proofread the finished product.
9) Use dark (black) ink.
10) Date and sign it.

Directions for Filling Out Applications

1. Identification
   - *Name:* Use full legal name, in order requested.
   - *Social security number:* Always provide your correct social security number (this is optional at the time of application and must only be provided upon employment).
   - *Address:* Provide full mailing address.

- *Telephone number:* Provide current number where it is easiest to reach you or leave a message.
- *Physical characteristics:* Some positions require this information for safety considerations. Provide if requested.
- *Citizenship:* Employers must ensure you have the legal status to be hired.
- *General health:* Your response to this area should be "good" or "excellent." If you have a health problem that will keep you from doing a good job, do not apply.
- *Disabilities and physical limitations:* Only applicable if they will affect your performance on the job. If not, do not list them.

2. **Education and/or formal training**
   - List all education and certification which applies to the position.
3. **Military experience**
   - List all required information and indicate responsibilities. Avoid using military terms not easily understood.
4. **Position desired**
   - *Job objective:*
     - Fill in the name of the job for which you are applying.
     - Do not put, "anything available."
     - If you want to apply for two jobs at the same company, fill out two separate applications.
   - *Salary:*
     - Use the terms "scale," "open," or "negotiable."
     - Do not state a specific salary.
   - *Hours:*
     - Indicate the hours you are willing to work. This tells employers how flexible you are willing to be.
5. **Previous work experience**
   - Think of this section as your mini-resume.
   - List all the skills you have that apply to the job.
   - Be prepared to go back as far as ten years.
   - Provide all requested information for every job listed.
6. **Reasons for leaving previous position**
   - Whatever the reason, never write "fired" or other negative reasons on an application.
   - Be truthful, but look for a positive way to express the reason for leaving.
   - If you can't say anything positive, then do not say anything at all.

7. **References**
   - Always have three good professional references.
   - Get permission to use and verify what they will say.
   - Do not use relatives as a reference; employers will not consider them to be objective.
   - It is best to select references with the same or similar background as the job you are seeking.
8. **Agreement**
   - At the end of every application is a statement that you must read, and, if you agree to the statement, you must sign and date the application.
   - A job application is a legal document.

Interviewing

You have sent your cover letter and resume and have been asked to interview for the job you have been dreaming of. Now what?

Practice, Practice, Practice

One of the best ways to prepare for interviewing is by "scripting" your lines in answer to key questions. Work with a friend, classmate, or coworker. Organize and review your answers to both basic and difficult interview questions. Remember, the more you prepare, the more relaxed you will feel during the interview. The more relaxed you feel, the better you will perform and the more likely you will be to get the job!

Opening Moves

Relax and project self-confidence. You are ready. Arrive about 10 to 15 minutes ahead of time so that you can make sure your appearance is professional. When you walk into the interviewer's office, smile, use direct eye contact, introduce yourself clearly, offer a firm handshake, and build a rapport as quickly as possible.

To build a rapport with the interviewer, look for the opportunity to socialize at the start. Use the interviewer's name. Use appropriate humor. Look for commonalties.

General Rules

- Answer all questions with a positive response.
- Do not say anything negative about anyone.
- Keep answers between 30 seconds and 2 minutes.
- Always talk about the three T's (Training, Transferable skills, and Traits) (Box 15-5).

● Use stories and specific examples where possible.
● Listen to and be sure you understand the question (it is acceptable to ask the interviewer to clarify the question).

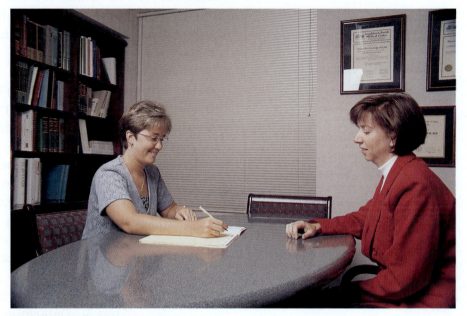

FIGURE 15-2: The interview

Question Response Techniques

The first key to answering interview questions is listening to be sure you understand what is being said. Also listen for the hidden or "true" meaning behind the question. Learn and use the following techniques to help answer interview questions:

1. Summary question: Interviewers normally start with a summary question. Be prepared to summarize your training, work history, and traits.
2. Specifying Question: If you did not hear or did not understand a question (need clarification), or you need a few seconds to think, ask:
   ● *Could you repeat that question?*
   ● *Could you rephrase that question for me?*
   If you want some information about something:
   ● Interviewer: *So tell me why you are qualified for this position?*
   ● Your response: *To help me answer that, could you tell me the main responsibilities of the position?*

If you need the interviewer to narrow the scope of the question:
- Interviewer: *Tell me about yourself.*
- Your response: *What exactly would you like to know about me?*

3. Substitution: If you cannot tell the interviewer exactly what he or she wants to know, then you should answer by substituting your strengths. This technique turns a disadvantage into an advantage.

a. Steps:
- Determine the real concern behind the question.
- Briefly acknowledge the surface question.
- Answer the concern if you can; if you cannot, substitute with other strengths.

Interviewer: *We are looking for someone with more experience in the field. Why should we hire you over someone more qualified?*

Your Response: Step 1: Ask yourself what is the real concern? Not years of experience, but whether or not I can do the job.

Step 2: Briefly acknowledge the surface question: *I'm sure there are people who have more years of experience.*

Step 3: Determine the strengths you do have and substitute those, such as: *However, I have several good traits that they might not have and that can't be taught. For example, I graduated from an accredited school with a GPA of _____%, which shows I am an extremely hard worker and I learn very quickly. What this means is that I will never say, "We used to do it this way at my last job."*

b. Story example: Give an illustration from your work or life experience when you used the particular skill or trait. Be sure to state the successes or results.

Box 15-13: Practice Interview Questions

- Tell me about yourself.
- In what type of position are you most interested?
- What challenges are you looking for in a position?
- Why do you want to be a phlebotomy technician?
- Why do you think you would like this particular type of job?

- How would you describe yourself? Your best friend?
- How would your previous employer describe you?
- What jobs have you held previously?
- What did you especially enjoy about your last job?
- What type of people were you working with last?
- Do you prefer working by yourself or with others?
- Do you like routine work?
- What did you enjoy least about your last job?
- What were the circumstances concerning your leaving your last position?
- Why are you looking for a change in employment?
- What do you plan to be doing five years from now in your career?
- What are you long-range goals? Short range?
- How does this job relate to your plans or goals?
- How long have you been planning for this type of work?
- In what ways do you feel your last/present job prepared you for this job?
- What kind of supervisor do you prefer?
- If I called your last/present boss, what would he or she tell me about your work ethics? Your job performance? Your dependability? Your interpersonal skills? Your quality of work? Your problem-solving skills?
- How would your peers describe your?
- Define teamwork. Define cooperation. Define communication.
- What types of work do you feel most comfortable doing?
- What sorts of things make you angry?
- What would you do if your supervisor made a decision with which you strongly disagree?
- What types of situations put you under pressure?
- How do you deal with pressure? Give an example.
- What was the biggest problem you personally confronted in employment? How did you solve this problem?
- What have you learned from your past mistakes?
- What shifts are you willing to work?
- What types of coworkers do you like working with?
- In your lifetime, what do you consider to be your greatest accomplishment?
- What is something you achieved that made you proud?
- Tell me about a time when you went out on a limb to help someone.
- Describe your strengths and weaknesses.
- What are you doing now to improve yourself?
- Do you intend to further your education?
- What do you think determines a person's progress/success in a company?

(continues)

Box 15-13: Practice Interview Questions *(continued)*

- What do you know about our company?
- Why are you interested in our organization?
- What do you expect from the company that hires you?
- Do you check with a supervisor for approval or do you operate with independent responsibility and authority?
- In past performance reviews, what were described as strong points and what areas were recommended for improvement?
- What was your most or least interesting subject in school? Why?
- How many days did you miss on your last job? Why?
- What is a good excuse for missing work?
- What are your salary requirements?
- How do you balance your professional and personal life?
- Do you predict needs before they arise? If so, how?
- What do you do to relax?
- What pace do you typically work at?
- Do you accept responsibility when mistakes occur?
- Do you have a drug or alcohol problem?
- Have you ever been convicted of a crime?
- What are your special abilities?
- At what age would you like to retire?
- What is the greatest asset you will bring to our company?
- Every company has its own quirks—what was dysfunctional about your previous/present employer?
- If we hire you, when should we expect you to be a fully productive member of the staff?
- Why should I hire you?
- If you had to choose among three factors: 1) the company, 2) the position you are applying for, or 3) the people you would be working with—which would you say plays the most significant role in your decision to accept our offer?

Closing the Interview

You will know when the interview is coming to a close by the interviewer's body language and comments. Prepare to accomplish the following:

- Summarize your qualifications.
- Ask two to three intelligent questions.
- End with a call-back closing.

You may be asked to summarize at the end of the interview with a question such as, "So, why are you the best choice for this job?" Be prepared to say, "I would like to summarize my qualifications for you."

Asking Questions

Employers like job applicants to ask intelligent questions. Often the last question will be, "Do you have any questions?" Be prepared for opportunities to ask good questions throughout the interview and always have three prepared questions that you plan to ask toward the end of the interview. You can write these down in your portfolio and refer to them when the time comes to ask questions. Do not ask questions about benefits, salary, compensation, or anything else the company can do for you. Ask questions like these:
● Will there be a second interview?
● What is the typical work schedule?
● Is there a training period? Length? Formal/informal?
● What are the major job responsibilities?
● Is there an overtime policy?

Call-Back Closing

A call-back closing is the same as the opening, but instead of introducing yourself, you are saying thank you. You are trying to find out what happens next. Remember the following:
● Make direct eye contact.
● Smile.
● Firm handshake.
● Say "Mr./Ms. _____, I enjoyed meeting with you today. Thank you for your time. I am very interested in this position. I know you are busy and I do not want to miss your call. When is a good time to call you and check on the status of this position?" (Get date and time.)

Follow-Up

This is the phase where applicants fail because they are shy, unsure, or forget to take the appropriate action. In this phase, you evaluate your interview performance, verify for the interviewer that you are a polite person, and remind the interviewer of your name.

Interview Evaluation

As soon as possible after the interview, open your portfolio and write down as many of the questions as you can remember. Jot down what you can do at the next interview. Use this information to prepare for future interviews.

Thank-You Letter/Note

Always send a thank-you card after *every* interview. Send it the same or very next day to avoid forgetting.

Telephone Call

For a call-back closing, ensure you make a note on your calendar to call at the scheduled time. If no agreement was made, wait a day or two, then call about the status of their decision.

Final Follow-Up Letters

1. Job rejection follow-up letter: If you are not selected for a position, send one more letter to the interviewer. In this letter, state:
   ● Your appreciation for the interviewer's consideration.
   ● Your continued interest in working for their company.
   ● Your request to be contacted should another position become available.

Box 15-14: Draft of a Follow-Up Letter

May 25, 20—

Laboratory Associates
8756 Nothern Lights Boulevard
Anchorage, Alaska 99504

Dear _____:

RE: PHLEBOTOMY TECHNICIAN POSITION

You have a resume on file that I delivered to your office on May 18, expressing my interest in a Phlebotomy Technician position within your lab. I want to express my continued interest in this position.

Your business is a highly respected one in the allied health industry. I want very much to be employed by your company. I believe I will be a contributing member of your staff by providing a standard of performance that is of the highest caliber.

I'm sure you have other qualified applicants; however, I urge you to again review my cover letter, resume, and letters of recommendation. You will find that in addition to my Phlebotomy Technician certification, I have:

- Outstanding letters of recommendation from my externship site.
- Substantial experience in administrative work and business correspondence composition (samples are available for your review).
- Proficient practical experience in my clinical skills.

Please call and allow me the opportunity to demonstrate and explain my qualifications more fully to you in an interview. You will be glad you made the call.

Respectfully,

Leah Marie Stapleton

2. Job Offer Acceptance Letter: If you are selected for a position, write a thank-you letter to relieve anxiety an employer may have about his/her hiring choice and to set the stage for developing a new and hopefully productive relationship. In this letter, state:
   - Your appreciation to the company for the confidence given to you by their selection.
   - Your interest, and that you look forward to working for their company.
   - The date you and the employer agreed upon as your start date.
   - Assurances to the employer that you are a quality employee.

SUMMARY

Finding the perfect job does not happen by chance—it takes dedication and hard work on your part. Finding that perfect job is a job in and of itself. You have the tools to make your job search successful. Set the goal, put it in writing, network, stay organized, dress for success, and follow through. Believe in yourself and remember to say thank you.

STUDY AND REVIEW EXERCISES
Defining Key Terms

Write the definition for each of the following key terms.

1) 3–T's _____

2) cover letter_____

3) market value _____

4) networking_____

5) referral_____

6) resume_____

7) traits_____

Reviewing Key Points

1) Identify three methods used to research potential employers.

2) Identify the three main steps in outlining a career marketing plan.

3) Define and describe networking.

4) List common networking errors.

5) Describe the steps of organizing your job search.

Sentence Completion

1) The first step in finding a job is setting a _____ to get a job.

2) Your _____ skills are what you acquire as a result of formal education or on-the-job training.

3) Your _____ skills do not change from job to job but go with you.

4) Your _____ are how you do things. Examples of these qualities include: cheerful, hardworking, enthusiastic, detail-oriented.

5) _____ to employment might be transportation, wardrobe, daycare, or illness.

6) One handy job-search tool you can create inexpensively for yourself is a _____ or mini-resume.

7) _____ is defined as talking with people you know about your career plans.

8) Think of your _____ as a sales brochure. It must be persuasive. It must excite the reader, arouse interest, and stimulate a desire to meet you in person.

9) Resumes are usually _____ page(s) in length and should never be more than _____ pages.

10) The _____ is the first formal "test" a potential employer will give, and often occurs before he or she meets you in person.

Multiple Choice

1) When writing a cover letter, a word grouping used to bring the message or text to a close is called:
   A. enclosure line
   B. signature line
   C. complimentary closing
   D. salutation

2) During an employment interview, you should do all of the following *except*:
   A. Answer only questions that you feel are important.
   B. Do not say anything negative about anyone.
   C. Keep answers between 30 seconds and 2 minutes.
   D. Use stories and specific examples where possible.

3) One of the three main steps in outlining your marketing plan is product analysis. Product analysis includes all of the following *except*:
   A. Identifying your skills or market value
   B. Networking
   C. Identifying your potential employment obstacles
   D. Presenting a professional image

4) Completing the application is which one of the following steps in outlining your marketing plan?
   A. Market analysis
   B. Product analysis
   C. Product presentation
   D. Transferable skills

5) Being friendly, outgoing, cheerful, and enthusiastic are examples of:
   A. education and training
   B. transferable skills
   C. employment obstacles
   D. personality traits

6) The best days and times to contact a future employer are:
   A. Tuesday through Friday mornings from 8:00–11:30
   B. Monday, Tuesday, Friday afternoons from 1:00–2:30
   C. Wednesday, Friday, Saturday from 7:00 AM–9:00 AM
   D. Tuesday, Thursday, Friday, Saturday from 6:00 PM–8:00 PM

7) Examples of networking groups are all the following *except*:
   A. Clergy
   B. People who sell you things
   C. Friends
   D. All of the above

8) Which one of the following would be inappropriate to wear or bring to an interview?
   A. Dark colored jacket or blazer
   B. Backpack
   C. 3 copies of your resume
   D. Sample application (completed)

9) Which of the following does *not* belong on your resume as part of the contact information?
   A. Social security number
   B. Complete name
   C. Permanent address
   D. Local telephone number

10) When writing your resume *do* all of the following *except*:
   A. Laser print on quality paper.
   B. Proofread carefully.
   C. Use action verbs.
   D. Include personal information.

Critical Thinking

During your interview with a prospective employer, she asks you the following two questions. How would you respond?
● What is something you achieved that made you proud?
● How many days did you miss on your last job? While you were in school?

Glossary

2-hour postprandial (2-HOUR PP): Collection of the specimen occurs 2 hours after the ingestion of the patient's last meal.

3-T's: Training—Transferable skills—Traits.

abandonment: A premature termination of the professional treatment relationship by the health care provider without adequate notice of the patent's consent.

accession number: A unique number given to each test request.

acid-base balance: The mechanisms by which the acidity and alkalinity of body fluids are kept in a state of equilibrium so that arterial blood is maintained at approximately a 7.35 to 7.45 pH level.

acidosis (**as**-ih-**DOE**-sis): An actual or relative increase in the acidity of blood caused by an accumulation of acids or an excessive loss of bicarbonates.

aerobic (er-**O**-bik): Living only in the presence of oxygen. Concerning an organism living only in the presence of oxygen.

afebrile (ay-**FEB**-ril): Without fever.

afferent (**AF**-er-ent): Carrying impulses toward a center.

agranulocyte (a-**GRAN**-u-lo-site): A nongranular white blood cell.

albinism (**AL**-bye-nizm): A partial of total absence of melanin pigment from eyes, hair, and skin.

aliquot (**AL**-ih-kwot): A portion of the specimen used for testing.

alkalosis (**al**-ka-**LO**-sis): An actual or relative increase in blood alkalinity caused by an accumulation of alkalies or reduction of acids.

alveoli (al-**VE**-o-lye): Air cells of the lungs.

anaerobic (**an**-er-**O**-bik): Pertaining to an anaerobe; able to live without oxygen.

analyte (**AN**-a-lite): A substance being analyzed, especially the method of chemical analysis.

anaphylactic shock (**an**-ah-fi-**LAK**-tik): An immediate allergic reaction characterized by acute respiratory distress, hypotension, edema, and rash. Anaphylactic shock can be life-threatening.

anatomy (a-**NAT**-o-me): The study of the structure of an organism.

antecubital (**an**-tee-**KU**-bi-tal): In front of the elbow; at the end of the elbow.

antecubital fossa: Triangular area lying anterior to and below the elbow, where the major veins for venipuncture are located.

anterior: Before or in front of; refers to the ventral or abdominal side of the body.

anticoagulant (**an**-ti-ko-**AG**-u-lant): An agent that prevents or delays blood coagulation (clumping).

antigen (**AN**-tih-jen): A protein or oligosaccharide marker on the surface of cells that identifies the cell as self or non-self; identifies the type of cell, e.g., skin, kidney.

antisepsis (an-ti-**SEP**-sis): The prevention of sepsis by preventing or inhibiting the growth of a causative microorganism.

anuria (ah-**NEW**-ree-ah): The absence of urine formation.

aortic semilunar valve (aye-**OR**-tik **sem**-ee-**LOO**-nur valv): The valve between the left ventricle and the ascending aorta, made up of three half-moon shaped cups.

apex: Distal tip of the heart, located between the fifth and sixth ribs just below the left nipple.

apnea (ap-**NEE**-ah): Temporary cessation of breathing.

arrhythmia (ah-**RITH**-mee-ah): Irregularity or loss of rhythm, especially of the heartbeat. An abnormal heart rhythm.

arterial blood gases (ABG): Literally, any of the gases present in blood. Clinically, the determination of levels in the blood of oxygen and carbon dioxide.

arterial line: A hemodynamic monitoring system consisting of a catheter in an artery connected to pressure tubing, a transducer, and an electronic monitor. It is used to measure systemic blood pressure and to provide ease of access for the drawing of blood for study of gases present.

arteriole (ahr-**TEER**-ee-ole): A small branch of an artery.

arteriosclerosis (ahr-**teer**-ee-o-skleh-**ROH**-sis): The hardening of arteries, resulting in thickening of walls and loss of elasticity.

arteriospasm (ahr-**TEER**-ee-o-spazm): *arteria* (artery) + *spasmos* (convulsion) = arterial spasm.

articulate: Distinct and clear enunciation of words, phrases, and sentences.

artifact: Interference in an ECG tracing.

assault (a-**SAWLT**): The act of intentionally causing someone to fear that he or she is about to become the victim of battery, or incomplete battery.

assay: The analysis of a substance or mixture to determine the components and relative proportion of each.

assignment of benefits: The transfer of one's right to collect an amount payable under an insurance company contract.

atherosclerosis (ath-er-o-skleh-**ROH**-sis): Pathogenic condition in which fat deposits accumulate in the lining of the arteries.

atrioventricular (AV) node: Pacemaking cells found in the right atrium of the interatrial septum.

atrium (**AY**-tree-um): An upper, collecting chamber of the heart. (*pl.* **atria**)

auscultate (**AWS**-kul-tayt): To examine by auscultation; to listen for sounds within the body.

autologous transfusion (aw-**TOL**-o-gus): Transfusion of blood donated by a patient before surgery or collected from a patient during surgery.

axon (**AK**-son): A process of a neuron that conducts impulses away from the cell body.

bacteriemia (**bak**-ter-**EE**-me-ah): Bacteria in the blood.

basophil (**BAY**-suh-fil): One type of granulocytic white blood cell. Basophils make up less than 1% of all leukocytes but are essential to nonspecific immune response to inflammation. They show an attraction for basic dyes.

battery: The act of intentionally touching someone in a harmful or offensive manner without the person's consent.

bevel (**BEV**-el): The point of a needle that has been cut on a slant for ease of entry.

bicuspid valve (bye-**KUS**-pid valve): Also called the mitral valve. Atrioventricular valve of the left side of the heart.

bilateral symmetry (bye-**LAT**-ur-al **SIM**-eh-tree) (**bisymmetric**): Relating to both sides of the body equally.

biohazardous: Anything that is harmful or potentially harmful to humans, other species, or the environment.

biohazardous waste: Any waste material that is harmful or potentially harmful to humans, or other species, or the environment.

bipolar: Composed of a negative and a positive pole; reflecting the difference in electrode potential between two poles.

blood banking: The process of collecting whole blood and certain derived components for processing, typing, and storing until needed for transfusion.

blood-borne pathogen: A term applied to any infectious microorganism present in the blood and/or other body fluids and tissues.

bolus (**BOH**-lus): A rounded mass; food prepared by the mouth for swallowing.

brachial (**BRAY**-kee-al): Pertaining to the arm.

bradycardia (**brad**-ee-**KAR**-dee-ah): A slow heartbeat characterized by a pulse rate below 60 beats per minute throughout one 10-min period.

bradypnea (**brad**-ip-**NEE**-ah): Abnormally slow breathing.

BUN (Blood Urea Nitrogen): Nitrogen in the blood in the form of urea, the metabolic product of the breakdown of amino acids used for energy production. BUN is a blood test that provides a rough estimate of kidney function.

bundle of His: Nerve fibers within the interventricular septum that carry impulses to the bundle branches located in the right and left ventricles.

burden of proof: A legal term used in conjunction with the terms malpractice and negligence. Must be proved by the client when an accusation of malpractice or negligence is claimed, rather than the health care provider proving that none existed.

butterfly infusion set: A ½- to ¾-inch stainless steel needle connected to a 5- to 12-inch length of tubing. It is called a butterfly because of its wing-shaped plastic extensions, which are used for gripping the needle.

calcaneous (**kal**-**KA**-nee-us): The heel bone.

calibrator (**KAL**-i-**bray**-tor): A material or device used to adjust the response or reading of an instrument.

capitation: A system of payment used by managed care plans in which physicians and hospitals are paid a fixed, per capita amount for each patient enrolled, regardless of the number of services provided over a specific period of time.

cardiac cycle: A single rhythmic repetition of the mechanical and electrical events that constitute the heartbeat.

carotid (kah-**ROT**-id): Pertaining to the right and left common carotid arteries, which comprise the principal blood supply to the head and neck.

carrier: A person who harbors a specific pathogenic organism, has no discernible symptoms or signs of the disease, condition, or infection, and is potentially capable of spreading the organism to others.

catheterization (**kath**-eh-ter-ih-**ZAY**-shun): Use or passage of a catheter into a part, chamber, or cavity. Cardiac catheterization is the percutaneous (through the skin) intravascular insertion of a catheter into a chamber of the heart or great vessels. It is the procedure used for the diagnosis, assessment of abnormalities, and interventional treatment and evaluation of the effects of pathology on the heart and great vessels.

causative organism: The organism responsible for causing an infection.

central venous catheter (CVC): A catheter inserted into the superior vena cava to permit intermittent or continuous monitoring of central venous pressure and to facilitate collecting blood samples for chemical analysis.

centrifuge (**SEN**-tri-fuj): A machine used for the process of separating substances of different densities, such as plasma and RBCs in the blood. The centrifuge spins substances at high speeds.

cerebrospinal fluid (seh-**ree**-bro-**SPY**-nul **FLEW**-id) (**CSF**): A water cushion protecting the brain and spinal cord from physical impact.

chain of custody: The procedure for ensuring that material obtained for diagnosis has been taken from the named patient, is properly labeled, and has not been tampered with en route to the laboratory.

chain of infection: A series of related events that lead to an infection.

chemoprophylaxis (**kee**-mo-**pro**-fi-**LAK**-sis): The use of a drug or chemical to prevent a disease (e.g., the taking of an appropriate medicine to prevent malaria).

cholesterol (**ko**-**LES**-ter-ol): The most abundant steroid in animal tissues. It serves many functions in the body including manufacturing of bile acids that allows the body to digest lipids and fats. Some cholesterol is used to manufacture hormones such as testosterone, progesterone, and estrogen. Cholesterol is broken into two factions: high-density lipoprotein (HDL) and low-density lipoprotein (LDL). In most individuals, an elevated blood level of cholesterol constitutes an increased risk of developing coronary heart disease.

chyme (kime): Food which has undergone gastric digestion.

claim: A billing sent to an insurance carrier.

clarity: The range of clearness to turbidity of a specimen.

code-blue: A coded message broadcast over a hospital's public address system. Code-blue indicates the need for an emergency team to respond to a patient in cardiac or respiratory arrest.

coinsurance: A cost-sharing requirement specified in a health insurance policy, providing that the insured will assume a percentage of the costs for covered services.

collateral circulation: A process allowing tissue to be supplied with blood from an accessory vessel.

communication: Transmission of a message from a sender to a receiver.

complexes: Groups of related, recorded waves.

contractility (kon-trak-**TIL**-ih-tee): Having the ability to contract or shorten.

copayment: A specified dollar amount that the patient must pay the provider for each encounter; also called copay.

coronary circulation: Blood supply to the myocardium of the heart from branches of the aorta.

courier sheet: A blank sheet of paper used to attach laboratory reports chronologically, in a shingled fashion.

cover letter: A letter of introduction accompanying your resume to prospective employers.

cranial cavity (**KRAY**-nee-al **KAV**-eh-tee): The cavity that houses the brain.

cultural diversity: The cultural identity of groups of people, their environments, ideas, values, traditions, institutions, and technologies.

culture and sensitivity (C&S): The process by which bacterial organisms are grown on media and identified, and an antibiotic susceptibility (sensitivity) test is performed to determine which antibiotics will be effective against the organism.

customer: A person, patient, or client to whom goods are delivered or services are rendered.

cytoplasm (**SIGH**-toh-plazm): Protoplasm of the cell body, excluding the nucleus.

database: A compilation of stored information in a unique software program that can be processed or produced by a computer.

deductible: Specified dollar amount that must be paid by the insured before a medical insurance plan or government program begins covering health care costs.

deep: Below the surface.

dendrite (**DEN**-drite): The nerve cell process that carries nervous impulses toward the cell body.

deoxygenated (dee-**OCK**-si-jen-ate-ed): The state of having oxygen removed from a compound or tissue.

depolarlization: A reversal of charges at a cell membrane; an electrical change in an excitable cell in which the inside of the cell becomes positive in relation to the outside; opposite of polarization.

dermis (**DUR**-mis): The true skin; lying immediately beneath the epidermis.

diaphoretic (dye-ah-for-**ET**-ik): Producing perspiration; sweating.

diastole (dye-**AS**-toh-lee): The normal "rest period" in the heart cycle, during which the muscle fibers lengthen, the heart dilates, and the cavities fill with blood.

differential (**dif**-er-**EN**-shal): The number and type of cells determined by microscopic examination of a thin layer of blood on a glass slide.

distal (**DIS**-tul): The farthest point of origin of a structure, opposite of proximal.

distress: Physical or mental pain or suffering. A term used to describe abnormal, unhealthy, or extreme stress.

donor unit: A specific amount of blood, approximately 1 pint, supplied by a volunteer as part of a blood-banking procedure.

dorsal cavity (**DOR**-sul **KAV**-eh-tee): The posterior cavity of the body which houses the brain and spinal column.

duodenum (**dew**-o-**DEE**-num): The first part of the small intestine, beginning at the pylorus.

duty of care: The responsibility not to infringe on another's rights by either intentionally or carelessly causing him or her harm.

efferent: Carrying away from a central organ or section, as efferent nerves.

elasticity (**e**-las-**TIS**-ih-tee): The quality of returning to original size and shape after compression or stretching.

electrocardiogram (ECG): A record of the electrical activity of the heart.

electrodes: Small, specially prepared tabs with conductive gel placed in direct contact with the skin to detect electrical current from within the heart.

electrolytes (ee-**LEK**-tro-lites): Substances that conduct electricity when dissolved in water. Acids, bases, and salts are common electrolytes, including potassium, sodium, and chlorine found in blood, tissue fluids, and cells.

empathy: Objective awareness of and insight into the feelings, emotions, and behavior of another person.

endocardium (**en**-do-**KAR**-dee-um): Membrane lining the interior of the heart.

endocrine gland (**EN**-doh-crin gland): A gland which secretes into the blood or tissue fluid instead of into a duct.

Environmental Protection Agency (EPA): The federal agency that regulates and monitors the inventory, storage, usage, techniques, and disposal of harmful substances to the environment.

eosinophil (**ee**-o-**SIN**-uh-fil): White blood cells whose granules stain a bright orange-red with eosin or other acid dyes. They increase in an allergic response.

epicardium (**ep**-ih-**KAR**-dee-um): External layer of the heart and part of pericardial sac.

epidermis (**ep**-ih-**DUR**-mis): Outermost layer of skin.

epiglottis (**ep**-ih-**GLOT**-is): Elastic cartilage which prevents food from entering the trachea.

erythrocyte (e-**RITH**-ro-site): A mature red blood cell (RBC).

ethics: A system of principles governing medical conduct. It deals with the relationship of the health care professional to the patient, the patient's family, associates, and society at large.

eustress: A term used to describe normal, healthy, or manageable stress.

excitability (ek-**sye**-tah-**BIL**-eh-tee): The ability to respond to stimuli.

exocrine gland (**EX**-o-crin gland): A gland that secretes into a duct.

explanation of benefits: An explanation of services periodically issued to recipients or providers on whose behalf claims have been paid.

extensibility (ek-**STEN**-sih-bil-eh-tee): The ability to increase the angle between two bones.

exudation (eks-oo-**DAY**-shun): Pathologic oozing of fluids, usually the result of inflammation.

false imprisonment: The intentional and unjustifiable act of preventing someone from moving about.

fasting blood sugar (FBS): The patient is required to restrict dietary intake for 12 hours prior to the collection of a specimen for testing for glucose levels in the blood.

febrile (**FEB**-ril): Feverish; pertaining to a fever. Abnormal elevation of temperature.

felony: A crime more serious than a misdemeanor, punishable by a sentence of more than one year in prison or death.

fimbria (**FIM**-bree-ah): The longest fringe-like extremity of a fallopian tube extending from the uterine tube to almost the ovary.

fomites (**FO**-mih-tez): Objects, such as clothing, towels, and utensils that possibly harbor a disease agent and are capable of transmitting it.

fraud: An intentional misrepresentation. A deliberate deception intended to produce unlawful gain.

frontal plane: A plane parallel to the long axis of the body and at right angles to the median sagittal plane. The frontal plane divides the body into anterior and posterior portions.

galvanometer (**gal**-van-**OM**-et-er): An instrument that measures electric current by electromagnetic action. The early ECG machine.

gamete (**GAM**-eet): A mature male or female reproductive cell; the spermatozoon or ovum.

gatekeeper: Primary care physician responsible for advising and coordinating the patient's health care needs.

glomerulus (gloh-**MER**-yah-lus): A part of the nephron; a tuft of capillaries situated within Bowman's capsule.

glucose tolerance test (GTT): A test involving multiple collections of blood and urine over time to evaluate the metabolism of glucose. It is performed by giving the patient a measured amount of glucose either orally or intravenously.

glucosuria (**gloo**-cos-**UR**-ee-ah): Sugar (glucose) in the urine.

granulocyte (**GRAN**-u-loh-site): A white blood cell having granules in its cytoplasm.

hard copy: A printed paper copy of a computer generated report.

hardware: Equipment used to process data (i.e., keyboard, disk drive, monitor, and printer).

health maintenance organization (HMO): A type of health care program in which enrollees receive benefits for services from authorized and preselected providers, usually a primary care physician. Generally, enrollees do not receive coverage, except for emergency services or for the services of providers who are not in the HMO network.

hematocrit (he-**MAT**-o-krit): Percentage by volume of red blood cells in whole blood.

hematoma (hem-ah-**TOE**-ma): A swelling or mass of blood (usually clotted), confined to an organ, tissue, or space that is caused by a break in a blood vessel.

hematuria (**heem**-a-**TOOR**-ee-ah): Blood in the urine.

hemochromatosis (he-mo-**kro**-ma-**TO**-sis): A genetic disease marked by excessive absorption and accumulation of iron in the body.

hemoconcentration (he-mo-**kon**-sen-**TRAY**-shun): A relative increase in the number of red blood cells resulting from a decrease in the volume of plasma.

hemoglobin (**HE**-muh-gloh-bin): The iron-containing protein pigment of the red blood cells, which carries oxygen from the lungs to the tissues.

hemoglobinuria (**he**-mo-glo-bin-**UR**-ee-ah): The presence in urine of hemoglobin free from red blood cells.

hemolysis (he-**MOL**-ih-sis): The destruction of the membrane of red blood cells and the liberation of hemoglobin, which diffuses into the surrounding fluid.

hemophiliac (**he**-mo-**FIL**-ee-ak): A person afflicted with a hereditary blood disease marked by greatly prolonged blood coagulation time, with consequent failure of the blood to clot and abnormal bleeding, sometimes accompanied by joint swelling.

hemopoiesis (**he**-mo-poy-**EE**-sis) (**hematopoiesis**): The production and development of blood cells, normally in the bone marrow.

hemostasis (**he**-moh-**STAY**-sis): An arrest of bleeding or of circulation. A stagnation of blood.

hepatitis B (HBV): A blood-borne pathogen that causes a severe acute infection and may progress to chronic infection and permanent liver damage. It is caused by the hepatitis B virus, an enveloped, double-stranded DNA virus.

high-density lipoprotein cholesterol (HDL): The "good" cholesterol.

homeostasis (**ho**-me-oh-**STAY**-sis): The state of dynamic equilibrium of the internal environment of the body.

hormone (**HOR**-mone): Chemical secretion, usually from an endocrine gland (e.g., insulin from the pancreas).

human chorionic gonadotrophin (HCG): A hormone produced by the placenta that appears in both urine and serum, beginning approximately 10 days after conception, the presence of which is an indication of pregnancy.

human immunodeficiency virus (HIV): A retrovirus that causes acquired immunodeficiency syndrome (AIDS).

hyperglycemic (**hi**-per-gly-**SEE**-mik): Pertaining to the condition in which the blood sugar (glucose) is increased, as in diabetes mellitus.

hyperkalemia (**hi**-per-ka-**LEE**-me-ah): An excessive amount of potassium in the blood.

hypertension (**hi**-per-**TEN**-shun): A condition in which the patient has a higher than normal blood pressure. For adults, this usually means a BP >140/90.

hypoglycemic (**hi**-po-gly-**SEE**-mik): Pertaining to a condition in which the blood sugar (glucose) is abnormally low, as in hyperinsulinism.

hypokalemia (**hi**-po-ka-**LEE**-me-ah): Extreme potassium depletion in the blood.

hypotension (**hi**-po-**TEN**-shun): A decrease of the systolic and diastolic blood pressure values which are significantly lower than normal.

hypothermia (**hi**-po-**THER**-mee-ah): The state in which an individual's body temperature is reduced below the normal range: <96.0˚ F.

ileum (**IL**-ee-um): The lower part of the small intestine, extending from the jejunum to the large intestine.

infection (in-**FEK**-shun): The presence and growth of a microorganism that produces tissue damage.

inferior (in-**FEH**-re-or): Beneath, lower, referring to the underside of an organ or indicating a structure below another.

informed consent: Agreement by the patient to a medical procedure or treatment after receiving adequate information about the procedure or treatment, risks, and/or consequences.

inpatient: A patient who is hospitalized overnight.

insured: Individual or organization covered for protection and loss under the specific terms of an insurance policy.

integrity: To adhere to a strict ethical code. To be in an undiminished or unimpaired state.

intentional infliction of emotional distress: The willful infliction of emotions or actions causing the patient to suffer duress.

interstitial fluid (in-ter-**STISH**-al): Fluid between the tissues; surrounding a cell.

intervals: A wave in addition to a connecting straight line.

intradermal (**in**-tra-**DER**-mal): Within the substance of the skin.

invasion of privacy: A tort involving one or more of the following four categories: illegal appropriation of another's name for commercial use, intrusion into a person's privacy, placing a person in false light, or disclosure of private facts.

invasive procedure: A procedure that requires penetrating intact skin or mucous membranes.

ischemia (ih-**SKEE**-me-ah): Inadequate flow of blood to the heart, leading to angina pectoris and, if untreated, to myocardial infarction.

jejunum (je-**JOO**-num): The section of the small intestine between the duodenum and the ileum.

ketonuria (kee-to-**NUR**-ee-ah): The formation or excretion of ketones in the urine.

kinesics (kih-**NEE**-six): Systematic study of the body and the use of its static and dynamic position as a means of communication.

lancet (**LAN**-set): A sterile, disposable sharp-pointed instrument used to pierce the skin to obtain droplets of blood used for testing.

lateral (**LAT**-ur-ul): Toward the side.

leukocyte (**LOO**-ko-site): A white blood cell or corpuscle (WBC).

libel: A written statement falsifying facts about someone that causes harm to that person's reputation.

low-density lipoprotein cholesterol (LDL): The "bad" cholesterol.

lumen (**LEW**-min): Passageway or opening to a tubular structure such as a blood vessel, phlebotomy, or hypodermic needle.

lymph (limf): Watery fluid in the lymphatic vessels.

lymphocyte (**LIM**-foh-site): A type of white blood cell; makes up less than 1% of the circulating blood cells.

malpractice: The misconduct or unprofessional treatment by someone in a professional or official position.

market value: What a product (you) is worth to the consumer (employer); characteristics and skills that are valuable in the employment market.

mastication (**mas**-ti-**KAY**-shun): Process of chewing.

means of exit: The route microorganisms can take to leave a host (i.e., eyes, mouth, nose, open wound, blood).

means of transmission: The method by which microorganisms can be transmitted from one host to another. The five main routes of transmission are: contact, droplet, airborne, common vehicle, and vector-borne.

medial (**MEE**-dee-ul): Toward the midline of the body.

mediastinum (**mee**-dee-as-**TIH**-num): Region of the thoracic cavity containing the heart and blood vessels, lying between the sternum and vertebral column and between the lungs.

melanocyte (**MEL**-an-o-**site**): A melanin-forming cell. Those of the skin are found in the lower epidermis.

meninges (men-**IN**-jeez): Membranes covering the spinal cord and brain: dura mater (external), arachnoid (middle), and pia mater (internal).

meniscus (men-**IS**-kus): The curved upper surface of a liquid in a container.

metabolism (meh-**TAB**-oh-**lizm**): Sum total of processes of digestion, absorption, and the resulting release of energy.

microbe (**MY**-krobe): A unicellular or small multicellular microscopic organism not visible to the naked eye.

microcollection container: Small plastic containers or tubes, often referred to as "bullets" because of their size and shape, that are primarily used to collect skin puncture blood specimens.

microorganism (**my**-kro-**OR**-gan-ism): A minute living body not perceptible to the naked eye, such as a bacterium or protozoan.

midsagittal plane (mid-**SAJ**-eh-tel plane): An imaginary line dividing the body into equal right and left halves.

misdemeanor: A crime less serious than a felony, punishable by a fine or imprisonment of up to one year in jail.

monocyte (**MON**-oh-site): Large mononuclear leukocyte with deeply indented nucleus and slate-gray cytoplasm.

myelin sheath (**MY**-eh-lin sheath): A phospholipids-protein of membranes forming an electrical insulator that increases the velocity of impulse transmission; found surrounding nerve fibers.

myocardium (**MY**-oh-**kar**-dee-um): Middle layer of heart muscle, responsible for pumping action.

needle gauge: A standard for measuring the diameter of the lumen of a needle.

negligence: The failure to act with reasonable care, resulting in the harming of others.

nephron (**NEF**-ron): A unit of structure of the kidney; contains glomerulus, Bowman's capsule, proximal distal tubule, loop of Henle, and distal tubule.

network: A group of microcomputers that are linked for the purpose of sharing resources and providing internal communication.

networking: Meeting with people you know, or have just met, to discuss your career plans.

neuron (**NEW**-ron): A nerve cell, including its processes.

neutrophil (**NOO**-trah-fil): Many-lobed nucleus, white blood cell that phagocytizes bacteria; sometimes called "polys or segs."

nonpathogenic: A microbe which is nondisease producing.

nosocomial (**nos**-o-**KO**-me-al): Infection acquired in a hospital.

occluded (o-**KLUDE**-ed): Closed or obstructed or joined together.

occult (uh-**KULT**): Obscure; concealed, hidden.

oliguria (**ol**-ih-**GOO**-ree-ah): Diminished urination.

osteochondritis (**os**-tee-o-**kon**-**DRY**-tis): Inflammation of the bone and cartilage.

osteomyelitis (**os**-tee-o-**my**-el-**EYE**-tis): Inflammation of the bone (especially the bone marrow) caused by a pathogenic organism.

ova (**O**-va): Female reproductive cell.

P-R interval: Time for electrical impulse to conduct through atria and the AV node.

P wave: Records atrial depolarization and contraction.

palpate (**PAL**-payt): To examine by touch; to feel.

palpation (pal-**PAY**-shun): Examination by feel or touch.

papilla (pa-**PIL**-uh): Small, nipple-shaped elevation (*pl.* papillae).

paresthesia (**par**-es-**THEE**-zee-ah): An unusual sensation of tingling, crawling, or burning of the skin for no apparent reason.

pathogen: An organism or substance capable of causing a disease, condition, or infection.

pathogenic: Capable of causing disease.

pCO$_2$: The symbol for partial pressure of carbon dioxide.

pericardium (**per**-ih-**KAR**-dee-um): The closed membranous sac surrounding the heart.

periosteum (**per**-ee-**OS**-tee-um): Fibrous tissue covering the bone.

peripherally inserted central catheter (PICC): Catheter inserted into the peripheral venous system (veins of an extremity) and then threaded into the central venous system.

periphery (**per**-**IF**-eh-rey): The outer part or surface of a body; the part away from the center.

peristalsis (**per**-ih-**STAL**-sis): A progressive wave of contraction in tubular structures provided with longitudinal and transverse muscular fibers, as in the esophagus, stomach, small and large intestine.

perpendicular (**per**-pen-**DIK**-yoo-lar): Being at right angles to the plane of the horizon.

personal protective equipment (PPE): Disposable gloves, lab coats or aprons, and/or protective face gear, such as masks and goggles with side shields, required by OSHA to be worn when handling body fluids.

pH: The degrees of acidity or alkalinity of a substance. The neutral point where a solution would be neither acid nor alkaline is a pH of 7. A number less than 7 would be acid and above 7 alkaline.

phagocytosis (**fag**-oh-sigh-**TOH**-sis): The ingestion of foreign substances or other particles, such as worn-out cells, by certain white blood cells.

phospholipids (**fos**-foh-**LIP**-ids): Fats containing carbon, hydrogen, oxygen, and phosphorous.

physiology (**fiz**-ee-**OL**-oh-jee): The study of the functions of the living organism and its components.

pneumatic tube system: A unidirectional, continuously operating vacuum system that transfers specimens in plexiglass carriers from the patient units to the laboratory.

point-of-care tests (POCT): Laboratory testing performed at the site of the patient, using portable or hand-held instruments.

polarized: Resting state of cardiac cells.

polycythemia (**pol**-ee-si-**THE**-me-a): A disease characterized by an overproduction of red blood cells.

posterior (pos-**TEER**-ee-ur): A location behind or at the back; opposite to anterior.

precordial leads (pre-**KOR**-dee-al leeds): Leads situated on the chest directly overlying the heart.

pre-existing condition: Any illness that began before the insurance policy was written.

preferred provider organization (PPO): A type of health benefit program in which enrollees receive the highest level of benefits when they obtain services from a physician, hospital, or other health care provider designated by their program as a "preferred provider."

professionalism: The conduct, behavior, and qualities that characterize a professional person.

prone: A position which is horizontal with the face downward.

proteinuria (**pro**-teen-**UR**-ee-ah): Protein, usually albumin, in the urine.

prothrombin: A plasma protein coagulation factor synthesized by the liver that is converted to thrombin in the presence of calcium ions.

proximal (**PROK**-sih-mul): A location nearest the point of attachment, center of the body, or point of reference.

pulmonary circulation: Flow of blood from right ventricle through the lungs, and back to the left atrium.

pulmonary semilunar valve (**PUL**-mo-neh-ree **sem**-ee-**LOO**-nar valv): The half-moon shaped valve between the right ventricle and the pulmonary artery.

pulse (puls): Rate, rhythm, and condition of arterial walls.

Purkinje fibers (pur-**KIN**-gee): Modified myocardial cells found in distal areas of the bundle branches. They conduct electricity from the bundle of His through the ventricles.

QRS complex: Represents depolarization or contraction of the ventricles.

QT interval: Measures from the beginning of ventricular depolarization to the end of ventricular repolarization.

radial (**RAY**-dee-al): 1) Radiating out from a given center. 2) Pertaining to the radius. 3) Pulse palpated over the radial artery of the arm.

reasonable fee: A charge is considered reasonable if it is deemed acceptable after peer review, even though it does not meet the customary or prevailing criteria. Reasonable fees include unusual circumstances or complications requiring additional time, skill, or experience in connection with a particular service or procedure.

referral: A name of a person or company given to you to contact as part of your career-marketing plan.

reflux (**RE**-fluks): A return or backward flow.

renal calculi: Kidney stones.

repolarization: Re-establishment of a condition or state in which the inside of the cell is considerably more positive than the outside of the cell.

reservoir host (**REZ** er-vwor host): Any person, animal, arthropod, plant, soil, or substance in which an infectious agent normally lives, reproduces, and depends on for survival, that allows transmission to a susceptible host. In essence, a reservoir host is the breeding ground for transmission or pathogens to others.

respiration (**res**-pir-**AY**-shun): The act of breathing (i.e., inhaling and exhaling), during which the lungs take in a fresh supply of oxygen and give off carbon dioxide and other waste products.

respondeat superior: A Latin phrase which means "let the master answer." In more common language, employers must answer for damage their employees cause within the scope of the employee's position.

resume (**REZ**-oo-**may**): A typed document describing your employment history, education, and objectives, given to prospective employers as a means of providing background information prior to or during an employment interview.

sagittal plane (**SAJ**-eh-tel plane): A longitudinal imaginary line dividing the body into equal right and left parts.

Schwann cell (shwon cell): One of the cells of the peripheral nervous system that forms the myelin sheath.

sclerosed (skle-**ROZT**): Hardened; having sclerosis.

sebaceous gland (seh-**BAY**-shus): An oil-secreting gland of the skin.

sebum (**SE**-bum): A fatty secretion of the sebaceous glands of the skin.

sediment (**SED**-i-ment): The substance settling at the bottom of a liquid.

segments: The straight lines connecting waves.

seizure (**SEE**-zhur): A sudden attack of pain, a disease, or certain symptoms. An epileptic attack; convulsion.

septicemia (**sep**-tih-**SEE**-me-ah): The presence of pathogenic microorganisms in the blood.

septum: A dividing wall between parts of the body. In the heart, the septum is located between the atria and also between the ventricles.

server: A computer in a network shared by multiple users, which serves as a central repository of data and programs. The terms may apply to both the hardware and software, or just the software that performs the service.

sharps container: A special puncture-resistant, leak-proof, disposable container used to dispose of used needles, lancets, and other sharp objects.

shingled: Attaching a report to a courier sheet in a layered fashion (like shingles on a roof), with the most recently dated report on top.

sinoatrial (SA) node (**sine**-oh-**AY**-tree-al): Natural pacemaker of the heart, positioned in the right atrium.

slander: The act of falsifying of facts which causes harm to a person's reputation. Slander is spoken as opposed to libel, which is written.

software: Coded instructions (programs) required to make hardware perform a specific function.

solute (**SOL**-yoot): A dissolved substance in a solution.

somatic interference: An artifact on an ECG tracing caused by the patient, for example, talking, sneezing, muscle tremors.

specific gravity: The weight of a substance compared with the weight of an equal volume of water. The specific gravity of water is 1.000.

spermatozoa (sper-**mat**-oh-**ZOH**-ah): A mature male sex cell.

sphygmomanometer (**sfig**-mo-man-**OM**-et-er): An instrument for indirectly determining arterial blood pressure. Two types are aneroid and mercury.

spinal cavity (**SPY**-nel **CAV** eh-tee): The cavity of the body that houses the spinal cord.

ST segment: Isoelectric line from the end of S wave to the beginning of T wave.

standards: That which is established by custom or authority as a mode or rule for comparison of measurement.

stratum corneum (**STRAH**-tum **KOR**-nee-um): The outermost horny layer of the epidermis.

stratum germinativum (**strah**-tum **jer**-mi-nah-**TIVE**-um): The innermost layer of the epidermis.

strike through: Contamination caused by pathogens being transported through a wet barrier from a nonsterile area to a sterile area.

subcutaneous (**sub**-ku-**TAY**-nee-us): Beneath the skin.

sublingual (sub-**LING**-wal): Beneath or concerning the area beneath the tongue.

superficial (**soo**-per-**FISH**-al): Pertaining to or situated near the surface.

superior (soo-**PEER**-ee-ur): In anatomy, higher; denoting upper of two parts, toward vertex.

supine (soo-**PINE**): The position of lying on the back with the face upward.

suprapubic (**soo**-pra-**PEW**-bik): Located above the pubic arch.

surfactant (sur-**FAK**-tent): A surface-active agent that lowers surface tension.

susceptible host: A person who has little resistance to an infectious disease.

sweeps: Hospital rounds (visiting each department or patient of the hospital) which occur at regular intervals throughout the day.

synapse (**SIN**-aps): The space between adjacent neurons through which an impulse is transmitted.

syncopal (**SIN**-ko-pal): A transient loss of consciousness resulting from an inadequate flow of blood to the brain, relating to or marked by syncope.

syncope (**SIN**-ko-pea): A transient loss of consciousness resulting from an inadequate flow of blood to the brain. The patient experiences a generalized weakness of muscles, loss of postural tone, inability to continue standing, and loss of consciousness.

systemic circulation: Flow of oxygen-rich blood to all body tissue and organs from the left ventricle via the arteries and the return of oxygen-depleted blood to the right atrium via the veins.

systole (**SIS**-toh-lee): Contractions of the chambers of the heart, in which blood is pumped from the chamber.

T wave: Represents repolarization (relaxation) of the ventricles.

tachycardia (**tak**-ee-**KAR**-dee-ah): An abnormally rapid heart beat. Usually defined as a heart rate greater than 100 beats per minute in adults.

tachypnea (**tak**-ip-**NEE**-ah): Abnormal rapidity of respiration.

therapeutic (ther-a-**PU**-tik): Pertaining to results obtained from treatment.

thrombocyte (**THROM**-boh-site): Platelet.

thromboplastin (**throm**-bo-**PLAS**-tin): The substance secreted by platelets when tissue is injured; necessary for blood clotting.

thrombosed (**THROM**-bosd): Denoting a vessel containing a thrombus.

topical (**TOP**-ih-kal): Pertaining to a definite surface area; local. Generally refers to the application of a substance to the skin.

tort: A private wrong or injury, other than breach of contract, for which the court will provide a remedy.

tourniquet (**TOOR**-ni-ket): Any constrictor used on an extremity to apply pressure over an artery and thereby control bleeding; also used to distend veins to facilitate venipuncture or intravenous injections.

traits: Personal attributes, characteristics, and/or behavior that you consistently demonstrate and that describe you (e.g., cheerful, outgoing, hard working).

transparency: In reference to urine, the ability or difficulty to see through a specimen.

transverse plane: A plane that divides the body into a top and bottom portion.

Tricare: Three options managed health care program offer to spouses and dependents of service personnel with uniform benefits and fees implemented nationwide by the federal government.

tricuspid valve (tri-**KUS**-pid valv): A three-part valve located between the right atrium and right ventricle.

tunica adventitia (**TOON**-ih-kah ad-ven-**TISH**-uh): The outermost fibroelastic layer of a blood vessel.

tunica intima (**TOON**-ih-kah **IN**-tih-ma): The lining of a blood vessel composed of an epithelial layer and the basement membrane, a connective tissue layer, and usually an internal elastic lamina.

tunica media (**TOON**-ih-kah **ME**-dyuh): The middle layer in the wall of a blood vessel composed of circular or spiraling smooth muscle and some elastic fibers.

turbidity: (tur-**BID**-i-tee): Opacity caused by the suspension of flaky or granular particles in a normally clear liquid.

U wave: Follows the T wave. Usually of low voltage; may become more prominent in some electrolyte imbalances, heart disease, or as an effect of medications.

unipolar lead: Measures absolute electrical force at the site of a positive electrode.

universal donor: An individual with type O blood which has no A or B antigens; can donate to all blood types.

universal recipient: An individual belonging to the AB blood group; can accept blood from all blood types.

uremia (yoo-**REE**-mee-ah): The presence of urea and excess waste products in the blood.

urethra (yoo-**REE**-thra): A canal for the discharge of urine extending from the bladder to the outside.

usual and customary fee: A method used by insurance companies to establish their fee schedules (specific amounts charged per procedure). It employs a complex system in which three fees are considered in calculating payment: the fee that is usually charged, the fee that is customarily charged by similar practices in the same geographic location, and the reasonable fee.

uvula (**YOO**-vew-luh): The projection hanging from soft palate, in back of throat.

vascular access devices (VAD): Indwelling catheters are also called vascular access devices (VADs). VADs consist mainly of tubing inserted into a main artery or vein. This main vein or artery is customarily the subclavian, which is located in the chest below the clavicle. VADs are usually inserted for administering fluids and medications, monitoring pressures, and drawing blood.

vasoconstriction (**vas**-oh-kon-**STRIK**-shun): A decrease in the caliber of blood vessels.

vector: Path or impulse representing the direction and magnitude of the heart's electrical current.

venipuncture (**VEN**-ih-**punk**-chur): Puncture of a vein for any purpose.

ventral cavity: Pertaining to the belly; the opposite of dorsal. The anterior portion or the front side of the body.

ventricle (**VEN**-trik-ul): A small cavity or chamber as in the heart or the brain. Lower pumping chambers of the heart.

villi (**VIL**-eye): Hairlike projections, as in intestinal mucous membrane (*sing*. villus).

vital signs (**VI**-tal sines): The traditional signs of life (i.e., heartbeat, body temperature, respiration, and blood pressure).

void (voyd): To evacuate the bowels or bladder.

waves: Deflections from the baseline of the ECG.

wheal (hweel): A more or less round and evanescent elevation of the skin, white in the center with a pale-red periphery, accompanied by itching.

Resources

A patient's bill of rights. http://www.aha.org/resource/pbillofrights.htm

Biopharm. Biopharm Copyright © 1996, 1997, 1998, 1999, 2000. http://www.biopharm-leeches.com/faq.htm. Most recent revision 15th February, 2002.

Blood transfusion. 2000. Microsoft® Encarta® Online Encyclopedia. http://www.aabb.org/All_About_Blood/FAQs/aabb_faqs.htm. http://encarta.msn.com © Microsoft Corporation. All rights reserved.

Brisendine, K. J. (1998). *Multiskilling Series, Electrocardiography for the healthcare provider*, Clifton Park, NY: Delmar Learning.

Career marketing. (2002). Anchorage, AK: Career Academy.

Courtesy Tox Talk. (1996). Phoenix, AZ: Sonora Laboratory Sciences.

Davis, B. K. (1997). *Phlebotomy: A client based approach.* Clifton Park, NY: Delmar Learning.

Erlich, A. (2001). *Medical terminology for health professions* (4th ed.). Clifton Park, NY: Delmar Learning.

Exposure to blood—What health care workers need to know. Department of Health & Human Services. This page last reviewed 10/23/02. http://www.cdc.gov

Flight, M. (1998). *Law, liability, and ethics for medical office professionals* (3rd ed.). Clifton Park, NY: Delmar Learning.

Flynn, J. C., Jr., (1999). *Procedures in phlebotomy* (2nd ed.). Philadelphia: W. B. Saunders.

Ford, G. *The Ancient Art of Blood Letting.* Museum of Questionable Medical Devices. Updated 8/19/00. http://www.mtn.org/~quack/devices/phlebo.htm.

Fordney, M. (1999). *Insurance handbook for the medical offices* (6th ed.). Philadelphia: W. B. Saunders.

Frengen, B., & Blume, W. (2001). *Phlebotomy basics, with other laboratory techniques.* Upper Saddle River, NY: Prentice Hall.

609

Garza, D., & Becan-McBride, K. (2002). *Phlebotomy handbook—Blood collection essentials* (6th ed.). Upper Saddle River, NY: Prentice Hall.

Handal, L. (2001). *Sensible application of the ECG—A pocket guide.* Clifton Park, NY: Delmar Learning.

Hoeltke, L. B. (2000). *The complete textbook of phlebotomy* (2nd ed.). Clifton Park, NY: Delmar Learning.

Hosley, J., Jones, S., & Molle-Matthews, E. (1997). *Textbook for medical assistants.* Philadelphia: Lippincott.

Keir, L., Wise, B. A., & Krebs, C. (1998). *Medical assisting administrative and clinical competencies* (4th ed.). Clifton Park, NY: Delmar Learning.

Kovanda, B. M. (1998). *Multiskilling Series, Phlebotomy collection procedures.* Clifton Park, NY: Delmar Learning.

Kovanda, B. M. (1998). *Point of care testing capillary puncture.* Clifton Park, NY: Delmar Learning.

Kubler-Ross, E. (1997). *On death and dying.* New York: Simon & Schuster.

Leland, K., & Bailey K. (1999). *Customer service for dummies* (2nd ed.). Foster City, CA: IDG Books Worldwide.

Lopez, V. (1993). *Business law and introduction.* Boston, MA: Mirror Press.

Marshall, J. R. (1999). *The clinical laboratory assistant/phlebotomist.* Orange, CA: Career Publishing.

McCall, R., & Tankersley, C. (1998). *Phlebotomy essentials* (2nd ed.). Philadelphia: Lippincott, Williams & Wilkins.

Monster Career Center Healthcare. htttp://www.monster.com

Needle phobias. On Health Network Company. Copyright 2000. http://www.onhealth.com

Nielson, R. D. (2000). *OSHA regulations and guidelines.* Clifton Park, NY: Delmar Learning.

Pendergraph, G. E., & Pendergraph, C. B. (1998). *Handbook of phlebotomy and patient service techniques* (4th ed.). Baltimore: Williams & Wilkins.

Ramuthowski, B., Barrie, A., Dazarow, L., & Abel, C. (1999). *Clinical procedures for medical assisting.* New York: Glencoe.

Removal of contaminated needles. OSHA Trade News Release. June 12, 2002. http://www.osha.gov. (Contact Frank Meilinger Phone # (202) 693-1999).

Scott, A. & Fong, E. (1998). *Body structures and functions* (9th ed.). Clifton Park, NY: Delmar Learning.

Sommer, S. R., & Warekois, R. S. (2002). *Phlebotomy worktext and procedures manual.* Philadelphia: W. B. Saunders.

Thibodeau, G. A., & Patton, K. T. (1997). *Structure and function of the body* (10th ed.). St. Louis, MO: Mosby.

Thomas, C. (2001). *Taber's cyclopedic medical dictionary* (19th ed.). Philadelphia: F. A. Davis.

UTHSC—http://www.utmem.edu/allied/MEd.Tech/WHATISA.html

Wedding, M. E., & Toenjes, S. A. (1998). *Medical laboratory procedures* (2nd ed.). Philadelphia: F. A. Davis.

Index

HCV. *See* Hepatitis C
HDL. *See* High-density lipoprotein
    cholesterol
Health care
    communication, considerations,
        536–537
    professional, stress, 544
    provider, health maintenance,
        545–548
    revisions, 212–213
    team, phlebotomist (interaction),
        11–15
Health Care Financing Administration
    (HCFA), 480
    HCFA-1500 form, 213
Health Maintenance Organization (HMO),
    definition, 212
Heart, 123–126
    anatomy, review, 275–278
    diagnostic tests, 126
    disorders, 125–126
    electrical conduction, 278–281
        system, 125
    electrophysiology, 279–281
    failure, 125
    function, 123
    layers, 125
    physiology, review, 275–278
    rate
        calculation, 286
        increase, 546
    structures, 123–124
Heartburn, 98
Heat. *See* Human body
Heels
    stick. *See* Infant
    usage, 357
HemaCheck, 504
Hematocrit (Hct), 482–485
    definition, 482
    reference value range, 485
    test, 145
Hematoma, 430–432
    definition, 430
    nonoccurrence, reasons, 431–432
    risk, 444
Hematopoiesis. *See* Hemopoiesis
Hematuria, definition, 107, 517
Hemoccult Sensa Test, 504
Hemochromatosis, definition, 4
Hemochron Jr., 493
Hemoconcentration, definition, 383
HemoCue Hemoglobin System (HemoCue,
    Inc.), 485
Hemogards™, 410
Hemoglobin (Hgb), 485–486
    A1c. *See* Glycosylated hemoglobin
    definition, 138, 485
    test, 145
    value ranges, 486
Hemoglobinuria, definition, 517
Hemogram, 145
Hemolysis
    cause, 398
    chance, 397
    definition, 25, 138, 335
Hemophilia, 144
Hemophiliac, definition, 427
Hemopoiesis (hematopoiesis), definition, 78
Hemorrhoids, 135
Hemostasis, 141–142, 494
    definition, 141, 491
HEPA. *See* High-efficiency particulate air
Heparin therapy, 492
Hepatitis, 98
    risk, 193

Hepatitis B (HBV), 189, 192
    carrier, identification, 194
    definition, 169
    prevention, 193–194
    transmission process, 193
    vaccination, 191, 193–194
Hepatitis C (HCV), 189, 192
    postexposure, 193
Hernia, 82. *See also* Hiatal hernia
Herniated disc. *See* Slipped/herniated disc
Herpes, 93. *See also* Genital herpes
Herpes zoster, 88
Hgb. *See* Hemoglobin
Hiatal hernia, 98
HICPAC. *See* Hospital Infection Control
    Practices Advisory Committee
High-density lipoprotein cholesterol (HDL),
    definition, 489
High-efficiency particulate air (HEPA) filter, 175
Hippocrates, 2–3
Hirudo medicinalis (medicinal leech), 5, 7
His, bundle (definition), 279
Histoplasma capsulatum, 504
Histoplasmosis (Histo) test, 504
History, 2–8
HIV. *See* Human immunodeficiency virus
Hives, 93, 427
HMO. *See* Health Maintenance Organization
Hodgkin's disease, 110
Iloffa, Ludwig M., 274
Homeostasis, definition, 68
Hook, Robert, 69
Hormones, 137
    definition, 99
Hospital Infection Control Practices Advisory
    Committee (HICPAC), 171
Hospital personnel, 12–14
Host. *See* Reservoir host; Susceptible host
Human body
    cavities, 66–67
    form/shape, 80
    functions, 68–69
    heat/temperature, 80
    introduction, 61–68
    movement, 80
    organization, 69–77
        levels, 62–63
    sections, 65–66
    substance isolation, contrast. *See*
        Universal precautions
    temperature measurement. *See* Core
        body temperature measurement
        tympanic thermometer competency
        check, 262
Human chorionic gonadotrophin (HCG)
    definition, 508
    test, 116
    urine test, competency check, 521
Human immunodeficiency virus (HIV), 111,
    189, 192
    definition, 169
    postexposure, 193
Hydrocephalus, 87
Hyperglycemic, definition, 486
Hyperkalemia, definition, 497
Hyperpnea, 121, 233
Hypersensitivity, 111
Hypertension, definition, 252
Hyperthyroidism, 103
Hyperventilation, 121, 233
Hypodermic needles, 337–338, 445
Hypoglycemic, definition, 486
Hypokalemia, definition, 497
Hypopnea, 233
Hypotension, 427
    definition, 252

Hypothermia, 235
Hypothyroidism, 101
Hypoxia, 121

I

ICD-9-CM. *See* International Classification of
    Diseases 9th Revision Clinical
    Modification
Ileum, definition, 96
Image, presentation. *See* Professional image
Immune system, 108–111
    diagnostic tests, 111
    disorders, 110–111
    function, 108
    structures, 108–110
Impetigo, 93
Implanted port, 469
Impotence, 115
Imprisonment. *See* False imprisonment
Indices, 145
Indirect contact, 163
Indwelling catheters, 468–470
Infant, heel stick
    competency check, 370
    usage, 360–361
Infant respiratory distress syndrome (IRDS),
    121
Infection
    chain
        breaking, 164–165
        definition, 162
    control, study/review exercises,
        195–199
    cycle, 162–164
    definition, 162
Infectious mononucleosis, 111
Inferior, definition, 64
Infertility, 115
Infiltrated IVs, 184
Infliction. *See* Intentional infliction
Influenza (flu), 121
Information, transference, 215
Informed consent
    definition, 20
    right, 537–538
Injury, sustaining, 21
Inpatient, definition, 355
Input, 215
Insulin test, 103
Insurance
    billing, 208–214
    company
        billing, 213–214
        laboratory billing, 211
Insured, definition, 209
Integrity, definition, 532
Integumentary system, 89–93
    diagnostic tests, 93
    disorders, 92–93
    function, 89–90
    structures, 90–92
Intentional infliction, definition, 18
Intentional tort, 18
Internal AV shunt, 470
Internal respiration, 118
International Classification of Diseases 9th
    Revision Clinical Modification
    (ICD-9-CM), 213
Internet, usage, 567
Interstitial fluid, definition, 69, 356
Intervals, 283–286. *See also* P-R interval; QT
    interval
    definition, 283
Interview questions
    asking, 589
    examples, 586–588